Communication Development and Disorders for Partners in Service

Communication Development and Disorders for Partners in Service

CHERYL D. GUNTER, PhD, CCC-SLP
MAREILE A. KOENIG, PhD, CCC-SLP

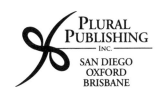

PLURAL
PUBLISHING
INC.

SAN DIEGO
OXFORD
BRISBANE

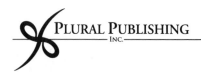

5521 Ruffin Road
San Diego, CA 92123

e-mail: info@pluralpublishing.com
Web site: http://www.pluralpublishing.com

49 Bath Street
Abingdon, Oxfordshire OX14 1EA
United Kingdom

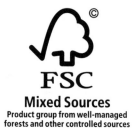

FSC
Mixed Sources
Product group from well-managed
forests and other controlled sources

Cert no. SW-COC-002283
www.fsc.org
© 1996 Forest Stewardship Council

Typeset in 11/13 Garamond book by Flanagan's Publishing Services, Inc.
Printed in the United States of America by McNaughton & Gunn

For permission to use material from this text, contact us by
Telephone: (866) 758-7251
Fax: (888) 758-7255
e-mail: permissions@pluralpublishing.com

Library of Congress Cataloging-in-Publication Data

Gunter, Cheryl, 1956-
 Communication development and disorders for partners in service / Cheryl D. Gunter, Mareile A. Koenig.
 p. ; cm.
 Includes bibliographical references and index.
 ISBN-13: 978-1-59756-025-2 (alk. paper)
 ISBN-10: 1-59756-025-1 (alk. paper)
 1. Language acquisition. 2. Language disorders. 3. Communication. 4. Communicative disorders. I. Koenig, Mareile A. II. Title.
 [DNLM: 1. Language Development Disorders. 2. Language Development. WL 340.2 G977c 2010]
 QP399.G85 2010
 616.85'5—dc22
 2010025461

Contents

PART III. COMMUNICATION DISORDERS AND CLINICAL SERVICE DELIVERY

Preface

We chose to pursue our studies and our careers —the discipline of communication sciences and disorders—because of our profound concern for individuals whose comprehension and/or conventional production of ideas and information has been compromised—individuals with communication disorders. Our primary aim always has been to do what we can with the time and the talent with which we have been blessed to enhance the quality of their communication and, as an extension, the quality of their day-to-day lives.

Some of our service to individuals with communication disorders occurs in our role as clinical service providers. We have been honored and humbled by the opportunities we have had to stand beside them as their clinicians, consultants, collaborators, and communication partners in their quest to more completely access the interactions that are such a valuable component of their lives. As a component of our clinical service provision, we incorporate information about normal and non-normal communication into our prevention, evaluation, and intervention endeavors. And over the course of our clinical service provision, we observe the need for a resource that both respects the depth and breadth of communication development and provides detailed information about communication parameters in an accessible format. We also observe the need for such a resource to inform our patients about the clinical process they are involved in when they seek our experience and expertise in the clinical context. Our sincere hope is that this book serves those particular needs.

Communication development occurs across the life span; conditions that can compromise communication development also occur across the life span. From the presence of syndromes that can influence the course of development from before birth, to the accidents that can alter the structural and/or functional status of the communication mechanisms, to the instantaneous and/or incremental deterioration of communication because of chronic medical issues, individuals can experience communication disorders that affect diverse combinations of skill areas with varied levels of severity. The impact of these disorders extends to family members—the parents, spouses, children, and other relations who comprise the intimate circle of support for our patients. These family members frequently query issues such as what a person learns who learns to communicate, what factors influence the development of normal communication, why communication disorders occur, and what conditions enhance the likelihood of positive clinical outcomes. We hope that this book addresses their diverse questions.

As speech-language pathologists, our experience and expertise are vital to the clinical service delivery process for individuals with communication disorders. However, we certainly are not solely responsible for their specialized clinical needs, but rather members of an expansive network of professional partners whose combined experience and expertise address various dimensions of the lives of those whom we serve. This network includes the providers of medical services, whose role in primary, secondary, and tertiary prevention of communication disorders is vital, as is the access to clinical services that their referral process provides. This network also includes the providers of educational and, when appropriate, vocational services, whose role in implementation of processes to enhance access of individuals with communication disorders to diverse personal and professional opportunities is vital. Our responsibility to our patients expands to educate their complementary service providers about communication. We hope that this resource enhances their professional development.

Individuals with communication disorders are members not only of their own family but also of the broader community of humanity. Unfortunately, this broader community is not always accurately and appropriately informed about the nature of normal and non-normal communication. Although some media sources strive for correct, complete, and consistent information provision, some sources of what members of the public come to believe reduce the richness of human communication to snippets and sound bites—approaches that disrespect the beauty and the bounty of this incredible human phenomenon. As speech-language pathologists, we have an ethical mandate to serve not only as clinical service providers but also as community educators—sources of current and conceptually sound details that expand and enhance public appreciation of the nature and nuances of communication. For those who wish to enrich what they know about communication development and disorders and the clinical needs of those with speech and/or language impairments, our sincere hope is that this resource enhances your interest.

Some of our service to individuals with communication disorders occurs in our role as clinical educators in our university faculty appointments. We cherish our various opportunities to prepare our students for their eventual clinical practice in speech-language pathology. We consider it particularly vital that our students in the undergraduate, preprofessional curriculum acquire the foundational information related to communication development and disorders that will become the basis for their continued appreciation for and application of theoretical concepts in the graduate, professional curriculum in the discipline—and certainly in their clinical practicum opportunities that prepare them for eventual independent clinical practice. Across

the academic classes for which we serve as instructors, we observe the need for textbooks that present concepts in a systematic fashion that allows students to create a conceptual framework that enhances the quantity and quality of the information they learn from classes. We hope that this book enhances their classroom experiences.

Our academic classes draw students from disciplines other than communication sciences and disorders. We welcome students from other health science disciplines, as well as from the natural sciences, behavioral sciences, social sciences, and education. We also welcome students from other disciplines who have an intellectual interest in the dimensions of communication we address. We consider it important for students from other disciplines that a textbook address both normal and non-normal communication to ensure that these students access a variety of concepts that they may not have the opportunity to access in other venues. We have constructed this book with three main areas of focus: the definition, description, and explanations for communication (Chapters 1 and 2), the development of communication (Chapters 3 through 5), and the clinical service delivery process for individuals with communication disorders (Chapters 6 through 8). We hope that this book provides the overview of communication that draws these students to further studies.

However you as a reader have become acquainted with our book, we wish you the very best as you study our words. Our shared quest to appreciate this treasure called communication is one that we cherish and one to which we wish to continue to contribute.

Cheryl D. Gunter, PhD, CCC-SLP
Professor of Communicative Disorders
College of Health Sciences
West Chester University, Pennsylvania

Mareile A. Koenig, PhD, CCC-SLP
Associate Professor of
   Communicative Disorders
College of Health Sciences
West Chester University, Pennsylvania

Acknowledgments

We wish to express our sincere appreciation to the staff of Plural Publishing, who have encouraged us and enabled us to pursue the preparation and publication of this book. We wish to particularly honor the memory of Sadanand Singh of Plural Publishing, whose commitment to the dissemination of information related to communication sciences and disorders was an inspiration to countless creators and consumers of such information. May he rest in peace. We also wish to thank specifically Stephanie Meissner, Sandy Doyle, and Lauren Narasky for their expertise in various phases of the production process of this book. We are indebted to you for your patience and your professionalism.

As we have prepared this book, at least in part, as a means to educate various populations about communication and communication disorders, it is only appropriate that we extend our sincere appreciation to those who shared their own experience and expertise with us as we started the process of our own professional education. Certainly, we count the influence of the faculty members from each university where we studied—Southern Illinois University, the University of Illinois, the University of Tennessee, the University of Memphis, and the University of Texas—as central to who we are today. Certainly, also, we treasure the contributions of our patients, our students, and the professionals whom we respect to our continued professional development, and we thank them sincerely, as well.

We dedicate this book to the children and families
whom we have been privileged to serve
and to our partners in service from across disciplines.

Cheryl dedicates this book with love to Easton Ray Walker, Jake Edwin Walker,
Avery Sloane Ritchey, Harper Sullivan Ritchey, and Sutton Truxel Ritchey.

Mareile dedicates this book with love to Bryan, Philip, Scott, and iBuddy Tim.

CHAPTER 1

Definition and Description of Language

INTRODUCTION

A father and a mother await the moment when their child produces that treasured word to be recorded for posterity in the milestones section of the "baby book." As the child babbles varied creative series of speech sounds, the parents debate with anticipation whether "dada" or "mama" is nestled in these productions or whether an alternate word ultimately will hold the place of honor as the earliest one. As the culmination of their anticipation, the moment arrives in which the child represents a developed concept with a conventional word in an appropriate context. No matter what the word, when this occurs the child has reached a milestone in his or her language development. We celebrate this accomplishment.

A teacher introduces language-related concepts to the students enrolled in his or her primary school classroom language arts curriculum. As the students focus their concentration on word classification, specific differential traits of nouns, verbs, and other words become clear. As their teacher separates sentences into their constituent phrases and clauses, concepts such as "subject" and "object" enter their consciousness. With practice and perseverance, the students learn to reflect on whether some aspect of sentence construction is correct, then to revise the elements to ultimately produce sentences that

are structurally and semantically intact. The use of language for reflection and correction is another accomplishment that we celebrate.

A reader relaxes in his or her favorite corner, curled up with a cup of tea and a recent local book club selection. As the author builds a case for a particular solution for a pervasive social problem, the reader becomes engaged in the argument in favor of this perspective. The author leads the spellbound reader through perceptive statements of the issues, abstracts of their possible resolutions, descriptions of the advantages and disadvantages of each of these proposed courses of action, and ultimate appeals for the reader to embrace the specific response for which the author has amassed seemingly irrefutable evidence. The use of language for information and persuasion is another accomplishment that we celebrate.

A consultant assists a local nonprofit association in formulating a strategic plan for the next five years. The consultant coordinates discussions in which the association leaders articulate the values that underlie the existence of their association. In these dialogues, the consultant helps the leaders envision which endeavors would best represent the mission of the association to the local community and, thus, translate their vision into productive action. The formulation of a mission statement, translated into action steps with measurable outcomes, reasonable timelines, and potential future directions, represents the use of language for problem solving and planning—another accomplishment that we celebrate.

A traveler approaches the advent of a dream come true—a tour of another country. In preparation, he or she views travel shows, visits travel Web sites, talks with others who have previously visited that area of the world, and consults books to become more familiar with the communication practices within that country. The quest to become sensitive to the myriad factors that can influence human interaction leads the traveler into such issues as the relative status of conversational partners, the boundaries of appropriateness for various topics, the criteria for successful interaction, and whether particular movements complement or contradict the content of what is said. Intercultural communication competence is yet another accomplishment that we celebrate.

These examples represent a multitude of ways in which language has a profound impact on the interactions of individuals every day. As we start to celebrate language, we believe that a shared view of language—between you, as our readers, and us, as the authors—is vital. Thus, this chapter presents information intended to establish a common frame of reference for language and includes a definition of the concept of language, a description of the properties of language, and an overview of the components (or skill areas) of language.

OVERVIEW OF COMMUNICATION

We start to construct our shared view with a description of communication. Definitions of *communication* center around the concept of exchange of information and ideas. Models of communication also abound (e.g., Adler & Rodman, 1991; Barker & Barker, 1993; Burgoon, Hunsaker, & Dawson, 1994; DeVito, 1994; Gibson & Hanna, 1992; Wood, 1992). The more recent models of communication were inspired by the seminal model from Shannon (1948), who conceptualized communication as the culmination of multiple components: the *source*, or the creator of the message; the *message*, or the ideas to be communicated; the *transmitter*, or the channels

that create and modulate a communication signal; the *signal*, or the parallel and/or serial channels that allow the message to travel through them; the *channel*, or the modalities which allow the message to travel; the *noise*, or the secondary signals that obscure or confuse the primary signals; the *receiver*, or the components capable of reception of ideas; and the *destination*, or the intended recipient who consumes and processes the message. However, the most common models of the process conceptualize communication as a three-component process.

Part 1 involves the *sender*. The sender is the source of the idea to be shared in this interaction. With the conception and formation of this idea, the process proceeds to Part 2, which involves the *channel*. The channel represents the means via which the sender converts the idea from an inward reflection to an outward representation. Upon the production of this idea, the process proceeds to Part 3, the *receiver*, or the recipient of the idea to be shared. A typical example of one of the thousands of day-to-day interactions will reflect this three-part process. Bill has information—the date, time, and site of an event—to share with Jill. His purpose is to help to enable her to attend this event. Either consciously or unconsciously, he considers various ways that he could express this information to her, and then selects one based on his own communicative style, his perception of her communicative capacity, or any other communicative considerations. He then conveys the information, which Jill then receives and to which she then responds. Although on a superficial level this process appears to be a linear, sequential three-part process, we note that the steps in the process are multifaceted. In reality, one is simultaneously a sender and a receiver. Although Bill conveys information to Jill, he simultaneously receives information from her about such aspects of communication as the extent of her attention and the depth of her comprehension. At the same time, he monitors his own interaction to determine whether he should offer clarification, specification, or elaboration of information. And, although Jill receives information from Bill, she simultaneously formulates her response to him. Thus, the process of communication is cyclical in nature and is complemented by the multichannel nature of the transmission of information. And the process contains both *interpersonal* and *intrapersonal* elements. In this example, both Bill and Jill communicate in ways other than only words to convey their ideas. Because of this, *communication* is considered a broader concept than *language*, one of multiple channels we can use to accomplish communication.

OVERVIEW OF LANGUAGE PROPERTIES

We continue to construct our shared view with a description of language. We know the word *language* from varied contexts. We studied English language arts in primary and secondary school, as well as international languages and literatures as we worked toward our undergraduate and graduate degrees. As children, we received reminders about which aspects of language were most appropriate for particular situations. As we developed as professionals in our discipline, we received constructive criticism about our language in such endeavors as writing literature reviews, practicing conference speeches, constructing grant proposals, leading committee discussions, and instructing clinical students. And, on a personal note, we continue to experience the lovely dimensions of language in the diverse books we explore, the artistic productions we appreciate, the interactions we savor, and the correspondence we treasure. The word *language* is one by which we are surrounded and we use with considerable frequency. We thus consider it vital that we devote some time to describe this remarkable phenomenon in detail.

The literature includes a variety of definitions of *language*. For our discussion, we present a definition from our national professional association. In 1982, the Committee on Language of the American Speech-Language-Hearing Association (ASHA) prepared a definition of language for our use as speech-language pathologists.

Language is a complex and dynamic system of conventional symbols that is used in various modes for thought and communication. Contemporary views of language hold that: (a) Language evolves within specific historical, social, and cultural contexts; (b) Language is rule-governed behavior and is described by at least five parameters—phonologic, morphologic, syntactic, semantic, and pragmatic; (c) Language learning and use are determined by the intervention of biological, cognitive, psychosocial, and environmental factors; (d) Use of language for communication requires a broad understanding of human interaction. (p. 1)

As do many statements, this statement defines language with a description of various properties that either implicitly or explicitly distinguish language from other concepts. Thus, an overview of some of the salient properties that are typically present across definitions of language follows.

Language as a Code

A code involves the use of one item to represent another item (or individual or idea) (Lahey, 1988). Codes serve a number of purposes. We use codes for camaraderie. Members of a particular association, for instance, may use a code—a uniform, an emblem, a motto—to indicate this relationship. We use codes for confidentiality, such as when we use a password to ensure that access to sensitive or protected information remains restricted. We also use codes for convenience. To represent phrases with simplified forms saves time and, in some cases, also enhances the camaraderie noted previously. We are familiar with many formalized codes, such as Morse code. We also are familiar with codes such as the expressions, movements, and other cues created by those in a close personal relationship that solidify their bond. We are aware of the present evolution of codes used in modern communication, such as the LOL abbreviation in chat room conversations, the <0) character incorporated into electronic mail, and shortened forms such as LUV2EAT on personalized license plates.

We can place codes on a continuum from *direct* codes to *indirect* codes. Take, for example, the idea of "earth." Suppose a child must create ways to represent this idea for a class science exhibit. The child could represent the idea of "earth" in very direct ways, or ways that reflect various physical properties of the idea. A clay model of the earth, embellished with various geographic elements, would represent the shape of the world and the relative sizes of the lands and waters it contains, as would a globe. However, the child also could represent the idea of "earth" in less direct ways—photos, sketches, movements, noises—that reflect some physical properties of the idea but not to the extent of the more direct ways. In some instances, the child may decide that the most appropriate representation of the idea is an indirect one, as is the case when he or she uses a word such as "earth." The word "earth," a combination of five written letters or two spoken sounds, does not share the basic physical properties of our world itself. Nonetheless, the word serves as a code for the idea of the earth, and other words combined with the word "earth" further serve to represent various concepts related to our world (Figure 1–1). Thus, language is a code that we use to represent ideas in a fashion that may be easier or more efficient than with other codes.

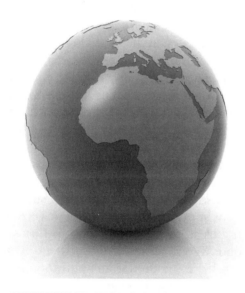

REPRESENTATIONS OF OUR WORLD

Soil-Leaf-Rock... Photo... Watercolor... Sketch... Globe Model... Sculpture... Gesture
WORD

FIGURE 1–1. Language is a code, or a representation of a concept in some fashion. Although some codes are direct (i.e., these codes share some properties with the concepts these represent), language is indirect, in that there is no inherent relationships between words and the concepts these represent. Image adapted from Shutterstock®. All rights reserved.

Language as Referential

The idea of referential, derived from the idea of *reference*, reflects that language serves not just as a code but also as a code for specific, identifiable referents (Matthias, 1999). That is, one who comprehends and/or produces language does so in reference to particular items, individuals, and/or ideas. Typical communicators sometimes use language that appears to be nonreferential. For example, productions such as "um" and "er" interrupt the flow of utterances, and the interjections of such words as "like" and "okay" into utterances serve more as "spoken punctuation marks" than as words to indicate specific referents. Atypical communicators often use language that, in the context used, does not appear to indicate referents. Their conversational partners do not easily relate their productions of echolalia, paraphasia, and other atypical behaviors to referents in the immediate or nonimmediate environments. With that said, however, note that intentional (nonautomatic) and sometimes even unintentional (or automatic)—language is referential. When we use words, we represent particular items, individuals, and/or ideas. Those who share our language expertise and language experience will comprehend the references we express, and our expertise and experience need not be identical for this to occur. Two communicative partners can use "cola" (the preference for the one) and "soda" (the preference for the other one) to refer to a brown, carbonated, nonalcoholic drink but comprehend what the other one means (Figure 1–2). One partner may prefer the term *clarity* to the term *perspicuity* and the term *history* to the term *provenance*, but communication breakdown need not occur if the other partner prefers the more sophisticated alternative terms. One partner may note that "the rain is very heavy" whereas the other notes that "it is raining cats and dogs" and yet continue to avoid communication breakdown because of the focus on a shared referent (present weather status).

In some definitions of language, the idea of language as referential is characterized as the *semanticity* of language, or the idea of the meaningfulness of language within a specific communication context. A typical abridged dictionary includes an estimated 10,000 words, whereas a typical unabridged dictionary includes an estimated 10 times that number. Even 10,000 words sounds like an enormous representational potential. However, even with a finite number of words in the language, one who learns that language has the potential to refer to an infinite number of items, individuals, or ideas.

Language as Arbitrary

Earlier, we described the idea of codes. The idea of language as *arbitrary* stems from the idea of language as an indirect code (Christiansen & Kirby, 2003; McNeill, 1979; Pinker, 1995). That is, a word and what that word represents are not the same (Figure 1–3). No inherent relationship exists between a word and its referents. Consider the concept of "cat." The animal, cat, has various physical properties—a purr, some whiskers, an adversarial relationship with mice, a preference for warm milk, and assorted feline mannerisms. The word, cat, does not share these properties. When written, the word has three letters—C-A-T. When spoken, the word has three sounds—[k], [æ], [t]. In the dictionary, the word appears in the "c" section. The word is primarily described as a noun but can be accurately labeled with other parts of speech. Over time, we have established a connection that the word stands for the referent. The arbitrary nature of language provides us with this power over the language we learn. Although it may be preferable to do so, we need not retain a particular connection between word and referent over an extended period of time. The English language contains words that we consider "archaic words" because we do not use them frequently, if ever. Either we have replaced them with newer words or we have decided that we do

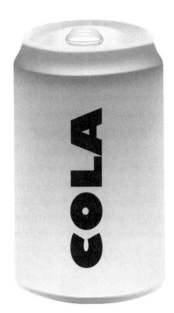

Is this

Soda? Pop? Soda Pop? Cola? Soft Drink? Flavored Water? Seltzer Water? Carbonated Water?

FIGURE 1–2. Language is conventional. Individuals who share a language share the words of that language. However, conventional does not indicate identical as multiple shared words can represent the same concept. Image adapted from Shutterstock®. All rights reserved.

THANK YOU VERY MUCH . . .

. . . Dankie . . . Faleminderit . . . Ashoge . . . Ngiyathokaza . . . Shukran . . . Mauliate . . . Ilakasugotia . . . Obrigadu . . . Soekoeria . . . Yrunyli . . . Medawagse . . . Ngiyabonga . . . Iwgwien . . . Yaqhanyelay . . . A dupe . . . Mila esker . . . Sas efharisto . . . Yewo chemene . . . Matu suksama . . . Nagyon köszönöm . . . Grazzi hafna . . . Tika hoki . . . Munchas gracias . . . Atkel bboxmu . . . Niwega muno . . . Fa'afetai tele . . . Ke itumtese . . . Maraming salamat . . . Kili so chapur . . . Ua tsaug ntau . . . Hawit basima chim raba . . . Amyaji chezu tinbade . . . Vrah bodah shukriyyaa . . . Ua koj tsaug ntau . . . Ah Dios mamexes dimo . . . Waaqni sii haa kennu . . .

FIGURE 1–3. Language has arbitrariness in that multiple words exist within a language to express the same concept and that varieties of languages have varieties of words to accomplish the same.

not need to represent the concepts the words once expressed. At the same time, the English language contains words that we introduce into the language on a periodic basis. Each year, for instance, the primary dictionary publishers announce the words now included (and excluded) from their volumes based on popular use in interaction. In addition to the exclusion and inclusion of words, some older words have newer interpretations. In short, the use of specific words for specific referents is based on tradition and consensus of a collection of language users, and as tradition evolves the language evolves in a complementary way.

Language With Cultural Transmission

In Chapter 2 of this book, we present an overview of the precepts of various theories of language development. What will become readily apparent is the relative value that various theorists ascribe to cultural influences on language development. However, even with these disputes in these explanations, it also is readily apparent that interaction with others is necessary for the process of language development to begin and/or to continue. Some theories that value *nature* (as opposed to *nurture*) confirm that some variation of external input is vital to stimulate the internal structures and/or processes responsible for subsequent language comprehension and production. And some theories that value *nurture* consider external input vital to stimulate and semantically, structurally, or functionally shape language comprehension and production in cultural contexts.

Culture is characterized as the values, beliefs, expectations, and customs that individuals in a shared area establish to enhance their existence (Jandt, 1998). The perpetuation of culture occurs in a vertical fashion, as elders transmit culture to subsequent generations, as well as in a horizontal fashion, as members of a present generation decide the elements of culture to retain or to reconceptualize. The influence of culture on language development is pervasive as the elements of culture permeate such aspects of language as the topics we address, the quantity and quality of information we reveal, the individuals with whom we communicate, the relative simplicity or complexity of our word combinations, our conversational style and proficiency, our bound-

aries for appropriate versus inappropriate communication, and numerous other considerations.

The influence of culture on language also is manifested in the specific dialect(s) of language we learn. The words we use to represent items or individuals (e.g., "sofa" vs. "davenport"), the combinations of those words and their modifiers (e.g., "blue car" vs. "car blue" or "running" vs. "a-running"), the productions of the speech sounds in those words (e.g., "[tiθ]" vs. "[tif]"), the patterns of conversations in small or large groups (e.g., to initiate a topic vs. to wait for others to initiate a topic), and even the incorporation of extralinguistic items into interactions (e.g., to look directly at another vs. to not look directly at another) all may be influenced in a systematic way by the language community that surrounds us in the process of language development and/or the language community in which we aspire to be considered a competent communicator.

Language as Conventional

The idea of conventional stems from the idea of *consensus*. When a collection of people arrive at a consensus, they accept some shared precepts or practices and consent to adhere to those as the basis for predictable, acceptable attitudes and actions. Language is conventional in that those who have learned that language have decided to share broadly the same code as others who have learned that same language (Bach, 1992; Bennett, 1976; Carruthers, 1996; Cummins, 1989). In some cases, our adoption of the code appears to occur without extended discussion. Consider the example of the child who learns his or her earliest words. When that child attaches the words "mama" and "dada" to favorite people and various action words to her favorite pastimes, he or she does so without sustained debate of the various implications or interpretations of these words. The child simply attaches the words from his or her environment to those referents.

In some cases, however, our consideration of the adoption of various aspects of the code is cause for considerable debate. Each of the authors pursued undergraduate and graduate degrees and subsequently served as a faculty member at multiple academic institutions. The names of these institutions have evolved over time as their academic missions have been redefined. The debate related to language conventions for individuals is as lively as the debate for institutions. Take names, for instance. Although some individuals retain their birth names and/or titles their entire lives, some individuals consciously decide to be known by other names and/or titles for a diversity of reasons. Individuals may select a new name to reflect a spiritual transformation. Couples who marry may decide to retain their birth names or adopt a new name to indicate a new marital status. In addition to institutional and individual debates, a society as a whole can deem some formerly appropriate language now unacceptable and vice versa. We note that conventional does not mandate identical. Those who share a conventional language certainly may have individual variation because of their own experiences. However, their language has conventional boundaries that enable them to share elements of the code with others.

Language as Dynamic

In our discussion of language as conventional, we noted that the conventional nature of language does not demand that those who learn a language learn an identical version of that language. Instead, language allows considerable individual variation within its broad confines. We echoed this idea in our discussion on cultural transmission, and we complemented this idea in our discussion of language as arbitrary. Because the words that we use do not equate the items, individuals, and ideas we use them to represent, language need not remain static over time. Instead, it is an alive, dynamic entity (Hockett, 1958, 1977). Consider words that we have used in everyday interaction but do not use now. The English language once included these words as viable ways to express various concepts. However, because of their decreased frequency of use over time, they evolved into archaic forms of interest primarily to those in historical linguistics and related areas. Consider words that we have used in everyday interaction and use now in an expanded fashion. These are familiar to us because of our frequent exposure to them. When asked to define them, we would be apt to state traditional definitions. However, in recent decades, we have broadened our appreciation of these words to include

alternative applications. Consider words that we have not always used in everyday interaction but do use now. In recent decades, these words have entered our vocabulary and have increased in both familiarity and frequency of use. In addition to words, combinations of words also are dynamic. And, in addition to words, the rules that dictate how we comprehend and produce those words are dynamic. In their own communication experiences, individuals can discern the evolution of their rules for interactions with others. The topics they discuss, the quantity and quality of information they provide, the adaptation of their communication based on their relationships with their conversational partners, and various other aspects of communication adapt as their own language evolves. In turn, individuals collectively across their shared experiences can influence the evolution of practices related to language. The relatively recent introduction of electronic mail, instant and/or text messages, voice mail, and Web cam avenues for communication are representative of shifts in communication norms and practices.

Language as Systematic

Definitions of language note the rule-based property of language with a variety of terms, which include *systematic*, *generative*, *creative*, and *productive*. No matter which perspective one prefers, it is evident that language reflects and results from intricate internal and external rules (Hockett, 1961; Pinker, 1984). We have rules that dictate which speech sounds English contains. We learn that such consonants as [f] as in "fad," [p] as in "pad," [m] as in "mad," and [s] as in "sad" typically are within the English language repertoire but that consonants such as those that are clicked or trilled, as well as those that are produced with the uvula, typically are not within the American version of English. We also learn which combinations of speech sounds the English language allows. We can combine the consonants [n] and [t] into the cluster [nt] and the consonants [t] and [w] into the cluster [tw]. At the same time, we understand that the appropriate production of these clusters restricts their position within words (Figure 1–4). The cluster [nt] can appear at the conclusion of a word such as "tent," but not at the start, whereas the cluster [tw] can appear at

**THESE CAN APPEAR IN WORD INITIAL POSITION,
BUT NOT IN WORD FINAL POSITION,
IN ENGLISH**

[h]

[pr, br, tr, dr, kr, gr]

[pl, bl, kl, gl]

**THESE CAN APPEAR IN WORD FINAL POSITION,
BUT NOT IN WORD INITIAL POSITION,
IN ENGLISH**

[ŋ]

[bs, fs, ks, ps, ts]

[dt, ft, kt, nt, pt]

FIGURE 1–4. Because language is systematic, rules of language dictate how children construct their utterances. In the English language, some elements can be combined, and some elements cannot be combined.

the start of a word such as "twin," but not at the conclusion. Other clusters, such as [st], can appear in either position of the word, as is the case for "stop" and "pest," and/or adjacent to each other at the start or conclusion of adjacent syllables in multisyllabic words. When we construct words from speech sounds, we learn which varieties of words the English language contains, as well as which words are appropriate to combine. We learn that, in contrast to some other languages, English typically reflects adjective + noun (rather than noun + adjective) combinations. We also learn that, although some varieties of words can be combined, these constructions do not necessarily convey information that we understand. And, as we create individual utterances, we learn the rules of cohesion that allow us to weave them into various forms of narratives. Because we produce much of our language in interpersonal contexts, we thus learn the intricate rules that dictate appropriate communication for various purposes and in response to the parameters of those contexts. How to introduce, maintain, switch, and conclude topics within interactions, as

well as when and for whom various topics are appropriate are examples of these rules. Our possession of the rules of a language allows us to both comprehend utterances to which we have never been exposed and construct utterances which we have never produced.

Language as Dual

The examples included in the description of the rule-based nature of language reflected the idea that learners of a language can combine the elements of that language into increasingly more sophisticated constructions. This represents the idea of the duality, or the hierarchical nature, of the language (Bickerton, 1981; Chomsky, 1965). We select from the speech sounds of our language those we need to create a meaningful word. The individual speech sounds do not contain meaning. In fact, even combinations of speech sounds do not necessarily carry meaning, as we observe in the child who produces various forms of coos or babble. However, some combinations carry conventional meaning. And we select from various affixes (prefixes and/or suffixes) to transform the word to the appropriate form. Once we have addressed the individual words, we move to the level of combinations of words. We select from the other words of the language those we can combine to enhance the quantity and quality of ideas we share. We can identify words that are subordinate (more specific) and superordinate (less specific) to those we select, such as *snickerdoodle*, which is more specific than *cookie*, which is more specific than *confection*. We consider the various sentences we could construct to convey those ideas with the clarity and consistency we desire. We also draw from our nonlinguistic contexts for the adaptations of our utterances to the perceived demands of our communicative partners and our communicative purposes. To a person previously unfamiliar with the topic of our conversation, we may provide more specific details than we would to a person familiar with the topic. We may provide more summary information in a short interaction than we would to a person with more time or we may provide fewer introductory details than to a person for whom this is a new topic. We can identify a hierarchy of our expectations for a communication encounter as we allow these expectations to influence our choices about the nature of that interaction.

Language as Discrete

When we combine the elements of language into increasingly more sophisticated constructions, as noted in the description of the duality of the language, the result is utterances that serve our communicative purposes. In the same way we can construct utterances, we can deconstruct utterances because of the discrete nature of the language (Chomsky, 1991; Hockett, 1960). Suppose a child produced the utterance, "Bill and Jill went to school, and Mom and Dad went to work." If this utterance is one of several utterances that comprise a narrative, we can identify the component to which this utterance corresponds—the initiating event, the responding event, or, perhaps, the coda. Within the utterance, we can identify the broad structure the child used. In this case, a compound sentence—the two sepa-

rate independent clauses of "Bill and Jill went to school" and "Mom and Dad went to work" connected with a conjunction. Within the independent clauses, we can identify the subjects, the predicates, and the prepositional phrases "to school" and "to work." We also can identify the parts of speech that characterize the individual words: noun, verb, conjunction, and preposition. Further, we can divide those words into the speech sounds that comprise them. "Bill" becomes [bɪl], "went" becomes [wɛnt], and "school" becomes [skul] (Figure 1–5).

With computer-based speech analysis, we can analyze the speech sounds even further for their acoustic properties—loudness, duration, harmonics, or even voice onset time, as well as the coarticulation influence of the speech sounds. We also can employ functional deconstruction to analyze this utterance, which serves the purpose of introducing characters, establishing locations, furthering plots, resolving crises, and so forth. An individual utterance, could serve an informative purpose with its clear statements of who went where, as well as a comparative purpose to contrast the actions of two sets of individuals.

Language as Specialized

Various physical structures and processes, when intact, increase the potential for typical language development to occur. A detailed discussion of neurologic structures and functions and their relation to language is outside the scope of this book. However, an example can illustrate the idea of specialization. Consider the occipital lobe in the brain. We currently attribute the reception and interpretation of visual information to the occipital lobe. Intact structure and function of this area contributes to our safety as we use visual information to avoid a variety of environmental threats, as well as to our security as we use visual information to locate food, shelter, apparel, and other necessities. Contributing to normal language development does not appear, at least on the surface, to constitute a primary or even a secondary function of the occipital lobe. However, this area contributes to the process of communication competence. Accomplishments such as visually relating words to their referents,

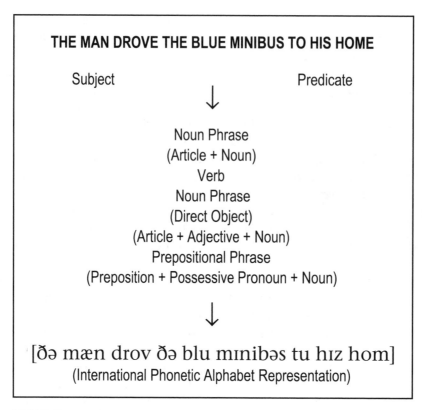

FIGURE 1–5. Because language is discrete, we can divide utterances into their constituent structural parts.

monitoring facial expressions and movements of conversational partners, determining appropriate distances for social and personal interactions, and producing and comprehending written language are possible because of the occipital lobe. In the same spirit, we describe the processes of hearing and speaking, which, although not mandated for learning language, enhance the quantity and quality of the spoken language one learns. A structure such as the tympanic membrane, which protects the middle ear structures, also serves the purpose of differential vibration in response to sound, which enhances the reception and interpretation of auditory information and increases the chance for intact speech production. This specialization of language can be conceptualized as an "overlaid function" of various physical structures (Chomsky, 1986). The use of hands for making tools and for writing and signing words and the use of oral structures for grinding and chewing food and for articulating words are only two of the special functions various structures perform.

Language as Displaced

When a child comprehends and produces the earliest words, he or she typically does so with reference to the immediate environment. This is characterized as the "here and now" aspect of language comprehension and production, which we can pair with the "out of sight, out of mind" aspect of language at this point in language development. These earliest words constitute valuable tools that allow a child to communicate even more effectively than by pointing, looking, or moving toward items or individuals the child wants to reference. As enhanced quantity and quality of language develops, however, a child does not restrict references to this context. In fact, to be considered competent in interactions with others, a child must not restrict his or her references only to what he or she can perceive in the immediate context. Instead, the child expands the scope of reference to that which is absent in time and/or space. This representation of the nonimmediate environment is known as *displacement* of language (Charlton, 2000). Some authors who have attempted to prioritize the most crucial properties of language have indicated displacement as central to the concept of language. Because of displacement, we need not restrict our language to represent that which we can perceive in the present time. We can express the immediate past. For example, in the moment after a snack, a child can note that he or she had juice and crackers. We also can express nonimmediate past. For example, several weeks after a field trip, a child can describe the presentations and the exhibitions at a local museum. We can express the immediate future. In the moment before a drive, a child can note that he or she will visit the store. We can also express the nonimmediate future. For instance, several weeks before a vacation, a child can indicate the states or areas the family will visit. Because of displacement, we need not restrict our language to the immediate physical context. Instead, we can indicate items and individuals absent from our immediate sensory ability, whether their distance from us is miniscule or monumental (Figure 1–6). We also can communicate from our imagination, in which we create the world in our minds.

Language as Interchangeable

Our earlier definition of the concept of "communication" described the roles of sender and receiver in the mutual transmission of information. The idea of language as *interchangeable* captures these roles as well. Those who have learned a language can send and receive that particular code (e.g., Barker & Barker, 1993; Burgoon, Hunsaker, & Dawson, 1994; Gibson & Hanna, 1992). Our roles of sender and receiver may be realized in an asynchronous fashion. Suppose two individuals, Dan and Jan, initiate a conversation and suppose that Dan has a sensitive idea to communicate to Jan. Because of the seriousness of the interaction, Dan may devote some time preparing his presentation to Jan. He may evaluate how best to formulate his utterances and how to enhance Jan's comprehension When appropriate, Dan speaks to Jan, then awaits her response, which she transmits to him as she shifts from receiver to sender. However, although superficially Dan and Jan may appear to shift their roles in actuality it is very hard to delineate an exact moment when the shift occurs. Because of that, our roles of sender and receiver are realized in an asynchronous fashion, with the acts of sending and receiving information occurring simultaneously. Dan, when he conveys ideas to Jan, monitors his own productions. He may rely on auditory feedback or on tactile feedback as he monitors placement of his articulators to evaluate whether he has formulated the correct sounds for his words. He also may rely on the expressions, movements, and other behaviors, both oral and nonoral, that Jan directs toward him even before she specifically

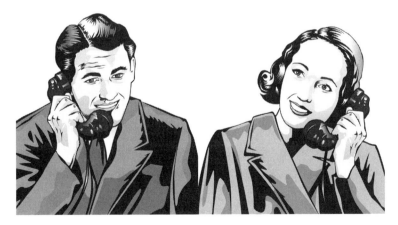

FIGURE 1–6. The trait of displacement allows language users to reference what is absent in time (temporal displacement) and in space (spatial displacement). Image from Shutterstock®. All rights reserved.

responds to the information he has shared. In turn, Jan monitors various dimensions of the interaction to enhance her participation in the encounter. The nature of the interchangeable relationship is easily apparent in the simultaneous occurrence of multiple communicative roles in day-to-day interactions.

In addition to these properties of language, some definitions of language contain properties which may or may not be present in language based on the circumstances at hand.

Language as Oral-Aural

Some definitions of language (Hockett, 1960) characterize language as *oral* (meaning that we produce language by speaking it) and *aural* (meaning that we monitor language by hearing it). We do not discount the value of spoken language for its convenience or for its contribution to clarity in communication. However, language need not be restricted to the spoken mode, as written and gestured modes of language also can be viable alternative expressions of language. English is available in each of these modes —spoken, written, and gestured (as represented in Signed English). Some languages are available in two of the three modes. Other languages are available in only one of the three modes. The modalities via which we can comprehend and produce language need not remain static over time. The language of Maltese, for instance, is a fascinating example of how language is evolving. The spoken form of Maltese has existed for millennia. However, the written form of Maltese has existed only since the early 1900s, whereas the signed form of Maltese has been systematically documented only in the past two decades.

Language as Transient

Some definitions of language characterize language as transient rather than permanent (Hockett, 1960). In many instances, this is certainly the case. Our day-to-day personal conversations typically are typically, with the exception of the portions of those interactions we retain in our memories. Our day-to-day professional conversations also typically are transient, with the exception of forms as corporate memos, medical records, or other documents. However, spoken language need not be transient due to the variety of media available to record our interactions. Some of those media also can preserve our signed interactions. Of course, these resources to capture our language cannot reproduce the complex nature of interactions. These may not represent the depth of the social, cultural, and emotional factors that influence our interactions. In a sense, the same is true for written language. Although we can treasure the printed word, we cannot easily recreate the impact of the writing on the ones composing and the ones comprehending the various available documents. However, we can preserve to some extent portions of the language for future appreciation.

Language as Broadcast

Some definitions of language characterize language as broadcast (that is, transmitted among those who share a language) (e.g., Adler & Rodman, 1991; DeVito, 1994; Hockett, 1960; Wood, 2002). As we noted previously, language certainly can enhance *interpersonal* communication. In interpersonal contexts, we use language to further interactions with others. We also may use language to initiate, expand, adjust, and/or conclude relationships with others. However, we should not restrict the description of language to the interpersonal dimension. Language certainly can enhance *intrapersonal* communication. We may, with language, think about various encounters and experiences. We choose whether we will convert these intrapersonal experiences with languages into interpersonal exchanges, as we report to others about our internal uses of language.

As a complement to our description of various properties of language, we now move to a description of the skills that children learn in the process of language development.

DESCRIPTION OF LANGUAGE SKILL AREAS

A traditional view of language presents six areas in which we develop language skills: lexicon, semantics, phonology, morphology, syntax, and pragmatics.

Lexicon

The lexicon of a language is the vocabulary of that language (Bloom, 1973). The lexicon is sometimes characterized as a "personal dictionary" a person develops. The words in the lexicon reflect "word knowledge." When we learn a word, we learn various dimensions of what that word means (Clark, 1979). Consider the word "stand" as an example of how a child learns these dimensions. When a child learns the referential meaning of "stand," he or she learns that "stand" represents a specific stand, typically within the immediate environment, with which he or she has had personal experience. This could be the music stand the mother uses for her sheet music, the plant stand the father uses for his floral plants, or the cake stand the local baker uses to display baked delicacies. When a child learns the extended meaning of "stand," he or she learns that "stand" represents every possible permutation of the concept, even if he or she had no experience with those variations. The child learns that he or she can appropriately represent all music stands, all plant stands, all cake stands, and all other varieties of stands with that term. The child also learns that, in addition to these variations on a theme of "stand" as a holder of items, he or she can represent alternate meanings for that word. "Stand" thus can expand to include the action of rising from a seated position, the action of supporting a person or a position, or the actual position supported. When a child learns the relational meaning of "stand," he or she learns that "stand" relates to other words that can be combined appropriately with it to convey additional information. The child can combine "stand" with various adjectives that describe "stand" as a noun and various adverbs that describe "stand" as a verb. When a child learns the categorical meaning of "stand," he or she learns that the word "stand" can be categorized in a variety of ways. Items of furniture, items constructed from particular substances, items possessed by specific individuals, and actions performed are only some of the many ways that a child could combine the word "stand" with others into collections of words with shared properties. The child learns the metalinguistic meaning of "stand." This occurs when the child reflects on the word as an entity itself: when spoken, the word contains five sounds and when written, the word

contains five letters. The child also realizes that the word can be characterized with multiple parts of speech, alphabetized in a particular fashion, and monitored as to its pronunciation and application. To a considerable extent, the development of the lexicon represents "world knowledge" in addition to "word knowledge." This is what intertwines lexical and semantic development.

Semantics

The semantic aspect of language centers around the meaning of the language—the meanings we learn for words and, subsequently, the combinations of words (Pinker, 1994, 1999). In the previous section on lexicon, we noted the variations of meanings that a child can learn for a word. To these, we add the *denotative meaning* and the *connotative meaning*. When a child learns a *denotative* meaning for a word, he or she learns the content that word represents. So, for the word "candy," the child learns that this word represents a small round white mint-flavored center coated in soft dark chocolate and numerous other varieties of sweet confections that vary in terms of shapes, flavors, and colors. The focus is on the physical properties of the item the word represents.

When a child learns a *connotative* meaning, he or she learns the implications associated with the word. If we return to the word "candy," we know that, based on the context of its production, the word carries an assortment of implications for the one who interprets it: whether it is tasty, desirable, healthy, pleasant, fancy, and other potential characteristics.

In addition to the denotative and connotative meanings, the semantic aspect of language encompasses the idea of *semantic networks*. When a child learns a word, he or she learns the properties of the referent which the word represents. Consider the word "bird." When child learns such properties as *beak*, *feathers*, *claw feet*, *chirp*, *wings*, and other salient components of a bird, he or she comes to realize that these properties can be components of other entities. As these properties intersect, the child establishes interconnected networks that form the bases for appropriate combinations of words, as well as appropriate inclusion of words into multiple classifications. In addition, the semantic aspect of language encompasses the skills involved in determination of whether a child should interpret an utterance in a literal or a nonliteral fashion, how a child should comprehend an utterance with multiple potential interpretations, whether a child should interpret the information or the implications in an utterance, and how a child appreciates the combined meaning of utterances that constitute a narrative structure.

Phonology

When we develop phonology, we acquire the rules for the perception and production of the smallest units of sound, phonemes, that can be combined into words with meaning (Ingram, 1974). We can differentiate nonspeech sounds from speech sounds and, with respect to these speech sounds, differentiate non-English from English sounds. We also can appreciate the concept of allophones. When we produce a particular phoneme within a word, we do not always produce that phoneme in the same fashion. This variation in production is due, in part, to the influence of the other phonemes in the word, as well as to the position of the phoneme in the word. Take, for example, the words "keep" (transcribed phonetically as [kip]) and "peek" (transcribed phonetically as [pik]). These words contain the same phonemes but combine them in a different order. Thus, a child who produces these words does not produce the consonants [k] and [p] and the vowel [i] in the same way because of the influence of some of the factors noted above. However, the varied productions of the consonants [k] and [p] and the vowel [i] (as well as the productions of the other consonants and vowels in the language) are sufficiently similar to represent the idea of the phoneme we perceive them to represent. We refer to these as allophones of that particular phoneme, and our rules of phonology allow us to categorize allophones into the phonemes these variations represent. Once a child comes to appreciate the relationship between spoken language and written language, he or she learns to discern the relationship between spoken phonemes and written graphemes, or letters. A most important distinction is the absence of a predictable 1:1 relationship between phonemes

and graphemes. One phoneme, for instance, is [ʃ]. We articulate that phoneme when we indicate to a person that we desire quiet, as in "shhhh." Certainly, when we write this phoneme with graphemes, we can spell it as "sh," as in the word "shoe." However, we can also spell it with "ch," and even as "ti," "si," and "ci." Another grapheme is "A." Certainly, when we speak this grapheme with phonemes, we can say [eɪ], as in "ache." However, that is not our only option. Consider the vowels in the words "action," "awful," "about," and "almond." Although the grapheme remains the same, the phonemes to represent the grapheme vary. This distinction, too, is a part of the development of the phonology of the language.

Morphology

When we develop morphology, we acquire the rules for the perception and production of the smallest units of meaning, morphemes (Berko, 1958). Each word a child learns is a morpheme, or a unit that carries meaning. Words such as *cat, cookie, car, candy*, and every other word in the lexicon of a child is a morpheme. These units are known as *free* (or sometimes *unbound*) morphemes. Although a child can convey a considerable amount of meaning with these free morphemes, it sometimes is necessary to refine the meaning of a word even further. For this purpose, a child learns *bound* morphemes, or morphemes that must be added to free morphemes to convey meaning. Some bound morphemes are *inflectional* in nature. When the child binds these to a free morpheme, that word remains intact. For example, when the child binds the plural morpheme to "cat," the word "cats" is simply the free morpheme plus and bound inflectional morpheme. The same pattern is apparent in the conversion of "walk" to "walks" (to indicate a third person present tense verb), the conversion of "her" to "hers" (to indicate possession), and the conversion of "smart" to "smarter" (to indicate comparison). However, some bound morphemes are *derivational* in nature. When the child binds these to a free morpheme, that word converts to a new form of the word, which often is characterized as a new part of speech. For example, "beauty" (a noun) becomes "beautiful" (an adjective), "quiet" (an adjective) becomes "quietly" (an adverb), and "restore" (a verb) becomes "restoration" (a noun). When the child enhances a free morpheme with a bound morpheme, he or she learns how to produce that combination of morphemes when speaking. The rules for how to produce a spoken morpheme are known as "morphophonological rules." Suppose a child needs to indicate a plural with the addition of a bound morpheme to a free morpheme. The word "cat" becomes "cats," but the word "dog" becomes "dogs," and the word "bus" becomes "buses." In "cats," the final phoneme in the word is [s], while in "dogs," the final phoneme in the word is [z]. In the word "buses," the child adds two phonemes in the syllable [ɪz]. Thus, the child produces the plural morpheme with phonemes that are influenced by the other phonemes in the word. In addition to the morphological rules related to combinations of free and bound morphemes, we learn the exceptions to those rules. Thus, with respect to plural morphemes, a child learns when a word remains the same (e.g., "moose" indicates both one and more than one moose), as well as when a word converts to a new word (e.g., "mouse" indicates one whereas "mice" indicates more than one mouse) and when both singular and plural forms of a word contain a bound morpheme (e.g., alumna indicates one whereas "alumnae" indicates more than one female graduate). The apprehension and application of varied morpheme rules is a vital part of morphological development.

Syntax

The area of syntax contains the rules for combinations of words to convey information and ideas (Garman, 1979). A child can convey ideas within individual words. For example, the word "cookie," accompanied by the staring at and reaching to the cookies on the kitchen counter, clearly indicates the child's desire. However, as the quantity and quality of the information a child accumulates increase, the need for more sophisticated forms in which to express these ideas increases. The rules of syntax allow the child to use a finite number of words for an infinite number of combinations of those words. Early word combinations include noun phrases (a noun plus words that modify it) and verb phrases (a verb plus words that modify it). Noun phrases

such as "red car," "nice house," and "sweet cake" would not be unexpected, nor would verb phrases such as "run fast," "smile nice," and "come quick." A child then expands various phrases into clauses, which we can describe as "independent" (i.e., the clauses that function independently as sentences) and "dependent" (i.e., the clauses that do not function independently as sentences and must be embedded into independent clauses). As a result, a child then produces what we characterize as "simple," "compound," and "complex sentences." A "simple" sentence contains one main noun (in the subject) in combination with one main verb (in the predicate), such as "Jim reads" or "Kim writes." A "compound" sentence, in the traditional sense, contains two or more conjoined simple sentences, such as "Jim reads and Kim writes." However, sentences can contain compound elements. The sentences "Jim and Kim read" and "Kim and Jim write" illustrate compound subjects. The sentences "Jim reads and writes" and "Kim writes and reads" illustrate compound predicates. Some sentences contain both compound subjects and compound predicates, as in "Jim and Kim read and write." Even objects within sentences can be compound. The sentence "Jim read a periodical and a paper" contains a compound direct object. The sentence "Kim read Jim and Tim the note" contains a compound indirect object. As a further example, the sentence "Tim stored books in the living room and the dining room" contains a compound object of the preposition "in." In language development, our expectation is that, in time, a child will not only increase structural complexity with conjoining but also with the embedding indicative of "complex" sentences, when the child, with some amount of elegance, inserts one clause into another rather than simply continue to produce the redundancy of added elements. Within the area of syntax, a child also realizes that he or she can express the same idea with multiple structures. The idea that Bill and Jill know each other, for example, can be conveyed in diversity of structures such as "Bill knows Jill," "Jill is known by Bill," "Jill, whom Bill knows . . ." and others. When individual sentences are insufficient to convey information and ideas, a child learns to combine multiple sentences into narrative structures that tell stories, describe events, or contain other variations of temporal and/or sequential information.

Pragmatics

The child who learns language skills related to pragmatics uses language appropriately for a variety of communicative functions across a variety of communicative situations (Griffiths, 1979; Wells, 1979). With respect to functions, a child learns that he or she can use language in an intentional fashion. A child may use language to inform, label, describe, request, persuade, entertain, and perform numerous other functions. Over time, a child may express these functions with increased sophistication. When a child starts to label, he or she may only use one word, such as *ball*. Over time, however, he or she may increase the quantity of information in his or her utterances with the addition of descriptions, as well as the sophistication of the structures in which the information is provided. To complement this, a child may produce utterances with multiple simultaneous functions. Suppose that a child produces the utterance, "Let's read this fun new book." Within that utterance, he or she may have informed (the child announced the book was available), labeled (the child named the item of interest), described (the child included two descriptions of the book), requested (the child invited another person to participate in an action), and perhaps even persuaded (the child intended that the attractiveness of the proposed action would convince another person to become involved in an interaction). In addition to the production of these multifunctional utterances, the child also learns to encode utterances on a scale of directness. For example, the child may encode a desire for a more comfortable room environment with such utterances as, "Please close the window?" or "May I close the window?" as more direct requests or with such utterances as, "Someone opened the window," or "Brrr, it's cold in here!" as more indirect requests.

The area of pragmatics also includes the array of conversational skills a child learns that allows him or her to initiate, maintain, switch topics within, switch turns within, and conclude conversations with others. The area of pragmatics also includes the appropriate responsiveness to both the linguistic and the nonlinguistic contexts that surround communication. With respect to *linguistic* contexts, the child learns to integrate his or her language with the language before and after his or her utterances, whether produced by the interactional partner(s) of the child or by the child. With respect to *nonlinguistic* contexts, the child allows factors in the situation (broadly defined) to influence the language that he or she produces. Such factors include participant variables (e.g., the participant linguistic level, how familiar the participant is with the topic at hand, how informed the participant is about the topic at hand, and how interested the participant is in this particular interaction) and situational variables (e.g., how conducive the environment is to communication, what time constraints are in place, what restrictions on the topic and/or the details are in place, and what influence of nonparticipant observers have).

In this textbook, three chapters provide detailed information about these six skill areas (lexicon, semantics, phonology, morphology, syntax, and pragmatics). Chapter 3 presents an overview of the advent of language skills in the prelinguistic level. Chapter 4 addresses the continued development of these skills in the earlier linguistic level, and Chapter 5 describes the continued increase in the quality and quantity of language skills in the later linguistic level.

DESCRIPTION OF EXTRALINGUISTIC AREAS

The skills of language development are known as "linguistic" skills. The development of these skills is complemented by the development of various "extralinguistic" skills, which are described below.

Nonlinguistic Skills

Nonlinguistic skills are various movements and positions that convey information simultaneously and/or sequentially with linguistic skills. These nonlinguistic skills serve multiple purposes: *repeating, substituting, complementing, deceiving/revealing, regulating,* and *accenting* (Barker, 1978). In *repeating*, people use nonlinguistic behaviors to convey the same content as the linguistic code. For example, those who accompany an affirmative response to a question with a head nod repeat the affirmation with that movement. In *substituting*, people use nonlinguistic behaviors to replace the linguistic code. For example, in America, various degrees of eye opening express various emotions, such as widened eyes that convey surprise and narrowed eyes that convey suspicion. In *complementing*, people use nonlinguistic behaviors to complete and/or to emphasize in an alternative form the content in the linguistic code. Those who teach dance, for instance, produce oral instructions combined with actual dance movements to emphasize the lesson for their students. In *deceiving/revealing*, people consciously or unconsciously use nonlinguistic behaviors that intentionally or unintentionally reveal information not contained in the linguistic code. For example, people who compliment friends on some aspect of appearance that they, in fact, do not find attractive, may contradict their words with movements such as shifts in eye contact or shuffles of extremities. In *regulating*, people use nonlinguistic behaviors to control various aspects of interaction. For example, the use of eye movements to initiate, maintain, and conclude conversations, as well as shift turns within these interactions, is common and allows a communicator to send cues to a partner that affect his or her participation at any specific point in the interaction. In *accenting*, people use nonlinguistic behaviors to punctuate or emphasize various aspects of the content in the linguistic code. Those who point, touch items, wave, or perform other hand movements use these to focus attention on the most salient aspect of the content they wish to convey. Various nonlinguistic skills are characteristic of the communication skills that children develop. These include gestures, postures, head movements, facial expressions, eye movements, proxemics, chronemics, and physical environment.

Gestures

Gestures are movements of physical structures, such as the hands, that replace, complete, complement, and/or contradict the linguistic information that a person shares (Mehrabian, 1972). These movements do not include the hand signals that constitute sign language. Gestures such as nods and shakes of the head, as well as shrugs of the shoulders, can indicate affirmative, negative, or inconclusive reactions to utterances. When gestures complete an utterance, they add information with a movement. For example, in response to the question as to which book he or she wants, a child who does not know the name of the book may point and say, "That one there." When gestures complement an utterance, they affirm information with a movement. When a child meets a friend on the street, he or she may wave while saying "Hi." When gestures contradict an utterance, they indicate that the words are not necessarily be true. If a child is asked whether he or she is scared, the child may contradict his or her denial of fear with hand movements that we associated with terror. In either case, gestures communicate a substantial amount of information in interaction. In addition to gestures, Mehrabian described various other movements.

Postures

Postures are relations of physical structures, such as the torso, to each other, as well as the position of a person within space. Postures can accomplish the same purposes as gestures. In addition, postures can indicate the level of a person's attention (e.g., leaning the torso forward to indicate particular interest in a topic). Posture also can convey a person's level of interest (e.g., positioning him- or herself at particular points in a space to commence or conclude interactions, as well as to promote or prohibit such contacts).

Head Movements

Head movements include forward, backward, and sideways movements of the head, as well as the fixed position of a head within space. Like gestures and postures, these movements can interact with linguistic information to cause a communication partner to interpret that information in a particular fashion. And, like postures, these movements can convey levels of attention and interest in the communication at hand.

Facial Expressions

Like gestures movements of facial structures, such as the brows and the lips can interact with linguistic information. The upward, downward, and inward movements of the brows can indicate various emotional reactions to the information. The pursed or retracted positions of the lips also can indicate emotional reactions, and the relative open position of the lips can convey the same. In addition, the positions of these structures can express the nature and the extent of attention to the interaction at hand.

Eye Movements

Eye movements include increases and decreases in the extent to which the eyelids are opened, as well as movements of the eyes upward, downward, and sideways. The position of the eyelids can transmit various reactions to interaction, such as fear or surprise. The movements of the eyes can indicate the extent of alertness or interest in the interaction at hand, as well as contribute to the start, continuation, end, and shifts of turns and topics within conversations.

Proxemics

Proxemics includes the relative distance of communicators from each other. Hall (1974) indicated that various distances can indicate the nature of the relationship between communicators. For instance, he characterized 0 to 1.5 feet as an *intimate distance*, 1.5 to 4 feet as a *personal distance*, 4 to 12 feet as a *social distance*, and over 12 feet as a *public distance*.

Chronemics

Chronemics includes the incorporation of time into interactions in terms of how communicators perceive, structure, and use time to convey information, as well as the relative status of the participants in an interaction. The influence of chronemics on interaction is apparent in attitudes toward what constitutes "on time," whether and under which circumstances one person waits for others, and how we allot time to participants to share information.

Physical Environment

The physical environment includes the information that an individual communicates by how he or she structures personal space, as in a room or a home. Choices such as colors, textures, shapes, and the relative positions of items within a space can speak to the aesthetic values of an individual. In addition,

his or her artifacts—photos, accessories, mementos, books, and other decorations—can provide information about personal and professional values and preferences.

In his seminal research on nonlinguistic communication, Mehrabian (1972) noted that our oral linguistic skills provide less than 10% of the information others derive in our interactions, paralinguistic elements provide between 35 and 40% of our content, and nonlinguistic elements provide over 50% of our content. Thus, as we stress in subsequent description of language development—in particular, the pragmatic aspects of language—the value of these complementary skill areas cannot be denied.

ADDITIONAL DISTINCTIONS

Before leaving this explanation and description of language, we note that exist multiple dichotomies in the literature to remind us that both learning to *understand* language and learning to *use* language are inherent and intertwined aspects of language development. This relationship is characterized as *language comprehension* versus *language production*, *receptive language* versus *expressive language*, *language encoding* versus *language decoding*, and *language competence* versus *language performance*. In addition to these divisions, in the literature, there is the framework of *formalist description* (with a focus on the structural elements of language) versus *functionalist description* (with a focus on the interactional elements of language. However, no matter which lens through which you choose to view language, we stress that the various aspects of language defined here are not independent but, rather, are interdependent. Our subsequent description of language development will elaborate on these distinctions.

CONCLUSION

In this chapter, we described language, beginning with an overview of the characteristics that distinguish language from other means of communication and continuing with an overview of the dimensions of language in which we learn an intricate collection of skills. We hope that this introduction enhances the appreciation for the elegance and the enormity of language development. In the next chapter, we expand the description of language with an overview of theories of language development.

REFLECTION QUESTIONS

1. Based on what you have learned about the properties of language, write your own definition of language that differentiates *language* from both *communication* and *speech*.

2. What trait(s) would you consider the most important trait(s) of language? What are your reasons for your decisions?

3. What trait(s) would you consider the least important traits to include in a definition of language? What are your reasons for your decisions?

4. One way to conceptualize language is to describe the skill areas within language (e.g., semantics). What is another way that you could conceptualize what children learn when they learn language?

5. With respect to the skill areas within language (e.g., semantics), define these, and provide examples of the specific kinds of language skills a child learns in each area.

APPLICATION EXERCISES

1. The parents of a child have been exposed to the term "language" across multiple contexts. However, they are uncertain as to whether this term is interchangeable with the term "speech" or if these are two distinct ideas. How would you explain the difference between these terms to these parents? And how would you describe the overlap that occurs between the language of a child and the speech of a child in some instances?

2. A child uses a particular word too broadly (e.g., the word "mom" to represent multiple women) and, in other cases, not sufficiently broadly

(e.g., the word "cookie" to represent only a chocolate cookie, the favorite of the child). How do these examples relate to such traits of language as *arbitrary*, *conventional*, and *dynamic*?

3. A child produces combinations of words that serve to convey information to other people, who understand what the child has produced with no difficulty. Reflect on the diverse areas within language in which a child acquires thousands of language skills. How does this accomplishment reflect the skill areas of *lexicon*, *semantics*, *phonology*, *morphology*, *syntax*, and *pragmatics*?

REFERENCES

Adler, R. B., & Rodman, G. (1991). *Understanding human communication.* Chicago, IL: Holt, Rinehart, and Winston.

American Speech-Language-Hearing Association. (1982). Definition of language. *Asha, 24*(6), 44.

Bach, K. (1992). Paving the road to reference. *Philosophical Studies, 67,* 295–300.

Barker, L. (1978). *Communication.* Englewood Cliffs, NJ: Prentice-Hall.

Barker, L. L., & Barker, D. L. (1993). *Communication.* Englewood Cliffs, NJ: Prentice-Hall.

Bennett, J. (1976). *Linguistic behavior.* Cambridge, UK: Cambridge University Press.

Berko, J. (1958). The child's learning of English morphology. *Word, 14,* 150–177.

Bickerton, B. (1981). *Roots of language.* Ann Arbor, MI: Karoma.

Bloom, L. (1973). *One word at a time.* The Hague, The Netherlands: Mouton.

Burgoon, M., Hunsaker, F. G., & Dawson, E. J. (1994). *Human communication.* Thousand Oaks, CA: Sage.

Carruthers, P. (1996). *Language, thought, and consciousness.* Cambridge, UK: Cambridge University Press.

Charlton, B. (2000). *Psychiatry and the human condition.* Oxford, UK: Radcliffe Medical Press.

Chomsky, N. (1965). *Aspects of the theory of syntax.* Cambridge, MA: MIT Press.

Chomsky, N. (1986). *Knowledge of language: Its nature, origins, and use.* New York, NY: Praeger.

Chomsky, N. (1991). *The sound pattern of English.* Cambridge, MA: MIT Press.

Christiansen, M. H., & Kirby, S. (2003). *Language evolution.* Oxford, UK: Oxford University Press.

Clark, E. (1979). Building a vocabulary: Words for objects, actions, and relations. In P. Fletcher & M. Garman (Eds.). *Language acquisition* (pp. 149-160). Cambridge, UK: Cambridge University Press.

Cummins, R. (1989). *Meaning and mental representation.* Cambridge, MA: MIT Press.

Devito, J. A. (1994). *Human communication: The basic course.* New York, NY: Harper Collins.

Garman, M. (1979). Early grammatical development. In P. Fletcher & M. Garman (Eds.), *Language acquisition* (pp. 177-208). Cambridge, UK: Cambridge University Press.

Gibson, J. W., & Hanna, M. S. (1992). *Introduction to human communication.* Dubuque, IA: William C. Brown.

Griffiths, P. (1986). Speech acts and early sentences. In P. Fletcher & M. Garman (Eds.), *Language acquisition* (pp. 279-306). Cambridge, UK: Cambridge University Press.

Hall, E. T. (1974). *Handbook for proxemic research.* Washington, DC: Society for the Anthropology of Visual Communication.

Hockett, C. F. (1958). *A course in modern linguistics.* New York, NY: Macmillan.

Hockett, C. F. (1960). The origin of speech. *Scientific American, 203,* 89-97.

Hockett, C. F. (1961). Linguistic elements and their relation. *Language, 37,* 29-53.

Hockett, C. F. (1977). *The view from language.* Athens, GA: University of Georgia Press.

Ingram, D. 1974. Phonological rules in young children. *Journal of Child Language, 1,* 49-64.

Jandt, F. E. (1998). *Intercultural communication: An introduction.* Thousand Oaks, CA: Sage.

Lahey, M. (1988). *Language disorders and language development.* Boston, MA: Allyn & Bacon.

Matthias, P. (1999). *Success in referential communication.* London, UK: Kluwer Academic.

McNeill, D. (1979). *The conceptual basis of language.* New York, NY: Lawrence Erlbaum.

Mehrabian, A. (1972). *Nonverbal communication.* Chicago, IL: Aldine Atherton.

Pinker, S. (1984). *Language learnability and language development.* Cambridge, MA: Harvard University Press.

Pinker, S. (1994). *The language instinct: How the mind creates language.* New York, NY: Morrow.

Pinker, S. (1995). The language instinct: The new science of language and mind. New York, NY: Penguin Books.

Pinker, S. (1999). *Words and rules.* New York, NY: Basic Books.

Shannon, C. E. A. (1948). Mathematical theory of communication. *Bell System Technical Journal, 27,* 379-423.

Wells, G. (1986). Variation in child language. In P. Fletcher & M. Garman (Eds.), *Language Acquisition* (pp. 109-140). Cambridge, UK: Cambridge University Press.

Wood, J. T. (2002). *Interpersonal communication: Everyday encounters.* New York, NY: Wadsworth-Thomson Learning.

CHAPTER 2

Theories of Language Development

INTRODUCTION

From very early in our existence as people we have pondered a variety of mysteries. The questions of "why" and "how" what happens in our lives are mysteries to which we have devoted considerable attention. As SLPs, whose very professional title contains the word "language," we have often wondered about the particulars of language. Why does the phenomenon of language occur? How does the intricate process of language development occur? We are not alone in our curiosity.

In the course of our clinical practice we have observed a theme in some of the questions we have received from the parents of our pediatric patients. A mother of multiple children wonders why the pattern of what ultimately can be characterized as typical language development has varied so widely from one child to another. A father whose child does not correctly articulate words or correctly formulate sentences desires advice on how to respond to these errors. Does he respond at all? If he responds, does he correct the errors or respond to the content rather than to the structure of what the child produced? When parents of children with suspected non-normal language development secure a language evaluation with an SLP, they wonder about the purposes of the various evaluation procedures and why multiple evaluations from multiple clinical practi-

tioners are not identical. And when these children receive a recommendation for intervention with an SLP to enhance their language development, their parents welcome assistance to discern which treatment options are most appropriate for their children.

To address their questions, we must accept that no complete explanation for the process of language development currently exists. Although various theories exist, there is no consensus as to the explanation that most truthfully explains this multifaceted phenomenon. We must be prepared to explain the tenets of the available theories to parents to help them understand the various principles on which evaluation and treatment protocols are based. We must be alert to contradictions, both within and across theories, that are potential sources of confusion in their quest for the most appropriate clinical services for their children. Although our primary concern is for our patients and their families, our interest in the theoretical explanations for language development extends even further. We pursue clinical practice that is based on internally consistent theoretical precepts. Rather than consider each clinical decision in isolation, we must view these with the lens that a unified framework provides. Even if the complete explanation of language development remains unavailable, we continue to consider those ideas that are available. We now shift our focus to an overview of various theories of language development.

THE CONCEPT OF THEORIES

A theory is a speculative explanation of a phenomenon that includes a set of principles, suppositions, and/or propositions. A theory of language development must explain both the nature of language and the development of a myriad of intertwined skills that constitute this phenomenon. In some cases, the creation of a theory may precede the conduct of research to confirm or not one or more of the precepts of the theory. For instance, a scholar may formulate a set of principles to explain the nature of language in children, then subsequently conduct a series of experiments to test various hypotheses that have stemmed from the theory presented. The outcome of this experimental inquiry subsequently may dictate revisions to the theory to enhance the extent to which it accurately describes the phenomenon in question. In some cases, however, the conduct of research may precede the creation of a theory. For instance, a scholar may conduct a series of descriptive studies to document the course of development in a specific aspect of language. The accumulation of information and the identification of patterns within development may stimulate the scholar to examine the philosophical explanations that would account for these patterns. Whatever the case—theory leads to empirical research, empirical research leads to theory, theory and experimental research proceed simultaneously—the creation of theories is not restricted to accomplished scholars. Any person with an interest in language development possesses his or her own explanation of this phenomenon. This individual theory may not be formalized, and may contain incomplete explanations of the input, output, or other aspects of language development. It even may contain contradictions in precepts. However, each of us has at least started to accept various principles that we believe to be the most appropriate explanations for language development.

Consider the scenario of a father who wonders how he should communicate with his child. Should he be careful to use complete, correct utterances? Should he select only vocabulary items that are comparable to the word choices of the child, or to the words that the child does not produce but comprehends? Or should he not be overly concerned about the perfection of his language structure or the sophistication of his language content? The person who responds to these queries reveals his or her own perspective on language. Consider another scenario: A mother wonders how she should respond when her child produces errors in communication. Should she call these errors to the attention of the child? Should she insist that the child practice these items to improve? Again, in answering these questions, one's perspective on language becomes clear. In addition to these scenarios, the issue of whether children are relatively active or relatively inactive in the course of language development further illuminates the conclusions people have reached about the nature of this phenomenon.

A variety of formalized language development theories are available for us to consider. In this chapter, rather than present the intricate details of specific theories, we present the central precepts inherent in various "families" of theories of language development. In our overview, we present what these families of theories posit about what a child learns when he or she learns a language, how the process of language development unfolds, what influences the process of language development, advantages and disadvantages of this kind of explanation, and clinical implications for those who hold to this particular viewpoint.

BEHAVIORAL THEORIES

We start our overview of theories with the principles of *behavioral* theories. On a *nature-nurture* continuum, these explanations of language development are placed within the *nurture* dimension of the continuum. This perspective reflects the considerable attention to and adaptation of the ideas of Skinner (1957). Although Skinner did not set out to explain language development in particular, theorists have applied his basic concepts to this phenomenon. Others who have used behavioral principles to describe language development include Mowrer (1954), Osgood (1964), and Staats (1963).

What a Child Learns

In the behavioral explanations of language, a child develops what Skinner characterized as "verbal behavior" or "verbal operants." These operants are verbal behaviors that a child produces in response to various kinds of stimulation, and are considered similar to other socially mediated behaviors that a child learns.

How Language Development Occurs

The traditional behavioral explanations for human behavior—which include language behavior—include a three-part process: stimulation, which leads to response, which leads to reinforcement. This process is known as the SRR process. In more recent literature this process is conceptualized as the ABC process, in which "A" represents antecedent, "B" represents behavior, and "C" represents consequence. In some cases, the addition of "O" for mitigation notes the influence of variables, such as the presence of an audience, on language behavior.

Stimulation

In this explanation, stimulation from the environment is crucial to shape the language that a child learns. We can conceptualize this stimulation on two levels. In one sense, the environment is the source of broad stimulation. From interactions with other people, the child can discern the relative value placed on his or her language development, as noted in the quantity and quality of interaction others provide. However, the environment also is the source of models of specific kinds of utterances to which the child attends. Other people in the environment can increase or decrease the complexity of the utterances they model based on various factors: whether they expect exact or approximated recreations of the utterances by the child, their perception of the skill level of the child, their perception of the needs of the situation, and other factors.

In addition to these levels of stimulation, we can describe variations of stimuli. An *eliciting* stimulus, for instance, is any stimulus, conditioned or unconditioned, that elicits a response. Then, within eliciting stimuli, the *unconditioned* stimulus is any stimulus that naturally elicits a specific response, whereas the *conditioned* stimulus is one that, although not naturally eliciting a specific response, acquires the capacity to elicit a specific response after it has been paired with an unconditioned stimulus. Consider the idea of food: A child may enjoy fruits with a harder rather than a softer texture. The harder texture fruits, then, would be unconditioned stimuli that naturally elicit a positive response from the child to their presence in a menu. The softer texture fruits would not naturally elicit a positive response. However, over time, if a parent introduced the softer fruits simultaneously with the harder fruits, the softer texture fruits could become conditioned stimuli that also would elicit a positive response from the child.

Other variations of stimuli occur in addition to these. A *discriminative* stimulus occurs when a language learner discriminates between closely related stimuli and responds positively only in the presence of that stimulus. This stimulus is also associated with reinforcement. And, with respect to reinforcement, an *adversive* stimulus is one which, when introduced after an occurrence of a response, decreases the intensity of a response on subsequent occurrences. Structured and unstructured stimuli also can appear in the course of interaction for language learners. A *structured* stimulus is organized and unambiguous, with its perception influenced more by stimulus traits than perceiver characteristics. An *unstructured* stimulus, in contrast, is ambiguous, with its perception influenced more by perceiver characteristics than stimulus traits.

Response

In this explanation, a child responds to stimulation in a variety of ways. An overview of some common responses follows.

A *mand*, also known as a command, a request, or a demand, is a verbal behavior that a child produces in response to a physical or psychological state. In a mand, a child specifies the reinforcer that he or she wants to receive in response to the mand. Suppose a child, who has crawled into bed for a nap, is cold. An utterance such as, "need blankie" is a mand that both responds to a state and specifies a reinforcer desired to address that state.

An *echoic*, also known as an imitation, an echo, or a reproduction, is a verbal behavior that a child produces in response to a verbal production of another person. In an echoic, a child reproduces the phonetic and acoustic properties of this stimulation, which may or may not include a request for a repetition on the part of the child. So, if a child, who is on a fieldtrip to a farm, hears an adult produce the utterance, "See the horsie run," he or she reproduces that utterance in response.

A *tact*, also known as a label, a description, or a name, is a verbal behavior that a child produces in response to a verbal production of another person. In a tact, a child comments on an item, an individual, an incident, or some kind of relationship between two of these. Suppose an adult, who enters a toy store with a child says, "a choo-choo train." The child produces a tact such as, "a red caboose," as a label for a complementary item in the store.

An *extended tact*, also known as overgeneralized language or figurative language, is a verbal behavior that a child produces in response to some form of stimulation. However, although the verbal behavior is one the child has previously produced, the stimulation is a new one to which the child has never before responded. So, if a child responds with, "want ice cream" to multiple verbal productions of another person, he or she has extended the tact into new communicative situations.

An *intraverbal*, also known as automatic language or routinized language, is a verbal behavior that a child produces in response to his or her own previous language use. So, a child may sing a favorite song or recite a favorite poem on multiple occasions. A child may also re-enact the script from a familiar social routine in multiple contexts that share similar interactional properties. The language of imaginative play, as well as routinized monologues, also constitute instances of intraverbal productions.

The behaviors described above share a focus on the use of language in response to internal and/or external stimulation. However, the concept of the *autoclitic* verbal production adds a focus on the structure of language. One variation, the autoclitic behavior, involves the imposition of phrase and sentence structure rules onto combinations of words, whereas the other variation, the autoclitic tag behavior, involves insertion of affixes onto words for additional refinement of utterance meaning. Thus, this explanation of language development encompasses both structural and functional aspects of interaction. Two additional concepts are noteworthy, *chaining* and *shaping*, which demonstrate the ability of the child to create even more sophisticated word combinations. The process of chaining occurs when a child appreciates interaction as a series of utterances that can influence the utterances to come and can be influenced from previous utterances. Thus, chaining enhances the appropriate, topic-relevant participation of a child in an interaction. The process of shaping occurs when a child appreciates the finer nuances that differentiate one production from another. As external reinforcement for behavior becomes more selective and relevant to more specific aspects of language, the child adjusts his or her language productions to reflect this polish.

Reinforcement

In this explanation, reinforcement is any reaction that either increases or decreases the likelihood that a child will reproduce a particular verbal behavior. The previous section on stimulation noted some variations of stimuli that can simultaneously encompass a reinforcement influence, namely the discriminative stimulus, in which the discrimination of the nuances across a collection of stimuli influences the proportion of productions of a particular response, and the adversive stimulus, decreases the intensity—if not the quantity—of a particular response over time.

Other variations of reinforcement appear in this explanation. Reinforcement that is *positive* indicates the introduction of stimuli that result in a pleasant experience to increase the frequency of a specific behavior. For instance, if a parent wants a child to request a cookie with the word "cookie" rather than with a noise or a point, on the production of the word, the parent rewards the child with the cookie. Reinforcement that is *negative*, in contrast, indicates the removal of stimuli that result in an unpleasant experience to increase the frequency of a specific behavior. If, in the previous example, the parent had placed the jar with the fresh homemade cookies behind a cupboard door, the move of the jar to an accessible place for the child who said the word "cookie" would constitute this kind of reinforcement. Another variation of reinforcement is *punishment*, or a stimulus that represses a behavior. For instance, if a parent wants the word "cookie," on the production of an alternative word or noise, the parent indicates the consequence of no cookies for a specified period of time in an attempt to repress this alternate. Reinforcement can also be characterized as *primary* (or reinforcement that is naturally reinforcing and without the involvement of learning) or *secondary* (or reinforcement that is not naturally reinforcing and with the involvement of learning). In addition to these distinctions, we can describe reinforcement as *periodic*, or administered with predictable intervals, or *aperiodic*, or administered with unpredictable intervals.

Factors That Influence Language Development

This explanation notes that although not innate per se, language development is influenced by some internal factors, such as the extent to which a child can receive and retain external input to imitate this model, as well as to habituate behavior and discern the relationship between the input received and the output produced. This explanation further notes that language development is influenced by environmental factors, such as the quantity and quality of input and the opportunities to receive reinforcement for his or her attempts to replicate this input.

Advantages to This Explanation

This explanation confirms the influence of the social context on the comprehension and production of language. This also accounts, at least to some extent, for individual differences in language development across children. This explanation also confirms the hierarchical nature of language, in which "easier" structures form the bases for expansion into "harder" structures. The presumption that language can be conceptualized in a hierarchical fashion is a popular one that has influenced clinical practice for decades. The preparation of long-term behavioral goals for clinic patients, then the breakdown of these into short-term goals, reflects a behavioral perspective, as do the inclusion of the criterion for success, the hierarchies for the presentation of both stimulation and reinforcement, and the roles of models and imitations of those models. That SLPs have continued to allow a behavioral perspective to influence clinical practice for several decades may reflect the convenience and the easily identifiable structure of a behavioral treatment approach; this also may reflect that

at least some elements of this explanation have proven valid in the course of clinical practice.

Disadvantages to This Explanation

A criticism of this explanation relates to the concept of what a child learns when he or she learns a language. This explanation conceptualizes the skill of a child as "verbal behavior" influenced by both internal and external factors. However, although this explanation may account for the individuality of the language of a child, this explanation does not account for the universality of the language of a child in relationship to other children. Although this explanation does value the hierarchical nature of language development, in that "easier" skills are the bases for "harder" skills, this explanation does not attest to a broader universal order of language development, nor for universal rules that children as a whole develop. A related criticism of this explanation relates to the classification system for utterances. As noted earlier in the description of mands, tacts, and other productions, we can label verbal behaviors with attention to the stimulation that precedes them. However, to date, no one has compiled a comprehensive list of the verbal behaviors a child has the potential to produce. We cannot capture utterances such as "hello" and "please" that serve as social rituals, for instance, with the classification system previously described. In this sense, this explanation captures some, but certainly not every, potential pattern of interaction. Another criticism of this explanation addresses the relationship between input and output. No consistent 1:1 connection exists between what is input (in the form of stimulation) from the environment and what is output (in the form of verbal behaviors) from the child. For certain, some utterances of children, particularly those at earlier points in the process of language development, are direct imitations of the utterances of others. However, even when children frequently employ imitation as a way to learn, only a minority of their utterances are direct imitations of the models others have produced. This explanation does speak to the processes of generalization and habituation. However, even these processes do not account for the language that does not appear to evolve from models. A further criticism of this explanation addresses the nature of reinforcement. Even the most well-intended communicative partners of children do not consistently reflect on or implement consistent patterns of reinforcement for the verbal behaviors of a child.

Clinical Implications

The behavioral view has had a considerable impact on clinical practice in SLP. Some of the impact has been on our evaluation methods. Suppose a child cannot correctly articulate the phoneme /r/. In an evaluation, we would collect information about the *stimulability* of that child, or how well that child could imitate our models at levels of increased phonetic complexity. Suppose a child cannot correctly formulate the sentence structure article + noun + verb + preposition + noun. In an evaluation, we would collect information about how well that child could imitate a hierarchy of sentence structures, then use that information to estimate the syntactic capacity of that child. Some of the impact has been on the formation of our treatment plan. When we establish long-term and short-term treatment goals, we typically write these as measurable, behavioral goals in which we specify the desired behavior, whether it is imitative or not, the context(s) in which we expect the child to produce that behavior, the criteria for its successful production, and other relevant factors. When we address these treatment goals, we often do so with careful attention to the stimulation we introduce, the responses we do and do not accept, and the reinforcement we provide for these responses. In addition, we discovered that of the diverse treatment methods available, the behavioral methods are the easiest to explain to family members, who subsequently find these the easiest to implement in home-based practice. The structure in behavioral methods is apparent to even those unfamiliar with clinical services. Parents who observe the participation of their child in a therapy session can easily identify and describe the stimulation an SLP provides, as well as the response the SLP desires from the child. Because of that, they also can easily identify the differentiated patterns of reinforcement and relate those to the quality of the response their child produced. An SLP who embraces the precepts of the behavioral explanations would offer a specific perspective in their advice to those who influence a child.

PSYCHOLINGUISTIC (SEMANTIC) THEORIES

In our description of *psycholinguistic* theories that attempt to explain the semantic dimension of language, rather than discuss a specific variation of these theories, we overview the concepts and/or principles that are common to this perspective on language development. On a *nature-nurture* continuum, these explanations of language development are placed in the midst of the *nature-nurture* poles. That is, these explanations posit that both internal (nature) and external (nurture) factors influence the development of the semantic aspect of language. This perspective reflects the considerable attention to and adaptation of the ideas of Piaget (1952). As was the case with Skinner, Piaget did not set out to explain language development in particular, but rather theories have applied his basic concepts to this phenomenon. Others who have advanced the psycholinguistic view of semantic development include Arbib, Conklin, and Hill (1987); Bloom (1970); Clark (1973); Nelson (1985); and Slobin (1973).

What a Child Learns

In this explanation, a child learns the content that he or she can express in words or in varied combinations of words. This content is most often characterized as "semantic features," "semantic relations," or "semantic categories." The focus in language development is not on words as parts of speech, but rather on words with respect to their relationship to other words. As a part of this process, a child moves from egocentric to nonegocentric perspectives in his or her interactions with the world, movement which further enhances the breadth and depth of content learned.

How Language Development Occurs

The process of language development commences with exploration of the environment. As a child explores the environment, he or she accumulates, then addresses, information from diverse sources. In this process, the child relates specific details to broader concepts.

Semantic Features

We can describe the process of language development with respect to semantic features. *Semantic features*, with the use of "+" or "−," indicate the presence or absence of semantic properties of words, or the aspects inherent in what words mean. Take the example of "cat." A child has some exposure to a cat, at which time he or she forms an initial concept of "cat." The child learns which features do and do not typically associate with that concept. We would characterize the cat as "+" for animal, feline, and whiskers, as well as for such traits as meowing, chasing mice, and consuming milk. In contrast, we would characterize the cat as "−" for traits the cat did not possess, such as human, canine, or bipedal. As the child has continued interaction with cats, he or she adjusts these semantic features to include additional features and/or to broaden appreciation of the features the cat shares with other creatures. This process reflects the hypothesis testing that is a substantial part of language learning. A child, consciously or unconsciously, formulates a hypothesis as to the correct name for a collection of features. To test that hypothesis, the child produces the name—the linguistic output—in a relevant communicative context. As others in that context react to that production, the child determines whether or not the reactions serve to support the hypothesis. He or she then refines the tenets of the hypothesis as appropriate. This reflects, in part, the perspective of Piaget in that this refinement can reflect the concepts of *assimilation* and *accommodation* of information to formulate concepts. We further elaborate on this process in subsequent chapters that describe early vocabulary development.

Semantic Relations

We also can describe this process with respect to semantic relations. That is, with respect to "cat," the child learns the relationships that this concept can share with other concepts, for which the child uses words and combines those words into utterances. Viewed alone, the word "cat" represents a noun. However, viewed in context, the word "cat" contributes assorted meanings to word combinations. In an utterance such as, "the cat sipped the cream," the cat is the performer of an action, but in an utterance such as, "the child stroked the cat," the cat is

the recipient of an action. There is no definitive, authoritative list of the semantic relations that children learn. In fact, there is no definitive approach to the construction of such a list, with perspectives that favor inclusion of universal relationships across concepts, as opposed to inclusion of varied levels of relationships. With that said, we include an example of one variation of the description of the semantic relations a child learns, with the reminder that this does not represent the only taxonomy of classification of these relationships.

An *active relation* describes a relationship between two concepts that expresses the performance of an operation that affects the other. Example: In the utterance, "mommy read book," the word *read* reflects that a person performed an action that had an effect on the item.

An *associative relation* indicates a relationship between concepts that individuals have, in their minds, associated and thus have made personal. Example: In the utterance, "baby like red binky," the word *binky* (as used for the pacifier) reflects that two individuals, perhaps a parent and a child, have associated this individualized word with specific content.

A *hyponymous relation* describes a relationship between concepts that relate in a hierarchical fashion, with some concepts subsets of others. Example: In the utterance, "want chocolate chip cookie," the word *chocolate* indicates that a person understands the idea of cookie to be broader than a particular flavor.

An *instance relation* indicates a relationship between a broad concept and the individual instances of that concept. Example: In the utterance, "drive car to store and to pool and to school," the specific locations provide evidence of the appreciation of the fact that the action, *drive*, can be applied to diverse situations.

A *locative relation* describes a relationship that indicates a location of an individual or information represented by yet another concept. Example: The utterances, "book on table," "book under table," and "book beside table" illustrate how one concept, *book*, can be described in terms of its various possible locations.

A *partive relation* indicates a relationship between a whole and its parts (that is, a broad concept and its constituent precepts). Example: The utterance in which a child names the parts of a car—wheels, doors, motor, windows—provides the constituent precepts of that concept, *car*.

A *passive relation* describes a relationship between two concepts, one of which is somehow acted on by the other concept. Example: In the utterance, "doggie petted by neighbor," the presentation of the object *doggie* before the action *petted* and the actor *neighbor* indicates an event in a grammatically passive fashion.

A *paradigmatic relation* indicates a relationship between two concepts that is evident or established after a natural relationship between these concepts has been widely verified. Example: Utterances that indicate, for instance, that foods are eaten, books are read, clothes are worn, trucks are driven, and other actions associated with specific items indicate this relationship.

A *possessive relation* describes a relationship between a possession and its possessor. Example: In the utterances, "doll mine," "mommy dress," "daddy shirt," and similar constructions, a child indicates what is owned by whom.

A *temporal relation* indicates a time or a time frame for events. Example: When a child describes an event, such as a birthday party, and tells whether this has occurred or, in contrast, is intended to occur, he or she indicates a temporal relationship.

We must stress that relationships between concepts are not the same as relationships between the words that express those concepts. However, there are terms used to describe the relationships between these words. Examples include: *synonyms*, or words with the same meanings; *antonyms*, or words with opposite meanings; *hypernyms*, or words that reflect meanings that are superordinate to those of related words; *hyponyms*, or words that reflect meanings that are subordinate to those of related words; *meronyms*, or words that name parts of a broader whole; *holonyms*, or words that name this broader whole; and *troponyms*, words that describe how to perform actions. Certainly the appreciation of these distinctions complements the development of semantic relationships.

Semantic Categories

We also can describe this concept with respect to semantic categories. That is, with respect to "cat," the child learns various categories of information,

then represents these categories in utterances with increased structural complexity. As with the semantic relations, there is no authoritative or exhaustive collection of semantic categories of information. However, some common entries in systems to describe semantic categories include existence, recurrence, attribution, possession, action, locative, state, epistemic, antithesis, and others.

Factors That Influence Language Development

This explanation asserts a relationship between cognitive development and language development. Whether the relationship is that of *cognition* preceded by *language*, *language* preceded by *cognition*, or an interrelated relationship between these two constructs remains unclear. However, the value of cognitive development is confirmed to, at least in some fashion and to some extent, contribute to language development. At the same time that this explanation supports internal variables, this explanation also supports external variables related to the environment. The language development of a child is enhanced by a diversity of opportunities for exploration and experimentation in the environment.

Advantages to This Explanation

This explanation confirms the value of both internal and external factors for language development. In terms of internal factors, this perspective attempts to relate cognitive development to language development. In addition, this perspective describes specific cognitive skills that can enhance the presence of specific language skills. In terms of external factors, this explanation attempts to relate the nature of the environmental input to the quantity and quality of language output of a child. In addition, this explanation values the natural inclination of a child to interact with his or her environment through experiments with items and other individuals. Besides the confirmation of the value of internal and external factors, this perspective considers that children do not simply learn words but, instead, learn what words mean both individually and in a myriad of relationships with each other. Thus, the content of the words, to some extent, dictates their functions within interactions, as well as their incorporation into structures that increase in sophistication.

Disadvantages to This Explanation

At the same time that this explanation confirms the relationship between cognitive and language development, it does not confirm the exact nature of that relationship. One possible relationship is a *determinist* one. In this view, the cognitive level of the child determines the language level and the ultimate potential for the level of language development a child can reach. However, one other possible relationship is an *interactionist* one. In this view, the cognitive level and the language level of a child need not be identical. At some points, the cognitive level may appear to be more advanced, and at others, the language level may appear to be more advanced. In some instances, these two domains may be so intertwined that the determination of a unidirectional influence of one on another is impossible. In addition, there is no indication of whether the role of cognition remains stable or, instead, adapts to the advanced language level of the older child. Because of the uncertain nature of this relationship, there is no explanation as to why the presence of "normal" cognition does not ensure the presence of "normal" language. Whether other factors interact with both cognition and language is unclear in this explanation. Another concern is with the actual parameters of this explanation and its focus on the semantic aspect of language. Although some proponents of this view do indeed note the relationship between semantics and the structural and/or interactional dimensions of language, semantics remains the primary focus.

Clinical Implications

The SLP who provides clinical services to enhance the language development of a child, because of the influence of this explanation, will consider the cognitive development as a child. If the SLP concludes that cognitive level is a predictor of eventual language level, then he or she can use it to determine the prognosis for successful remediation of language challenges. If the SLP concludes that cognitive skills precede language skills, then he or she will plan a course of treatment that includes the establishment of cognitive foundations of language development prior to work to address specific language challenges. However, if the SLP concludes that cognitive skills and language skills develop simultaneously—in either an independent or an interdependent fashion—then he or she will plan a course of treatment that addresses concept development in its broadest sense that includes words to label collections of information. In either case, the focus of treatment is semantic. The SLP need not entirely focus the treatment on the semantic dimension of language, however. This explanation is sufficiently broad to allow the SLP to integrate the semantic components with the structural and/or interactional dimensions of language. With respect to the structural elements, the SLP could aim to enhance the sophistication of the structures that a child uses to encode semantic information. And, with respect to the interactional elements, the SLP could aim to enhance the extent to which a child accomplishes his or her communicative intentions with the presentation of semantic information across diverse contexts.

PSYCHOLINGUISTIC (STRUCTURAL) THEORIES

In our description of *psycholinguistic* theories that attempt to explain the structural dimension of language, rather than discuss a specific variation of these theories, we overview the concepts and/or principles that are common to this perspective on language development. On a *nature-nurture* continuum, these explanations of language are placed within the *nature* dimension of the continuum. This perspective reflects the considerable attention to and adaptation of the ideas of Chomsky (1957). Others who have advanced the psycholinguistic view of structural development include Fodor (1983), with the *modularity theory*, and Gleitman (1990), with the *bootstrap theory*.

What a Child Learns

In this explanation, a child learns—or at least provides observable evidence of the presence of—universal language rules that underlie the combination of phonemes into words, then those words into phrases, clauses, sentences, and narratives. These rules are hierarchical in nature and dictate not simply the kinds of phonemes and words that can be combined but also the structures into which phonemes, words, and sentences can be incorporated. A child demonstrates both these "deep" rules and the "surface" manifestations of these rules in the combinations that he or she eventually produces.

How Language Development Occurs

In this explanation, a child possesses an intricate network of linguistic rules that govern the structure of his or her language. Chomsky conceptualized this network as the language acquisition device (LAD). What exactly is the LAD? Is it an actual anatomical structure? Is it an intricate neural network that represents connections within the central nervous system? Is it an intricate cognitive network that represents hierarchical executive functions? Or is the LAD another kind of structure or system? Chomsky did not provide these details; however, he did provide an overview of its function: the extraction of linguistic rules and linguistic transformations from the language input to which others expose the child. He subsequently broadened the idea of the LAD into the concept of *universal grammar*, which is the presumption that languages share a set of universal principles that lead to common structural elements. The process of language development as described by the LAD unfolds in a series of linguistic operations. The child receives, from his or her environment, linguistic input which, by its very nature, is often incomplete (e.g., the adult who says "give mommy book" to a toddler) and often incorrect (e.g., the adult who says "walk good" to a toddler). On this receipt, the LAD analyzes the structure of the input. If the input matches the expected output from a specific linguistic rule, the LAD recognizes a match; if not, the LAD recognizes a mismatch, and a more detailed analysis is necessary. The LAD searches the available linguistic database for potential matches between the input and the rules, which involves the formulation of hypotheses as to which rules are the most suitable matches for the input. Ultimately, the LAD forms a conclusion as to compatibility and activates the rules involved. Access

to those rules then allows a child to interpret the nature of the input and, subsequently, to apply the extracted rules to his or her own linguistic productions. Thus, if a child interprets the structure subject + verb + object from input, then he or she will apply that rule to subsequent utterances.

Central to this explanation of language development is the nature of language structure—*deep structure* versus *surface structure*. The *deep structure* of language indicates the semantic content the language user wishes to share. Like the principles, or language universals, inherent in this explanation, semantic content is shared across languages. The deep structure of language becomes observable in the *surface structure* of language, or the utterances a language learner produces. A specific deep structure can be realized in multiple surface structures. Picture this scene: parent-child book time. The *deep structure* that captures this event includes the content that represents this interaction. The *surface structures* that capture this deep structure include, "The parent read the book to the child," "The parent read the child the book," "The book was read by the parent to the child," "The child was read the book by the parent," and others. This process of representation is conceptualized as *transformational grammar* or *generative grammar* (Chomsky, 1966).

Central to this explanation of language development is also the nature of *language operations*. These operations serve to transform deep structures into varieties of surface structures to create not only simple but also compound and complex sentences. Multiple elementary operations contribute to transformations. We can describe some operations with respect to the specific action on a deep structure. Operations of *addition* expand the surface structure to reflect more semantic content, *deletion* reduces the surface structure to reflect less semantic content, and *transposition* shifts the order of elements in a surface structure to reflect a change in deep structure. Operations of *substitution* replace elements in a surface structure to reflect another shift in deep structure.

In addition to these, language learners can employ *generalized* operations to multiple deep structures to create compound and complex sentences. The operation starts with the creation of a *simple* sentence, one that contains one subject and one predicate verb, for example, "John ate the pizza." A child converts this *simple* structure to a *compound* structure with the operation of conjoining, which involves adding elements to the original structure with the purpose of adding meaning. This results in sentences such as, "John ate the pizza, and Mary ate the pasta" (two simple sentences conjoined into a compound sentence), "John and Mary ate the pizza" (a compound subject), "John ate and drank" (a compound predicate verb), "John ate the pizza and the pasta" (a compound object), and even sentences that reflect compound subjects, verbs, and objects within a compound sentence. An alternative conversion occurs when a child converts this *simple* structure to a *complex* structure with the operation of embedding, which involves blending—and sometimes even deleting for the purpose of language elegance—elements from the original structure for the purpose of adding meaning. The *simple* sentence, "Mary eats the pizza," becomes a gerund form (e.g., "Mary likes eating the pizza"), an infinitive form (e.g., "Mary likes to eat the pizza"), a complemental form (e.g., "Mary thinks that she is eating the pizza"), or a relative clause (e.g., "Mary, who likes to eat, has a pizza"). Additional operations that a child applies to structures include statement to question transformation, active to passive transformation, positive to negative transformation, and several others.

In some explanations of this view, the concept of *bootstrapping* becomes relevant as a link between the structural and the semantic dimensions of language. This concept reflects the process via which a child uses the structure of an utterance to determine what individual words within that utterance mean. In addition to *bootstrapping*, the concept of *binding* becomes relevant. In a revision of his earlier explanations of language, Chomsky (1981) indicated that two additional aspects of language development can occur. One is the restriction on which elements of language structure can occur at specific points within utterances, whereas the other is the imposition of a hierarchy of elements to indicate variety in the level of interpretation needed to extract their rules.

Factors That Influence Language Development

This view underscores the importance of the neurolinguistic status of the child, or the presence of intact neurologic structures that either comprise the LAD or provide the neurologic basis for the intact function of the LAD. Before the process of extraction of language rules occurs, the child must be able to receive the actual language input that contains these rules. To ensure that the LAD extracts the most extensive range of linguistic rules available, the child somehow must be exposed to diverse language input.

Advantages to This Explanation

This explanation attempts to explain how children can produce utterances that they have never before constructed, as well as how children can comprehend utterances to which they have never been exposed. The idea of a sophisticated linguistic—perhaps neurolinguistic—network that houses a substantial assortment of linguistic rules that enable this production and comprehension accounts for the creative nature of language described in Chapter 1. This explanation attempts to account for *language universals*, or rules that are present to some extent across the languages of the world. At the same time, newer variations of this explanation note that structural rules can be organized into hierarchies, as well as bound to specific points within utterances that allow a child to more accurately interpret the semantic elements of those utterances. The focus on universals also accounts for the similarities across the language structure of children from distinctive environments, whose utterances develop from simple to compound to complex in a similar fashion.

Disadvantages to This Explanation

Although this explanation affirms the value of input for the child, the focus is on the presence of the input, not on its nature. Because of this, there is minimal value placed on the role of interaction for purposes other than to "awaken" the LAD. The contributions of input to the content and the function of language for a child are thus discounted. The interactional modifications that adults demonstrate in the presence of the child, namely, the adaptation of adult language to the language that the child comprehends and produces, are not considered vital for the language development of the child. While this explanation describes the rules that are present for children across languages, the focus is on shared rules, not on how these rules are manifested in the personal styles that children display in their interactions. In addition, this explanation is silent with respect to the issue of what constitutes an acceptable level of individual variation in typical language development as opposed to what indicates atypical language development. Although this explanation accounts for "immature" linguistic rules, it provides no criteria by which SLPs can determine whether immature rules will eventually mature into adultlike language structure or, instead, dictate the need for remediation. In addition to these considerations, because this explanation focuses on language structure, by definition, it limits this view. Although newer versions of this perspective have incorporated some reference to semantic content and how the presence of structural rules can enhance interpretation of content, the focus remains primarily on structural elements of language.

Clinical Implications

With a focus on the hierarchical nature of language structure, this explanation provides a blueprint for SLP clinical services that address the need to enhance the sophistication of utterances. This view posits the presence of rules that increase in terms of the quantity and quality of their constituent parts. This allows the SLP to plan a course of treatment that starts with simple constructions, then adds elements to result in compound and complex constructions. The addition of elements involves transformations that build on previous, less advanced structures. This explanation also provides a framework for the interpretation of what adults could otherwise perceive as language errors on the part of a child. It posits that productions of a child that do not match the productions of an adult are immature productions rather than an indication of a clinical problem. Rather than start with the idea that an adult production is a standard to which a child production is compared, and thus rendered deficient, this view starts with the idea that a child builds on his or her own previous constructions. Thus, the focus is on what the child *has* acquired thus far, not on what

the child *has not* acquired. Supposed "errors" are not to be corrected but rather are to be celebrated as typical steps in language development. In addition to this consideration, the focus on maturation is central to this explanation. The SLP whose clinical practice is influenced by this view would consider whether a child possessed intact neurologic structures and processes that this explanation presumes are vital for language. If these were present, then the SLP would trust that maturation of language would be possible and thus would focus treatment on the presentation of input to stimulate and enhance the maturation process.

SOCIOLINGUISTIC THEORIES

In our description of *sociolinguistic* theories, rather than discuss a specific variation of these theories, we overview the concepts and/or principles that are common to this perspective on language development. On a *nature-nurture* continuum, these explanations of language are most often placed within the *nurture* dimension of the continuum. However, elements of *nature*, such as the readiness to accept and ascertain the nature of input, as well as to adapt interaction to cues within this input, are also central to this explanation. This perspective reflects the considerable influence of Vygotsky (1962). Others who have advanced the sociolinguistic view of language development include Bloom (2000), with the *intentionality model*, and Tomasello (2003), with the *use-based model*.

What a Child Learns

In this explanation, a child learns the routines that comprise a substantial portion of day-to-day social interactions. To learn these patterns of communication, a child adapts the *form* of his or her communication to its *function* to enhance the effectiveness of his or her language across communicative contexts.

How Language Development Occurs

In this explanation, over the course of repeated social interactions, a child assumes increased responsibility for the completion of social routines. As noted in Chapter 1, one of the properties of language is its creative rule-based nature, which allows children to produce utterances to which they have not produced before and to comprehend utterances to which they have never been exposed. Although we celebrate this creative nature that ensures production and comprehension of unique utterances, we also note that a substantial proportion of day-to-day communication is routinized. A social routine is an interaction with repetitive, predictable elements that are apparent even in variations of the situation. A *social routine* contains a *social script*, or the linguistic output that, when combined with the nonlinguistic output in an appropriate fashion, constitutes successful participation in that predictable situation. The road to success can be conceptualized as a process in which the child assumes the leadership in a routine for which the adult once served as the leader (Gunter, 1986, 1987). We can describe this process as a series of steps, and for the purposes of explanation we select the routine of a visit to a fast food restaurant.

Step 1: Observation

In this step, a child receives an introduction to the social routine that he or she has started to learn. This introduction comes from direct observation of the situation. In a visit to a fast food restaurant, the child will see the enactment of the components of the routine: the entrance, the review of the menu, the placement of the food order, the receipt of the food, the provision of the cost, the selection of a table, the completion of the meal, the clearance of the trash, and the departure. The adults in the situation may complement these elements with not only scripted comments but also unscripted comments about various components of the routine that stimulate the child to reflect on. In addition to this direct observation, the child can be exposed to this routine via such media as advertisements and interactions as reports of others about their own experiences. At this step, the adults do not expect the child to be an active participant in the routine, as in one who completes one or more components in an independent fashion. However, the adults do structure the situation to stimulate the interest of the child.

Step 2: Scaffolds and Simulated Participation

In this step, a child has opportunities for simulated participation in the social routine. This participation, in part, comes from scaffolded interaction in the situation. When an adult uses *scaffolds*, he or she structures the interaction to ensure the best possible level of success for the child with respect to participation in the social routine. The adult models a component of the situation, except for a final act, then allows the child to attempt the completion of that particular component. Take the review of the menu, for instance. At this point, rather than scan the menu and select the items to order, the adult leads the child in this review with closed-ended questions (e.g., "Would you like one drink or the other drink?"), then with open-ended questions (e.g., "Which drink would you like?"). The child then responds with a choice, an act which the adult confirms with a response appropriate to the context. For other aspects of the situation, the adult provides cues as to how and when to participate. Take the placement of the order. The adult provides such cues as, "Tell the clerk what you want," or, "Ask the clerk what you owe." Take the clearance of the trash. The adult provides such cues as, "Where should you take this trash?" and, "What items should you return?" Whenever the child completes a component of the routine with this support, the adult, as before, responds in a noncontrived fashion to stress the contribution of the child to the interaction.

Step 3: Participation and Natural Consequences

In this step, a child demonstrates more independence with respect to the completion in the social routine. Rather than depend on the scaffolds of an adult, the child extracts information about the quality of his or her performance from the *natural consequences* within the situation. Consider the review of the menu. Instead of dependence on adults to provide cues as to how to complete this act, the child shows more initiative in this component of the routine. Instead of dependence on adults to structure an interaction to increase his or her interest and success, the child attends to the salient aspects of the natural consequences. So, the clear presentation of his or her selections to the clerk reaps the natural reward of the service of the food the child indeed selected. On the other hand, the unclear or confused presentation of selections reaps the natural response of a request for clarification, specification, and/or elaboration of the request. By this experimentation with the content and the format of the social routine, the child acquires a more sensitive appreciation for the appropriate linguistic and nonlinguistic elements that are linked with predictable, scripted interactions.

Step 4: Generalization

Once the child has demonstrated competence with respect to a particular social routine, he or she can broaden application of the principles to similar routines. After a child has learned to review the menu, this can be expanded to include other menus from other restaurants. After a child has learned to complete the meal, he or she can expand this to include meals with multiple courses, creative utensils, and other variations. After participation in diverse variations of this routine, the child can extract elements for application in nonrestaurant situations. For instance, the child can extend the act of calculation of cost and remission of cash to other situations that involve purchases of items. In addition to continued experiences with this particular routine, the child serves in the role in which the adult once served. As a model for other, less competent children or as a person whom others observe to be introduced to the routine, the child can now act as performer and instructor.

Because social experiences are not identical, even children from similar environments may not demonstrate a comparable level of proficiency for a specific social routine. In addition, a specific child may demonstrate a variety of levels of proficiency across the social routines to which he or she has been introduced. However, the attainment of a level of sophistication in the completion of routines follows this predictable sequence of steps.

While the maturation of social routines is of paramount importance for success in interpersonal communication, the sociolinguistic viewpoint does not restrict the explanation of language development to these situations alone. Within the sociolinguistic viewpoint is the concept of *speech acts* (Searle, 1969), which consists of three components:

the *illocution*, the *locution*, and the *perlocution*. The *illocution* reflects the intention of an individual, in this case a child, or what he or she hopes to accomplish in a specific interaction. For instance, the child may wish to inform, request, or complete another purpose. The *locution* reflects the manner in which the child transmits this intention to an interactional partner. This transmission may consist of linguistic and/or nonlinguistic elements and, to some extent, represents the sophistication of the language structure of the child. The *perlocution* reflects the interpretation that the interactional partner imposed on the locution. In many scenarios, the aim of the child is to construct the locution in such a fashion that the intention and the interpretation of that intention are consistent. Instances in which a mismatch between these occurs provide information from which the child can draw implication for future constructions.

Factors That Influence Language Development

This view centers around the opportunities a child has for exploration and experimentation in a diverse assortment of social interactions. To benefit from these experiences, a child must be exposed to both appropriate and inappropriate variations within interactions in order to observe the natural consequences that result. The child must be able to appreciate the connection between communication choices with these consequences, as well as to discern from situational cues, initially explicit, then implicit, that reveal the norms and needs within these situations.

Advantages to This Explanation

The sociolinguistic perspective focuses, in a more extensive fashion than other perspectives, on the social dimension of communication. With the emphasis on *social routines*, this perspective incorporates the idea that one does not produce linguistic and nonlinguistic behaviors in isolation but, instead, in response to the communication demands of a particular situation. Thus, the relationship between "form" and "function" is explicit and is further promoted in the emphasis on *speech acts*. The sociolinguistic perspective also focuses on natural rather than contrived influences on language development.

The natural reactions, in relevant contexts, to the behaviors of a child focus only on the content and the structure of the language as these enhance the function of the language. These reactions, which address communication effectiveness, note the correctness or incorrectness of content and structure as these increase or decrease the successful completion of an interaction. The simultaneous development of content, structure, and function spares a child from the difficult transition between contrived and noncontrived day-to-day situations.

Disadvantages to This Explanation

This explanation of language development presumes that a child is exposed to a diverse collection of social experiences. However, for some children, this is not the case. This explanation does not account for how children extract language rules from restricted quantity and/or quality of interactions, nor what potential deficiencies in language development could result. It also does not note the extent to which exposure to social experiences is sufficient to facilitate language development, nor the reasons that some children require more exploration and experimentation than others. In addition to these concerns related to exposure, this explanation of language development places as much value on the "end result" of language use as on the means to accomplish that end. The minimized demand for language use that is semantically and structurally correct raises the question of how deficiencies in these areas could be addressed when present. In addition to this concern, this explanation of language development draws conclusions from the information in day-to-day interactions. The nature of these interactions has a substantial impact on what children learn. However, because these skills are so context dependent, we can know the pattern of development (as in the description of social routine development) but not the detailed norms that we have available for the structural elements of language. Thus, we are forced to use descriptive evaluation methods rather than normative evaluation methods, which would allow us to compare the performance of children from comparable environments. Although not necessarily a concern, this may prove problematic in the instances in which we must describe the language development in a normative fashion.

Clinical Implications

The SLP who believes that this explanation is the most appropriate description of language development will affirm the interdependence of the areas in which children develop language skills. The SLP can use the concept of social routines as a framework for the provision of clinical services. In this approach, a child learns which behaviors are most apt to result in successful interaction and that these behaviors represent relationships across areas. The SLP also can use the concept of speech acts as a framework. In this approach, a child learns to construct locutions, then to evaluate whether these most clearly convey the intention of the child so that the interpretation of this aim is accurate. Adherence to this explanation also colors the view toward what can be perceived as "errors" in social interaction. Rather than consider these on a continuum of correct versus incorrect, the SLP interprets these with respect to the extent that they cause a breakdown in communication and provides feedback to the child about the relative effectiveness of his or her attempts. Although the applications of this explanation to clinical practice are valuable, the SLP does not focus on the output of the child alone. Instead, the SLP considers the extent to which a child can observe situations, extract relevant details about the nature of the interaction, evaluate what constituted effective attempts, consider which modifications would increase the chances for a positive interaction, and revise the content and/or the structure of his or her own language to achieve this end. Should the SLP note the need for intervention to address these skills, then the focus of clinical service delivery can expand to encompass these areas.

CONCLUSION

Quite an assortment of explanations of language development exist. In addition to the broad families of theories presented in this chapter, explanations of specific aspects of language, such as lexicon, also exist. We present some of these in our subsequent discussions of language skills in Chapters 3, 4, and 5. Even with our access to these theories in their earlier and present forms, still there is no comprehensive, authoritative explanation of how language development occurs across the life span. For each advantage that we can describe for each of the available theories, we can present a companion disadvantage. Because of that, we are motivated to continue to collect information about children that could enhance and expand our appreciation of the language development process with the hope that, at some future point, we have captured the conditions and processes that dictate this development. In that respect, each and every interaction that we share with children becomes a research opportunity for us, as children cause us to question, revise, expand, blend, and otherwise deal with theoretical information with the ultimate aim of a unified explanation of a wonderful phenomenon.

REFLECTION QUESTIONS

1. What are the central questions you have regarding why and how children develop language? What prompted these questions—what you have read, observed, or experienced?

2. Based on the information you have reviewed in this chapter, which of the theories of language development mirrors your own views? What commonalities can you observe between this explanation and your own? If none of the theories is consistent with your own views, then write your own explanation for how language development occurs.

3. Currently, no explanation of language development exists that is a complete, correct, and consistent account of how this complex area of skill comes to be for a child. How would you resolve the limitations of the presently available theories?

4. What does it mean for a theory to be "internally consistent" in nature? Why is the formulation of a noncontradictory theory so vital in clinical practice and day-to-day interaction with children?

5. How could you use the information about theories to advise parents and professionals, such as teachers, about their role in the language development of a child?

APPLICATION EXERCISES

1. The parents of a child present a question to you: "How should we interact with our child?" They wonder whether they should be very careful to always speak correctly to their child, as well as whether they should speak as if to other adults. How would you respond to the concern of these parents, who want to do their best to enhance the language of their child? How would each of these broad explanations of language development inform your response to that question?

2. The teachers of a child are uncertain how they should respond when that child communicates in an imperfect fashion. Sometimes the child has produced the sounds incorrectly, and sometimes the child has incorrectly selected the words to convey information. The teachers are not sure whether to respond to the structure of what the child said, to the content, to both, or to neither. How would you respond to their uncertainty? How would theory influence your response?

3. A child with a communication disorder receives clinical services from multiple practitioners. The parents are concerned about the possibility of contradictory practices. How would the application of theory to clinical practice contribute to the prevention of contradictions? If the parents asked you for an opinion as to whether services that stem from multiple theoretical perspectives hurt, help, or have no impact on the child, how would you respond? How would theory influence your response?

REFERENCES

Arbib, M. A., Conklin, E. J., & Hill, J. (1987). *From schema theory to language*. New York, NY: Oxford University Press.

Bloom, L. (1970). *Language development: Form and function of emerging grammars*. Cambridge, MA: MIT Press.

Bloom, L. (2000). The intentionality model of word learning. In R. M. Golinkoff, K. Hirsh-Pasek, N. Akhtar, L. Bloom, G. Hollich, & L. Smith (Eds.), *Becoming a word learner: A debate on lexical acquisition.* New York, NY: Oxford University Press.

Chomsky, N. (1957). *Syntactic structures.* The Hague, The Netherlands: Mouton.

Chomsky, N. (1966). *Topics in the theory of generative grammar.* The Hague, The Netherlands: Mouton.

Chomsky, N. (1981). *Lectures on government and binding.* Dordrecht, The Netherlands: Foris.

Clark, E. V. (1973). What's in a word? On the child's acquisition of semantics in his first language. In T. E. Moore (Ed.), *Cognitive development and the acquisition of language.* New York, NY: Academic Press.

Fodor, J. (1973). *The modularity of mind.* Cambridge, MA: MIT Press.

Gleitman, L. (1990). The structural sources of verb meanings. *Language Acquisition, 12,* 299–311.

Gunter, C. D. (November, 1986). *A model of the social transmission of language behavior.* Annual Convention, American Speech-Language-Hearing Association, Detroit, MI.

Gunter, C. D. (April, 1987). *Language learning in situation-specific activities.* International Symposium on Specific Speech and Language Disorders in Children, The University of Reading, England.

Mowrer, O. (1954). The psychologist looks at language. *American Psychologist, 9,* 660–664.

Nelson, K. (1985). *Making sense: The acquisition of shared meaning.* New York, NY: Academic Press.

Osgood, C. (1963). On understanding and creating sentences. *American Psychologist, 18,* 635–751.

Piaget, J. (1952). *The origins of intelligence in children.* New York, NY: International Universities Press.

Searle, J. (1969). *Speech acts.* Cambridge, England: Cambridge University Press.

Skinner, B. F. (1957). *Verbal behavior.* Englewood Cliffs, NJ: Prentice-Hall.

Slobin, D. (1973). Cognitive prerequisites for the development of grammar. In C. Ferguson & D. Slobin (Eds.), *Studies of child language development.* New York, NY: Holt, Rinehart, and Winston.

Staats, A. W. (1963). *Complex human behavior.* New York, NY: Holt, Rinehart, and Winston.

Tomasello, M. (2003). *Constructing a language.* Cambridge, MA: Harvard University Press.

Vygotsky, L. S. (1962). *Thought and language.* Cambridge, MA: MIT Press.

CHAPTER 3

Language Development: Prelinguistic Skills

PRELINGUISTIC DEVELOPMENT: PARAMETERS

The prelinguistic period is the time between a child's birth and the production of his or her first real word at about 12 months. The milestones achieved during this time form the infrastructure for later language development.

PRELINGUISTIC DEVELOPMENT: PURPOSES

Language is a tool for communication, but it is not the only tool. As mature communicators, we also send messages nonverbally through facial expressions, gestures, body posture, and even deliberate silence. However, prelinguistic infants are restricted to nonverbal signals alone. Initially, these signals occur in response to biological states or sensory stimulation, and their meanings are partly dependent on the interpretations of caregivers. As infants mature, their perceptual skills and motor control become increasingly sophisticated. They develop concepts about the world. They begin to understand language, and they learn the social skills needed to communicate intentionally through vocalizations and gestures. This progress unfolds gradually through interactions between infants and their caregivers. Milestones in this process are considered with an eye toward these components of future language development: lexicon, semantics, phonology, morphology, syntax, and pragmatics.

PRIMARY ACCOMPLISHMENTS: LEXICON AND SEMANTICS

Background

Semantics is the system of rules that determine the meanings of words and the meaningful relationships between words. Words in a language can be divided into two types: lexical words and function words (Werker & Tees, 1999). Lexical words are content words such as nouns, verbs, adjectives, and so forth. Most early words are lexical. Function words serve a grammatical purpose. They include articles, prepositions, auxiliary verbs, and others. Within a broader framework, the word lexicon refers to an individual's vocabulary. Here, we address three important influences on future lexical growth: child-caregiver interactions, the development of lexical comprehension, and the development of protowords.

Child-Caregiver Interaction: The Contributions of Infants

Language is a conventional social skill, and the experiences needed to learn a specific language are embedded within the context of social interaction. During the prelinguistic period, this interaction is typically dyadic, consisting of the infant and one of his or her caregivers. Below is a description of what an infant and a caregiver contribute to the interactive process.

Right from the start, infants exhibit many behaviors that draw their caregivers to them. During the first week of life, they show a preference for looking at faces, especially the angular features of faces and the eyes. They move their bodies in synchrony to speech (**interactional synchronization**). They show a preference for speech versus nonspeech sounds and especially for the speech produced by their mother. If they hear speech, they will search for the source; and when they see the face of the speaker, their eyes may widen, their body may tense, and they may pause as if expecting a response. Infants produce an array of facial expressions reflecting the appearance of joy, anger, fear, sorrow, discomfort, and others. Although there is no evidence that infants experience these emotions in the manner attributed to older children, caregivers notice these expressions and respond to them. Infants also produce a number of vocal patterns. Most mothers report that they can distinguish their own infant's cry from that of other infants in the nursery; and infants will often stop crying when they hear their mother's voice. These are but a few of the infant behaviors that normally engage caregivers and launch a loving, interactive relationship that continues throughout life.

Over the course of the prelinguistic period, stunning changes occur in an infant's physical maturation, perceptual awareness, motor control, social skills, and cognitive growth. Each change brings new abilities and new opportunities for child-caregiver interaction. A thorough description is beyond the scope of this chapter but can be found elsewhere (e.g., Bremmer & Fogel, 2001; Lamb, Bornstein, & Teti, 2002). However, changes in cognitive development are directly relevant to future lexical growth and will be summarized here.

Cognition

Cognition is defined here as the processes and products of mind. It is an important precursor to lexical growth because (among other things) a caregivers' perceptions of an infant's moment-by-moment cognitive status influences the content of speech addressed to the infant and therefore the language that is acquired. It is also important because some theories of language acquisition assume that the acquisition process itself (including the initial lexicon) is based on domain-general (as opposed to domain-specific) cognitive processes (e.g., Saffran & Thiessen, 2007). **Domain-general theories** propose that the cognitive processes involved in language learning are the same as those involved in learning any other type of problem-solving skill. In contrast, **domain-specific theories** propose that language acquisition is made possible by a module in the brain that is specific to language. Whether language development is domain-general, domain-specific, or some combination thereof awaits final determination. However, it is clear that language and thought are intimately connected.

It is challenging to study cognition because mental processes are not directly observable. This is especially true in the case of infants, who cannot verbalize what they know or how they think. However, as in any other science, knowledge about infant cognition is guided by theories and evidence that either supports or questions theoretical stands.

Currently theories of infant cognitive development vary according to assumptions about an infant's innate abilities and about the nature of subsequent development (Meltzoff & Moore, 1999). For example, Jean Piaget (1952) assumed that infants are born with sensory-motor reflexes but that the capacity for mental representation and other cognitive processes develops gradually, in qualitatively distinct substages, through systematic interaction with the environment over the first two years of life. Piaget based these assumptions on detailed observations of his own three children. More recently, researchers have found evidence of rudimentary cognitive skills much earlier than reported by Piaget, sometimes even within days of an infant's birth (e.g., Baillargeon, 1987; Baillargeon & DeVos, 1991; Baillargeon, DeVos, & Graber, 1989;

Baillargeon, Graber, DeVos, & Black, 1990; Meltzoff, 1988, 1990). These findings suggest that fundamental cognitive abilities actually may be present at birth and that subsequent development may be continuous rather than stage-based. Unlike Piaget, current researchers have had the benefit of observing a larger number of infants under carefully controlled laboratory conditions with sophisticated instrumentation. Differences in findings are due, in part, to differences in the observation procedures and assessment tasks (e.g., Moore & Meltzoff, 1999). However, although Piaget may have underestimated the ages of emergence of particular abilities, his estimates regarding the ages of mastery remain relatively stable. With this in mind, we present the following brief summary of the processes and products associated with infant cognitive development from a Piagetian perspective.

Piaget (1952) viewed cognition as a trait that evolves with physical maturation and environmental experience through a series of four stages. At each stage, a child uses characteristic **schemes**, which are organized ways of making sense of experience. At first, schemes are sensorimotor actions such as sucking, grasping, dropping, throwing, poking, and so forth. Eventually, schemes include mental representations such as images and concepts. Development is made possible through the process of adaptation and organization as infants interact with the environment. **Adaptation** involves the complementary processes of assimilation and accommodation. **Assimilation** is the process by which individuals recognize similarity between new experiences and existing knowledge, whereas **accommodation** is the process by which individuals modify existing knowledge to include the novel features of a new experience. Most experiences involve a balance of assimilation and accommodation. Too much familiarity (assimilation) is boring and too much novelty (accommodation) is difficult to process. In fact, Piaget proposed that children naturally seek **minimally discrepant stimulation**. For example, when playing peek-a-boo with her infant, a caregiver may notice that the infant eventually tires of repeated rounds that are exactly the same (too much assimilation). So, to maintain the infant's interest, the caregiver may vary some feature of the game (e.g., the speed) to add a small element of novelty and surprise (increasing the infant's need for accommodation).

Another way in which schemes change over time is through the process of **organization**. This takes place internally and independently of direct environmental manipulation. It is a process of building connections between schemes. For example, infants will eventually relate the "dropping" scheme to the "throwing" scheme and to later mental representations of "nearness" and "farness" (Berk, 2006).

In addition to the above developmental processes, Piaget (1952) described a number of cognitive products that are acquired by infants gradually during the first two years of life. We highlight three of these here, including object permanence, object play, and means-ends development. Another product (i.e., imitation) is considered in the section of this chapter on the precursors to phonological development. As indicated above, a caregiver's perception of these and other aspects of cognitive development is likely to influence the content of child-addressed speech. Additionally, Bates, Camaino, and Volterra (1975) showed that tool use, imitation, and means-ends abilities at 9 months are correlated with word use at 12 months. Furthermore, object permanence is included because of its link with the acquisition of words for object states, such as "all gone," "more," and others (e.g., Gopnik & Meltzoff, 1986). The following descriptions of object permanence, object play, and means-ends are based in part on tasks used to measure these skills as described in Uzgiris and Hunt (1975).

Object Permanence. Object permanence is the understanding that objects continue to exist even if they are not within sight. It can be measured in various ways (e.g., Meltzoff & Moore, 1999). One way is to observe whether an infant tracks or searches for an object that is moving or disappearing under a cloth. When measured in this way, object permanence develops gradually and may not be fully mastered until 24 months. However, significant growth can be observed during the prelinguistic period. For example, infants between birth and 1 month of age will track a slowly moving object for a short distance if they are positioned in supine and if the object is of interest. Between 1 to 4 months, infants learn to track objects across a 180° arc, again, if the object is of interest. Between 4 to 8 months, infants will recognize and retrieve a preferred object if it is partially hidden (e.g., a teddy bear partially covered by a blanket), and by 8 to 12 months they can find an object hidden in one of two places, alternately as long as they see it being hidden. Early within the 8- to 12-month period they may make a "place error" by searching in the location where they found the toy the first time rather than searching in the new location where they observed it being hidden. However, with practice in playing object-search games, they become quite successful at finding objects hidden in one of two places alternately. The permanence of objects appears particularly interesting to infants at this age, and it is not surprising to note that "peek-a-boo" games become particularly frequent between 8 and 12 months (Gustafson, Green, & West, 1979).

Object Play. Object play is another important area of growth. This too can be measured in various ways. Here, we summarize object manipulation patterns observed when an infant is playing independently. During the first month of development, infants may track slowly moving objects but they do not yet grasp toys volitionally. During the period between about 1 to 4 months, there is a gradual increase of interest in toys. Initially, infants engage in incidental object use. So, if an object (e.g., a rattle) is placed in the palm of an infant's hand, the infant may close his or her fingers around it. If the infant then moves his or her arm the rattle will make a sound. Infants at this stage are also increasingly interested in toys presented to them by others. Between 4 to 8 months, infants develop systematic object use. This involves systematic repetitive actions with objects (e.g., mouthing, banging, patting, poking, waving, etc.). The action applied to an object is not specific to the object. For example, any object may be patted, poked, or mouthed, regardless of its conventional function. Between 8 to 12 months, infants begin to demonstrate combined systematic object use as well as some functional object use. Combined systematic object use may involve banging a spoon on the edge of a bowl or banging two blocks together. Functional object use involves the manipulation of an object in a way that is specific to the object (e.g., rolling a ball, hugging a teddy bear, patting a bunny). As infants begin to categorize objects by object-specific actions, they are perceived as increasingly social and there is increasing motivation (on the part of caregivers) to label

objects to which an infant is attending and to label the actions that the infant is performing.

Means-Ends Behavior. Means-ends (goal-oriented) behavior is the third key area of growth with some important implications for language. During the first month there is no evidence of means-ends behavior. From 1 to 4 months, infants engage in primary circular reactions but these behaviors are not planned in advance. Primary circular reactions consist of the repetition of an action that occurred spontaneously involving some part of the infant's body. For example, if the infant's hand comes in contact with his cheek, a rooting reflex may result, the infant's thumb may then come in contact with his mouth, and this will trigger a sucking reflex. Given this sequence, the infant may continue to engage in thumb-sucking thereby sustaining the pleasurable sensation of sucking that occurred initially by chance. Between 4 to 8 months, there still is no clear evidence of planned goal-oriented behavior. However, infants may engage in secondary circular reactions. These patterns are similar to primary circular reactions except that they involve an object rather than the infants own body. For example, the child may contact a rattle by chance and then continue to shake the rattle repeatedly if the chance contact was accompanied by a sound that was interesting to him or her. The beginnings of planned goal-oriented behavior emerge between 8 and 12 months. For example, if an infant sees a toy that he or she wants to manipulate, and if another toy is in the way, the infant may push the interfering toy aside in order to access the desired toy. Similarly, an infant may pull a string to access a desired toy that is out of reach but attached to it. Some infants may demonstrate tool use, which is the use of one object (e.g., a spoon) to access a completely different object that is out of direct reach (e.g., a toy). As with functional object manipulation, the emergence of goal-oriented behavior reflects increasing maturity and provides caregivers with increasing information about the objects and activities in which their infants are interested. This, in turn, affects the way in which caregivers communicate with their infants.

Categorizing

We now turn to the topic of categorization, which is a crucial cognitive process, consistent with Piaget's ideas about assimilation and accommodation. We define it here as the process of grouping similar objects and events into a single representation. Categorization is an important adaptive ability because it enables humans (including infants) to reduce an overwhelming amount of information to a manageable level (Cohen, 2003; Oakes & Madole, 2003). Categorization is also a crucial lexical precursor, since categories of meaning are later linked with linguistic forms. Furthermore, categorization foreshadows the development of cause and effect because it enables children to learn that the appearance of one kind of thing predicts the appearance of a related kind of thing (Payne & Wenger, 1998).

Infant categorization has been studied by many researchers and results have varied depending on the methods used to observe the infant's performance. Based on observations of sorting tasks, Vygotsky (in Rieber, 1987) noted that very young children may use several different criteria for sorting objects during the same sorting task. For this reason, he characterized very young children's categorizations as complexes rather than concepts, which are categories based on consistent criteria. On the other hand, studies of visual perception using a habituation paradigm indicate that infants can categorize objects and events into an impressive array of meaningful categories, including food items, furniture, birds, animals, vehicles, kitchen utensils, plants, spatial location ("above," "below," "on," and "in") and others (Berk, 2006).

Problem Solving

Another important cognitive process is analogic problem solving, or the ability to find solutions to a novel problem based on previous experience with a similar problem. Recent studies suggest that infants between 10 to 12 months can use this strategy. For example, Chen Sanchez, and Campbell (1997) presented 10- to 12-month-old infants with a sequence of three similar problems. To solve each problem, they had to overcome a barrier and pull a string to obtain a desired toy that was attached to the string. However, the specific barrier, toy, and string were different in each task. Prior to the first attempt, the infants were provided with a model of how to solve the problem. Results indicated that infant performance improved with each successive problem,

suggesting that these 10- to 12-month-old infants represented and accessed the solution rather than having to rely on trial and error to solve each problem individually.

Additional examples of cognitive processing will be discussed in the section on phonological precursors to language. However, the above sampling of prelinguistic cognitive skills is quite impressive, and it is not surprising that caregivers support their infants' acquisition of these skills by scaffolding (see below) and by commenting on moment-to-moment examples of their infants' attention to these skills.

Child-Caregiver Interaction: The Contributions of Caregivers

Caregivers treat their infants as communication partners from birth on. In addition, the behavior of caregivers is influenced by an intuitive curriculum (Kaye, 1979) reflecting cultural expectations as well as the caregiver's visions for his or her own particular child. As the more mature and flexible communicative partner, and in consideration of the infant's state of arousal at any given point in time, a caregiver assumes the role of a tutor, enabling the infant to succeed at skills just above his current level of independence. This is consistent with Vygotsky's (1930–1935/1978) concept of the **zone of proximal development (ZPD)**. Vygotsky noted that at every point in development there are some skills that a child can perform independently and some skills that he or she can only perform with the support of a more experienced and knowledgeable caregiver. The ZPD refers to those skills that are the next level up from the child's current independent performance level, which are supported by caregivers in the interactive process. Interestingly, these patterns appear to "fit" with Piaget's (1952) suggestion that children seek minimally discrepant stimulation.

Scaffolding

As indicated above, the patterns of support provided to infants serve to scaffold their development, and in this context our focus is on the development of interactions. At the most general level of scaffolding, caregivers engage their infants in repeated and predictable **joint activity routines** (e.g., feeding, bathing, dressing, play). Within these activities, caregivers weave their own behaviors around the bursts and pauses of the infant's behavior, moving the infant toward the goal of the joint activity routine. For example, Kaye and Wells (1980) observed that infants demonstrate a burst-pause sucking pattern when nursing. Mothers respond to this pattern by remaining relatively still when the baby is sucking and by stimulating the baby (e.g., jiggling the nipple, stroking the infant's cheek) when he or she is pausing. This results in a kind of **turn-taking structure** between the baby and the mother. A similar pattern is observed in other contexts as well (e.g., face-to-face engagement; object-oriented play). As an infant learns to use more mature behaviors within a joint activity routine, caregivers adjust their scaffolding to accommodate and expand the more mature levels of participation.

Scaffolding: Interpreting Behaviors

The creation of a turn-taking structure within joint activity routines is but one aspect of scaffolding. Another important scaffolding pattern involves the systematic interpretation of an infant's behaviors. For example, Snow (1977) conducted a longitudinal study in which she periodically observed two infants interacting with their mothers from 3 months old to each infant's second birthday. Initially, their mothers interpreted almost every behavior as a communicative signal. For example, if an infant burped, his mother might say, "excuse you." Interactions generally were short, and the mothers were careful to pause and wait for the infants to take their behavioral turns. However, as the infants matured, they produced a larger variety of sounds, and mothers became more selective about the sounds to which they responded. For example, mothers responded more to social vocalizations than to biological sounds.

Scaffolding: Adjusting Speech

Another aspect of scaffolding involves adjustments in the speech and language used by caregivers when speaking to their infants. This has been studied in depth (e.g., Kaye, 1980; Matychuk, 2004; Snow & Ferguson, 1977; Waterson & Snow, 1979). In fact, the style of language used by caregivers when interacting with infants and young children has come to

be known as "baby talk," "motherese," "adultese," "infant-addressed speech," "child-addressed speech," and others. We use the term **motherese** to characterize adjustments in speech addressed to infants. However, please note that motherese does not refer to caregiver utterances that appear to imitate children's speech production errors (e.g., "Div mama a gweat bid tiss.") Instead, we are referring to adjustments in the form, content, and use of language that serve to attract an infant's attention and (later) to support the comprehension of words. Specifically, motherese tends to involve a higher pitch, more extreme pitch variations, more exaggerated stress patterns, a reduced speech rate, and longer pauses than speech addressed to adults. Utterances are generally shorter, with simpler syntax. Vocabulary is restricted, and the same words are used repeatedly in successive utterances (e.g., "See the bunny? Nice bunny. Pat the bunny"). Motherese also involves the use of paralinguistic features such as exaggerated facial expressions and a high frequency of gestures (e.g., pointing, showing, and demonstrating actions on objects). As infants mature, there is a tendency to pronounce labels more distinctly (Kuhl et al., 1997) with exaggerated stress and higher, more variable pitch. Overall, these features of motherese can be considered ideal for evoking an infant's attention and leading him or her to discover the meanings of words within joint activity routines. Moreover, research indicates that infants prefer motherese over adult-addressed speech beginning as early as in the first month of life (Fernald, 1985; Cooper & Aslin, 1990). Although research has not demonstrated that motherese is necessary for language acquisition per se, the data suggest that it at least enhances the language acquisition rate (Clarke-Stewart, 1973).

The features of motherese discussed so far were identified in studies involving middle class American mothers and their infants. However, some of these features may differ across cultural groups and between classes within a culture. For example, higher pitch and exaggerated intonation is not characteristic of motherese in rural African families in North Carolina, Kaluli families in New Guinea, or Quiche-Mayan families in Guatemala (Sachs, 2005). Some variations in motherese reflect differences in the values and beliefs of a group. For example, although motherese spoken to middle class North American children includes a high proportion of questions, motherese to children from lower socio-economic groups includes a higher proportion of imperative forms, and in some groups infants may be expected to learn language by observation rather than by interacting (Owens, 2008). Additionally, there is evidence that features of motherese may vary depending on the gender of the infant. For example, mothers may address longer utterances to their daughters than to their sons.

Singh, Morgan, and Best (2002) have questioned the assumption that infants prefer motherese. Through laboratory observations utilizing carefully controlled stimuli and preference tasks, they found that 6-month-olds prefer speech with positive affect (i.e., "**happy talk**") regardless of whether it has the structure of motherese or of adult-addressed speech. However, as motherese typically is spoken with positive affect whereas adult-addressed speech is not, it is not surprising that infants prefer it.

Scaffolding: Sharing Attention and Reference

As infants and caregivers learn to interact with each other, one of the most important patterns in their interaction is the achievement of joint attention and joint reference. During the prelinguistic period, **joint attention** typically involves the coordinated visual regard of an infant and his or her caregiver to a particular object or event (e.g., Morales et al., 2000). For example, joint attention may be achieved when the infant looks at a toy and a caregiver follows the infant's line of regard, manipulating and commenting on the toy to which the infant is attending. **Joint reference** occurs when the caregiver or the infant performs an action that is intended to achieve joint attention. For example, joint reference is initiated when an infant points to an object which he then expects the caregiver to notice. Similarly, joint reference occurs when the caregiver deliberately activates, points to, or names a toy that she or he wishes the infant to notice. Although infants use nonverbal gestures to initiate joint reference during the prelinguistic period, joint reference is also a crucial feature of verbal conversations. Arguably every conversational turn involves an effort of one conversational partner to influence the attention of the other in relation to a topic.

The influence of joint attention and joint referencing on early semantic development has been studied by numerous researchers (e.g., Brooks & Meltzoff, 2005; Campbell & Namy, 2003; Carpenter, Nagell, & Tomasello, 1998; Markus, Mundy, Morales, Delgado, & Yale, 2000; Morales, Mundy, & Rojas, 1998; Rollins, 2003; Smith, Adamson, & Bakeman, 1988; Tomasello, Mannle, & Kruger, 1986; Tomasello & Todd, 1983). One of the major findings of these studies is that infants who spend more time engaged in joint attention with their caregivers learn to comprehend words sooner and acquire larger expressive vocabularies by 18 months. Caregivers tend to name and talk about the objects of joint attention, which creates an ideal opportunity for infants to recognize the correspondence between an object and its label. But how do infants learn to engage in joint referencing?

Owens (2008) described four phases in the development of joint reference. Phase I takes place between 0 and 6 months. At this time, an infant learns to look at objects and events in the environment while his mother is looking at them too. This is joint attention, and a caregiver's efforts to encourage joint attention are positively correlated with later language development (Karrass, Braungart-Rieker, Mullins, & Lefever, 2002). Initially, caregivers encourage joint attention in the context of face-to-face interaction. Later (at about 4 to 6 weeks) objects begin to be introduced. At this time, caregivers may jiggle an object to which an infant is already attending, or they may move an object into their infant's visual field while activating it. Either way, attention to the object typically is marked by language (e.g., calling the child's name or using a phrase like "Oh look") and then by words related to the object itself (e.g., "kitty"). These joint attention patterns gradually become a routine part of infant-caregiver interaction. An infant comes to expect this pattern and eventually learns to extend and expand his or her participation. For example, by 8 weeks infants can typically follow their caregiver's movements visually, and by 4 months they can follow the direction of their mother's pointing gesture. Additionally, responses to verbal signals (e.g., "Look") become increasingly quick and accurate. By 6 months, infants can typically respond to several cues (gestural, speech, intonation) quite fluently.

Phases II, III, and IV take place between 7 to 12 months. At this time, typical infants learn to take an increasingly active role in initiating and regulating joint attention with others. Between 7 and 8 months

(Phase II) they first learn to establish joint reference by pointing to or showing objects or events, but they do this without looking at the caregiver for confirmation. Later, they learn to use an abbreviated reach to signal requests while shifting their gaze between the desired object and the caregiver. Between 8 to 12 months (Phase III), typical infants begin to use gestures together with vocalizations; and by 12 months, they begin to use words, with and without gestures, to establish joint reference.

As with other aspects of infant-caregiver interaction, there are cultural differences in the pattern of joint attention to objects. Sachs (2005) described two sets of studies illustrating this point. One set of studies highlighted differences between American and Japanese caregivers in their patterns of organizing joint reference routines. Specifically, if infants looked away from them, American mothers were more supportive than the Japanese mothers. For example, the American mothers would say things like, "Want to look around? There you go," compared to Japanese mothers, who would make comments like, "Say, look at me," and "What's wrong with you?" (Morikawa, Shand, & Kosawa, 1988, pp. 248–249). Additionally, American mothers were more likely to name objects of joint attention while Japanese mothers were more likely to use the objects to initiate social routines. Another study addressed cultural differences in object play (Bakeman, Adamson, Konner, & Barr, 1990). In contrast to findings involving American and Japanese mother-infant dyads, this study indicated that object play is not a frequent context of interaction among !Kung San caregivers in Botswana and their infants. In fact, these caregivers were more likely to interact with their infants when the infants were not attending to an object than when they were.

Scaffolding: Ritualizing Interactive Games

We indicated, above, that caregivers scaffold their infant's behaviors in part by exposing them to joint activity routines with predictable elements in which word-meaning correspondences are relatively transparent. Ritualized interactive games have been recognized as a special type of joint activity routine with particular potential to scaffold communication development, including lexical knowledge (e.g., Bruner, 1981; Bruner & Sherwood, 1976; Gustafson,

Green, & West, 1979; Ninio & Bruner, 1978; Platt & Coggins, 1990; Ratner & Bruner, 1978; Snow, 1977, 1978). Examples of specific games include "This Little Piggy," "Gonna Get You," "Horsie," "So Big," "Peek-a-Boo," "Copy Cat," "picture-book reading," "pat-a-cake," and others, including many that are unique to particular infants and their caregivers. Some of these games are initiated by the caregiver during the first month of an infant's life, and there is a gradual increase in the frequency and variety of games throughout the prelinguistic period. Ritualized interactive games are considered particularly effective in scaffolding language because, as a form of social play, they are highly motivating for infants and because they are structured within the child's ZPD. Specifically, ritualized games are short, repetitive, and predictable. A relatively small number of words mark key events within each round. The roles of the participants are well defined, and they are reversible.

As with any other activity, caregivers monitor their infants closely when ritualized games are in progress. Given the limited attention spans of very young infants, initial games tend to be extremely short. For example, the earliest form of peek-a-boo may simply involve looming a small toy over a short distance within an infant's visual field and saying "boo" at a stopping point. Caregivers will adjust successive rounds of the game to evoke the infant's maximal attention and pleasure. Over time, as the infant participates in repeated episodes of the same game, she or he will come to anticipate the routine and to participate more actively, perhaps by vocalizing when an expected event is about to occur. And as caregivers observe their infants' emerging skills, they make further adjustments in the game to maintain or encourage more advanced levels of participation. Peek-a-boo may eventually involve covering a toy with a cloth and then quickly removing the cloth while saying "boo." Eventually, the infant may initiate the game thereby reversing his or her typical role from observer to director of the ritualized routine.

Joint picture-book reading is a ritualized routine with special potential to set the stage for the acquisition of lexical skills. The books incorporated into this routine are typically short, made of sturdy material with bright pictures on glossy pages with inserts providing opportunities for direct manipulation. For example, some pages may present textures for the infant to touch, tabs which can be pulled to move objects, buttons which can be pushed to activate sounds (e.g., music, environmental sounds, utterances of characters), and others. Joint picture-book reading, particularly when the same book is used in successive sessions, can provide infants with repeated exposure to a script with consistent images, consistent models for how to talk about the images and events, and with encouragement to assume an increasingly active role.

Despite the prevalence of ritualized games among middle class American families, such games are not a part of infant-caregiver interaction in all speech communities (e.g., Heath, 1983). In fact, play itself is not a routine activity between mothers and infants in some cultures (Ochs & Schieffelin, 1983; Schieffelin, 1990). However, caregivers in all cultures structure their infants' experiences in other routine activities of daily living (bathing, diapering, feeding, going down for a nap, etc.) and the structure of these routines can help infants discover the same word-meaning correspondences as does the structure of ritualized interactive games (Sachs, 2005).

Lexical Comprehension

Observation of Comprehension

To understand a spoken word, infants must recognize its acoustic form (speech perception) and associate that form with meaning. The development of speech perception is discussed in the next section of this chapter. In the current section, we focus primarily on the emergence of word-meaning relationships.

To appreciate what is known about this aspect of prelinguistic development, it is helpful to consider the procedures that have been used to assess infant language comprehension. Unlike language production, language comprehension is a private act. Since understanding occurs within a person's brain, we can only measure it indirectly. Three general strategies have been used. The first is parent report, which can be accomplished through interviews or structured checklists. However, these are indirect measures. Examples include the *McArthur-Bates Communicative Development Inventories* (Fenson et al., 2007) and the *Language Development Survey* (Rescorla, 1989).

A second strategy for assessing language comprehension is direct observation of responses to language in the natural environment or under controlled conditions. For example, an infant can be asked to point to items (e.g., "touch your nose"), to perform actions (e.g., "kiss Mommy"), or to act out relational concepts (e.g., "make the dog chase the cat") within the natural context of mother-infant interaction. However, the results of this procedure may reflect communicative rather than linguistic comprehension. In **communicative comprehension**, the infant uses nonlinguistic contextual cues in addition to the linguistic signal to decode the message. **Linguistic comprehension**, on the other hand, involves the use of language alone to interpret meaning. For example, a child could be presented with a set of unrelated objects (e.g., bottle, teddy bear, shoe, and book) by an unfamiliar observer outside of a typical interactive routine. The observer could then ask the child to "touch [object]" without any joint referencing cues to signal the correct item.

The third and most recently developed strategy is the Intermodal Preferential Looking Paradigm (IPLP) (Hirsh-Pasek & Golinkoff, 1996). In this procedure, an infant is seated on a parent's lap in front of two video monitors. While the parent is blindfolded, the infant watches short videos that are accompanied by a recorded voice, making comments about what is being shown on one of the screens. If the infant focuses for a significantly longer period on the screen that matches the voiceover, it is assumed that she or he understands the language. Various experimental controls ensure that external factors, such as differences in lighting or timing between the two videos, do not bias the outcome. By using this method, it has been possible to study more complex issues than would be possible with a direction-following task.

Milestones in Comprehension

At the most general level we find, not surprisingly, that infants typically understand a variety of words before they begin to talk. However, their level of understanding grows slowly, with word recognition emerging before word comprehension, and associative comprehension possibly preceding symbolic representation (Bates, 1979).

Specific milestones are suggested by the results of several studies. Mandel, Jusczyk, and Pisoni (1995) observed that 4½-month-old infants preferred to hear the sound of their own names rather than other words with similar stress patterns. However, these results reflect auditory perceptual preferences rather than an understanding of word-meaning relationships. Word-meaning relationships develop later, but the reported ages of emergence vary depending on observational methodology. Results based on IPLP procedures reveal earlier ages of comprehension than results based on parent interview. Using the IPLP methodology, Tincoff and Jusczyk (1999), found that 6-month-olds systematically looked at pictures of their own mother or father when they heard "mommy" or "daddy," respectively. Studies using parent interview procedures found evidence of comprehension at about 8 to 10 months. Among the earliest words comprehended are words for the names of caregivers ("mommy," "daddy"), "bottle," and words associated with ritualized interactive games (e.g., "peek-a-boo"). Studies of subsequent development place the acquisition of a 50-word comprehension vocabulary between 11 and 13 months (Benedict, 1979; Fenson et al., 1994; Menyuk, Liebergott, & Schultz, 1995). However, Fenson's results may be an overestimate owing partly to the nature of the instructions given to the parents before completing the interview form (Tomasello & Mervis, 1994).

Protowords. Shortly before they begin using their first real words, infants sometimes use protowords, which are phonetically consistent forms referring to a specific meaning (Dore, Franklin, Miller, & Ramer, 1976). For example, the infant son of a colleague said "ee-yo-ee-yo-ee-yo" (with stress on "ee") when he wanted his mother to turn the pages of a picture book they were reading together. He used this sound sequence deliberately while shifting his eye gaze between the book, and his mother, and when his mother turned the page, he stopped. He did this consistently every evening during their joint book-reading routine, and he did not use this sound sequence in other contexts. The infant grandson of another colleague said, "da-ya-ya" (stress on "da") to refer to compact disks (CDs) with which he enjoyed playing. For example, if he wanted access to a CD that was out of reach, he pointed to it, looked at his parent, and said "da-ya-ya." When the disk was given to him, he stopped. Infants typically do not generalize their use of a protoword to other

referents. However, this child did. When he visited his grandparents' home he pointed to a circular pattern in the living room rug (which resembled the appearance of a CD) and said "da-ya-ya."

To qualify as a word, a sound sequence must meet two criteria: (a) It must resemble a word that is used by speakers in the linguistic community, and (b) it must refer to a meaning that resembles the meaning of the word used in the speech community. For example, Helen Keller's famous first word "wawa," resembled the sound of the word "water" and it referred to water coming out of a spout (Keller, 1905). Similarly, when an infant says "baba" to request his or her bottle, we hear a sound sequence in reference to a meaning that resemble those of the conventional word, "bottle." Neither of these characteristics (conventional form, conventional meaning) apply to protowords. However, the use of protowords is significant because it reflects the infant's understanding that a sound sequence can be used as a tool for referring to a referent.

PRIMARY ACCOMPLISHMENTS: PHONOLOGY

Background

The phonological component of language is a system of rules that shape the segmental features and the suprasegmental features of speech. Segmental features include (a) the set of **phonemes** (also known as phonetic categories or speech sounds) that are used in a particular language and (b) **phonotactic rules** which limit the ways in which phonemes can be sequenced to form syllables and words. An example of a phonotactic rule in English is that no English word can begin with "ng." The suprasegmental features of speech (also known as prosody) include speech rate, pause patterns, variations in pitch, stress, and intonation contour. Intonation contour refers to the melodic structure of an utterance. For example, say the following sentences: "She's gone." and "She's gone?" Speakers of **General American English (GAE)** should notice a difference in the melodic contour of the statement versus the question.

To describe the sounds and syllables that infants gradually acquire, we need a way to represent them on paper. Our system of orthography is insufficient for this purpose for several reasons: First, the number of speech sounds is greater than the number of letters in the alphabet. In fact, GAE includes about 45 speech sounds but the alphabet includes only 26 letters. Therefore, some letters must represent more than one speech sound. For example, consider the different sounds represented by "s" in the words "sing," "laser," and "treasure." Furthermore, different spellings are used to represent the same speech sound. For example, consider the words "elf," "cliff," and "laugh." These words end with the same speech sound but the sound is represented by different spellings. In the interest of clarity, therefore, we will use the symbols of the **International Phonetic Alphabet (IPA)** to represent the set of English speech sounds. Table 3–1 lists the IPA symbols for the basic sounds in GAE and in other dialects spoken in the United States. Each symbol is accompanied by an orthographic example to illustrate the sound to which it refers.

Two important features of the IPA should be noted. First, each IPA symbol represents a phoneme (also known as a phonetic category). By definition, a phoneme is the smallest unit of sound that makes a difference in meaning. For example, /p/ is a phoneme in English because if we replace it with another speech sound, the replacement will change the meaning of the words in which it occurs. Consider the word "pin." If we replaced /p/ with /b/, we would have the word "bin," which refers to something different than "pin." Second, note that each phoneme actually represents a category of individual phonetic units (also known as allophones). For example, if you were to say /p/ five times in a row, each production would have subtle but acoustically measurable differences. Similarly, if you were to say /p/ in five different words (e.g., "pin," "sip," "apt,"

TABLE 3–1. International Phonetic Alphabet

	Consonants				
Symbol	**Example**	**Symbol**	**Example**	**Symbol**	**Example**
/p/	**p**at	/f/	**f**un	/h/	**h**at
/t/	**t**ap	/θ/	**th**umb	/m/	**m**at
/k/	**c**ap	/s/	**s**um	/n/	**n**ut
/b/	**b**at	/ʃ/	**sh**un	/ŋ/	si**ng**
/d/	**d**ab	/v/	**v**at	/l/	**l**ed
/g/	**g**ap	/ð/	**th**at	/r/	**r**ed
/tʃ/	**ch**ap	/z/	**z**oo	/j/	**y**et
/dʒ/	**j**ab	/ʒ/	gara**ge**	/w/	**w**et
	Vowels				
Symbol	**Example**	**Symbol**	**Example**	**Symbol**	**Example**
/i/	f**ee**d	/ɔ/	t**au**ght	/ɚ/	bett**er**
/ɪ/	f**i**t	/ow/	c**oa**t	/ai/	b**i**te
/ei/	m**ai**d	/ʊ/	f**oo**t	/aʊ/	b**ou**t
/ɛ/	f**e**d	/u/	f**oo**d	/ɔɪ/	t**oy**
/æ/	f**a**d	/ʌ/	f**u**n	/ə/	**a**bout
/a/	h**o**t	/ɝ/	b**ir**d	/ai/	b**i**te

"poor," "spot"), there would again be subtle but measurable acoustic differences in each production of /p/ due in part to the affect of the other phonemes surrounding /p/. However, mature listeners ignore those subtle acoustic differences and recognized each allophone of /p/ as a member of the /p/ category. In other words, listeners within the same speech community have a range of tolerance for subtle acoustic variations in the production of phonemes. This helps us to (among other things) recognize consistent features of speech across acoustic differences due to age, gender, speech rate, and prosodic variations. For notational purposes, we differentiate phonetic categories (phonemes) from phonetic units (allophones) by placing phonetic categories within slash marks (e.g., /p/) and phonetic units within brackets (e.g., [p]).

Prelinguistic Speech Perception

In our earlier discussion of semantic precursors, we noted the importance of infant-caregiver interaction as a context for language acquisition. Within these interactions, children are exposed to an enormous sample of motherese, a style of language structured to attract their attention. We now consider prelinguistic milestones in the perception of these utterances.

Perception is the process by which organisms interpret sensory information in reference to previous experience. Since speech is an auditory signal, its perception involves the recognition of sound patterns, including individual speech sounds, word segments, stress patterns, and intonation contours. Therefore, to understand the precursors to phonological development we must first consider the perceptual skills of infants. To appreciate the perceptual challenge facing infants during the first year of life, consider the fact that human languages (combined) make use of some 600 consonants and 200 vowels (Cheour, Caponiene, Lehtokoski, Luuk, & Allik, 1998), and that there are no spaces between the sounds or words in flowing speech. How do infants identify the subset of phonemes used in their particular speech community during the first year of life, and how to they extract words from the continuous stream of sound in the speech signal?

Although infants cannot tell us directly what they hear, carefully controlled observational methods allow scientists to make reliable inferences about infant auditory preferences and perceptions. What they have found so far is that, within the first two months of life, when infants are given a choice, they prefer to listen to speech rather than to other environmental sounds (Voulomanos & Werker, 2004). Moreover, they prefer motherese over adult-to-adult speech (Fernald, 1985; Fernald & Kuhl, 1987), and they prefer their mother's speech over the speech of other caregivers (DeCasper & Fifer, 1980; Krasnegor, Rumbaugh, & Studdert-Kennedy, 1991). Overall, these studies of infant auditory preferences indicate that infants pay active attention to speech, but how do they perceive what they hear?

A technique known as **high amplitude sucking (HAS)** has enabled scientists to examine infant auditory perception beginning in the first month of life (Menn & Stoel-Gammon, 2005). In this procedure, an infant sucks on a pacifier that is connected by a long, narrow tube to a sound-generating computer system. Each time the infant sucks, the system generates a speech sound. For example, an infant may hear [ba] immediately following each suck. When the infant first notices that sucking produces a sound (in this case, [ba]) his or her suck rate typically increases. This is interpreted by researchers as a sign that the infant is interested in hearing the sound. However, after a certain number of [ba] repetitions, the infant's suck rate typically decreases, reflecting a loss of interest in hearing the same sound. This loss of interest is known as habituation. When habituation occurs, the experimenter changes the particular sound triggered by the suck. So, in our example, instead of continuing to hear [ba] following each suck, the infant now hears [pa]. If this change in sound then triggers a return to a high rate of sucking, it is inferred that the infant recognized /p/ as being different from /b/. In other words, it shows that the infant recognized a phonetic contrast between /p/ and /b/.

The results of experiments involving HAS procedures have shown that infants are capable of **categorical perception** beginning within the first month of life (Eimas, 1975; Eimas, Siqueland, Jusczyk, & Vigorito, 1971). What this means is that they recognize individual phonetic units (e.g., [b]) as members of a phoneme category (e.g., /b/), and they can identify phonetic contrasts that differ by only a single acoustic feature. For example, the difference between /b/ and /p/ is based on the single feature of voicing (vocal fold vibration): /b/ is produced with simultaneous voicing whereas /p/ is produced without voicing. By putting your hand on your throat while making each sound, you will notice a vibration in your throat when you say [b] but not when you say [p]. The infants observed by Eimas and colleagues perceived that difference acoustically during the first month of life. In fact, unlike adults, one-month-old infants can discriminate all the phonetic categories in human languages (e.g., Jusczyk, 1997), including those that do not even occur in their own linguistic environment (Trehub, 1976). This is an impressive skill, since it can help infants identify the segmental features of any language to which they are exposed. Interestingly, this same perceptual skill has also been observed among chinchillas and macaque monkeys (e.g., Kuhl & Miller, 1975, 1978; Kuhl & Padden, 1983), indicating that categorical perception, although supporting speech development, is not a species-specific trait.

The categorical aspect of infant speech perception is of particular interest because it shows that infants are able to overlook subtle acoustic variations in specific phonetic units and to treat those units as functionally equivalent members of a single phonetic category. To appreciate this, notice that the sounds to which infants are exposed during the course of a day vary along many dimensions. Some words are produced more quickly than others, some are spoken by women, others by men, and others possibly by cartoon characters or other children. Furthermore, the same caregiver may produce a particular utterance repeatedly but with variations in rate, overall intensity, and intonation contour. Also, as indicated above, the acoustic features of allophones will vary slightly depending on the phonetic context in which they occur. For example, when /b/ is produced in the word-initial position (e.g., "boo") it sounds different than when it is produced in the word-final position (e.g., "tub"). Try saying each word with the palm of your hand held open within an inch of your mouth—you should feel a puff of air when you say "boo" but not when you say "tub." This puff of air accompanying word-initial [b] is known as aspiration, and it creates a feature of sound that is not heard when /b/ is pro-

nounced without aspiration. Yet, mature English-speaking listeners perceive both allophones as members of the same phonetic category: /b/.

The process of categorization requires us to determine which examples are members of category and which are not. Studies in cognitive science have shown that the categorization of objects is based on the degree to which a particular object resembles the **best example (prototype)** of the category (e.g., Mervis & Rosch, 1981; Rosch, 1975). Examples that share the greatest number of features with the prototype are classified as category members while those that share only a few or no features with the prototype are excluded from membership. Similar processes are believed to apply in the perceptual classification of individual phonetic units (allophones) (Kuhl, 2000). In other words, phonetic units are included within a phonetic category depending on the number of acoustic features they share with the category's prototype. In this way, the phonetic prototype within each phonetic category functions as a "**perceptual magnet**" Kuhl, 2000, p. 833) for categorizing phonetic units (allophones). However, the phonetic categories of different languages have different prototypes, even when there is an apparent overlap between categories (e.g., English /t/ vs. French /t/). Therefore, mature listeners of each language will have slightly different degrees of tolerance for the range of acoustic variability in phonetic units (allophones) to be classified within a similar phonetic category (e.g., Kuhl, Williams, Lacerta, Stevens, & Lindblom, 1992). These cultural differences gradually affect infant perception. In fact, after repeated exposure to a specific language, the categorical perceptions demonstrated by infants at one month of age become "warped" at 6 months of age in the direction of the category boundaries specified by the phonetic prototypes of the language they hear (Kuhl, 2000, p. 11853). This **perceptual magnet effect** is uniquely human and does not occur in the case of other mammals (Kuhl, 1991). Moreover, infant perceptual abilities at 6 months predict language performance (i.e., word understanding, word production, phrase understanding as measured by the MacArthur Communicative Development Inventory) at 13, 16, and 24 months (Tsao, Liu, & Kuhl, 2004).

As indicated above, the perceptual magnet effect helps to constrain or narrow down an infant's attention to the specific phonetic categories used in his or her language. In fact, as development progresses between 6 to 12 months, and as infants are awake for longer periods of time, they are increasingly bombarded with motherese, including only the subset of phonetic categories relevant in their language. This constraint in language input combined with the perceptual magnet effect eventually results in a kind of native language filter that predisposes infants to ignore phonetic contrasts that are not relevant in their native language and to focus instead on the phonetic patterns that their language uses (Kuhl, 2004). So, by the time they are 10 to 11 months old, infants exhibit the same decline in foreign language consonant perception that is observed in native speakers of their language (Werker & Tees, 1984). For example, 10-month-old Japanese infants (like Japanese-speaking adults) will no longer respond to the difference between /l/ and /r/, because the difference between these phonetic categories does not create a difference of meanings in Japanese words. It has been proposed that selective attention to the sound segments in the infant's own language requires the infant to tune out sounds unique to other languages (Bates, 1997).

It must be noted here that our discussion of infant perception has been organized within a developmental framework to match the linguistic organization of this chapter. For a compelling alternative interpretation of these data from a behavior analytic perspective, readers are encouraged to read Schliger's (2010) treatment of this topic.

Prelinguistic Phonotactic Rules

In our discussion of the precursors to semantics, we noted that language comprehension skills emerge for most infants at about 9 months. Word comprehension requires infants to recognize word boundaries in the speech stream and to recognize the phonological sequencing constraints unique to their language. The problem is, there are no spaces between the words. To appreciate this challenge, try figuring out how many words are included in the following utterance: "Ichmöchtewissenwaskinder-hören." Without knowing something about German semantics and orthography, it is impossible to make a reasonable guess. Sometimes even adults have difficulty segmenting words from nursery rhymes they memorized as children. Below is a rhyme whose words are often missegmented:

Maresey Dotes (missegmented version)	**Mares Eat Oats (correctly segmented version)**
Maresey dotes	Mares eat oats
And dosey dotes	And does eat oats
And liddle lambsey divey	And little lambs eat ivy.
A kiddley divey too	A kid will eat ivy too,
Wooden ewe?	Wouldn't you?

During normal conversational speech, mature listeners automatically and fluently use their stored knowledge of words to identify the words they hear. This use of existing knowledge for making sense of incoming sensory information is known as top-down processing. Until recently, it was assumed that prelinguistic infants did not have access to this strategy. However, Bortfeld, Morgan, Golinkoff, and Rathbun (2005) found that infants as young as 6 months typically do recognize at least two frequently used words (i.e., "mommy" and the child's own name). Moreover, infants can use their knowledge of these words to segment words occurring next in sequence to the familiar word. For example, after listening to the utterance, "The girl laughed at Mommy's feet," 6-month-old infants demonstrate recognition of the word "feet." However, it is unclear how long the paired word will remain in the infant's memory, and it is clear that the lion's share of **word segmentation** must be accomplished through bottom-up processing—that is, searching for patterns in the sensory information provided by the speech signal itself. How do infants solve this pattern detection puzzle?

Fortunately, the phonotactic rules of a language limit the phonetic sequences allowed within words. Additionally, there are statistical regularities associated with sound sequences within words that do not apply to sound sequences across word boundaries (Saffron, Newport, & Aslin, 1996). For example, consider the phrase "pretty baby." In English, the probability of a transition from "pre" to "ty" is greater than the probability of a transition from "ty" to "ba." These statistical features within the speech stream can help infants to identify word segments. In fact, research shows that infants are adept at **statistical learning** (i.e., detecting phonetic patterns based on the kinds of transitional probabilities just described). For example, in a carefully controlled study, 8 month olds discriminated patterns in the distribution of sounds within and across the words of an artificial language after only 2 minutes of concentrated listening and without the benefit of prosodic cues (e.g., Saffran, Aslin, & Newport, 1996). Similar results are reported by others (e.g., Aslin, Saffron, & Newport, 1998; Goodsit, Morgan, & Kuhl, 1993). Furthermore, English-learning infants become sensitive to phonetic patterns that can occur at the end of a syllable or word (e.g., /pt/) but not at the beginning. Interestingly, patterns of statistical learning also have been observed in monkeys, so this is not a species-specific trait (e.g., Hauser, Newport, & Aslin, 2001).

In addition to statistical learning, infants also use **prosodic cues** to identify potential words. Recall that prosody refers to the suprasegmental features of speech, such as intonation, stress, and others. Once again, each language is organized according to phonological rules that limit the number of prosodic patterns. For example, during conversational speech, about 90% of multisyllabic English words begin with stress on the first syllable (e.g., "pretty," "baby," and "birthday," Cutler & Carter, 1987). This strong-weak (trochaic) stress pattern does not occur in every language. Some languages (e.g., Polish) have the weak-strong (iambic) pattern and others (e.g., Japanese) have a pattern in which short syllables are spoken with nearly equal stress and time. Infants can discriminate their own language versus a foreign language based on such prosodic cues shortly after birth (Mehler et al., 1988; Nazzi, Bertoncini, & Mehler, 1998). By 5 months, they can discriminate their own language from other languages with similar prosodic patterns, presumably by using a combination of prosodic and segmental cues (Bosch & Sebastian-Galles, 1997; Nazzi, Jusczik, & Johnson, 2000). By 8 months, English-learning infants can segment words with a trochaic stress pattern but not words with an iambic stress pattern (Kuhl, 2004). In fact, they would segment a phrase like "guitar is" as "taris," because "guitar" does not follow the trochaic stress pattern (Juscyk, Houston,

& Newsome, 1999). In sum, prosodic features can help infants discover word segments (Echols, Corhurst, & Childers, 1997; Jusczyk, Houston, & Newsome, 1999; Morgan, 1994; Morgan & Saffran, 1994); and by 8 months, infants can retain familiar word segments in memory even though they may not know the words' meanings (Jusczyk & Hohne, 1997). Later, sensitivity to word segments may actually help infants to map meanings (e.g., Graf Estes, Evans, Alibali, & Saffron, 2007).

Although the segmental and prosodic pattern detection strategies are helpful in highlighting potential words, infants could not succeed at word segmentation without the scaffolding provided by their caregivers. Clearly, the acoustic structure of motherese helps direct an infant's attention to word segments (Thiessen, Hill, & Saffron, 2005). Exaggerated stress, loudness, and pitch variations make selected words more noticeable. Placing a new word at the end of an utterance, prior to a pause, highlights the word (Fernald & Mazzie, 1991), and repetition of newly introduced words in the final position of stereotyped phrases can further enhance the salience of word segments (e.g., "That's a ball.," "See the ball?," "Where's the ball?"). Finally, exposure to words in the context of joint attention also supports the segmentation process, as infants are sensitive to the social intent of speakers in a word-learning context (Baldwin & Meyer, 2007). In these ways, the perceptual preferences and biases of infants combine with the acoustic characteristics of motherese within the context of communication to support an infant's acoustic perception of word segments.

Prelinguistic Vocal Patterns

The gradual development of universal to language-specific speech perception is paralleled over the first 12 months by the gradual shift from universal to culture-specific babbling patterns. In this section we summarize stages of babbling development and patterns of infant-caregiver interaction that support it.

Vocal Patterns: The Contributions of Infants

Infant vocal production has been studied by various researchers with general agreement in findings (e.g.,

Holmgren, Lindblom, Aurelius, Jalling, & Zetterstrom, 1986; Koopmans-van Beinum, & van der Stelt, 1986; D. K. Oller, 1978; Stark, 1980; Stoel-Gammon & Otomo, 1986). One point of agreement is that not all vocalizations are equal. During the first month of life, sounds can be classified as reflexive (e.g., fussing, crying, groaning, sneezing), vegetative (e.g., burping, grunting, coughing) and nonreflexive (e.g., cooing, squealing, babbling, etc.). The reflexive and vegetative sounds are fixed vocal signals in the sense that their meanings remain stable and lack the potential flexibility of the nonreflexive forms (D. K. Oller, 2000). For example, the squeals of a 5-month-old may accompany anger or joy. However, crying is a relatively fixed biological signal for one or another kind of discomfort. As infants mature, reflexive and vegetative sounds decrease in frequency while nonreflexive sounds (also known as **protophones**) expand increasingly to include the acoustic features of "speechiness" or the infrastructure of adult speech (D. K. Oller, 1978; 2000).

Another point of agreement among researchers is that protophones develop in a sequence of stages (D. K. Oller, 1980). Each stage is marked by features that appear with regularity for the first time at that stage; however, the stages overlap. Protophones characteristic of a given stage may have been produced at very low frequencies in the previous stage and may continue to be used for a period of time in the next more advanced stage. There also is considerable variability among infants in the ages at which they reach each stage, and researchers vary slightly on the age ranges they associate with each stage. A summary of the stages is provided below, based on the work of several researchers (Menn & Stoel-Gammon, 2005; D. K. Oller, 1978; Stoel-Gammon & Otoma, 1986) with age ranges based on J. W. Oller et al. (2006). Finally, as the production of protophones at successive stages requires increasingly sophisticated motor control, we supplement information about protophone development with information about development in related domains.

Stage 1 (~0–2 months)—Quasivowels

Early in this stage, infants produce mostly vegetative and reflexive sounds. However, protophones do occur, often in response to smiling or talking by the caregiver. Typically, they consist of vowel approximations (quasivowels) without any deliberate shaping of the articulators (e.g., tongue, lips, and cheeks). The infant simply vocalizes while his mouth remains in a relaxed or smiling position. However, there is variability across infants. We have observed some infants who appear, by the age of about 6 weeks, to actively move their articulators while producing vocalization and sometimes approximating features of the adult model during proto conversations. Still, their vowel productions have a nasal quality and lack consonants.

To appreciate the acoustic quality of quasivowels (also known as quasiresonant nuclei, or QRN) it is helpful to consider the anatomic structures involved. During the first two months of life, an infant's oral cavity is relatively small and almost completely filled with the tongue. The larynx, a cartilaginous structure that houses the vocal folds, is positioned high in the infant's short neck, and there is little separation between the oral and nasal cavities (Kent, 1992; Lieberman, Crelin, & Klatt, 1972). Consequently, sound is directed partially through the mouth and partially through the nose, resulting in a slightly nasal quality. In adult speech, vowels serve as the nucleus of a syllable. In that sense, semivowels may be considered the raw material of what will later contribute to the syllable structure of adult speech.

By the second month, reflexive vocalizations include fewer stress sounds, and quasivowels are produced with slightly better control. At times, the back of the tongue may come in contact with the soft palate, creating an acoustic effect resembling /g/ or /k/, a pattern is known as Gooing (Oller, 1978).

Stage 2 (~2–3 months)—Primitive Articulation

During the second month, crying has become less frequent, laughing (another reflexive vocal form) is becoming more frequent, and protophone development now includes a primitive type of articulation. Articulation refers to the shaping of the airway by movements of the jaw, tongue, and lips. For example, in adult speech, the articulation of /p/ requires us to bring both lips together, build air pressure, and release the airflow in a quick burst. By the second and third month of life, an infant has had many opportunities to exercise oral musculature through feeding and exploration (e.g., sucking on bottles, pacifiers, fingers, etc.), and has heard and seen many speech models in the form of motherese. As a result, movements of the tongue, lips, and jaw are somewhat more controlled. Quasivowels sound more like vowels in the local language, and several vowel forms can be identified among an infant's vocal productions. In fact, infants between 12 and 20 weeks can produce vocalic sounds that resemble vowels just produced by a model (Kuhl & Meltzoff, 1996).

Stage 3 (~3–6 months)—Expansion of Protophones

Motorically, infants are continuing to gain control over their bodies, including their oral musculature and patterns of respiration. By 4 months, they spend up to 4 hours per day engaged in nonnutritive sucking as they explore their fingers and other objects (Owens, 2008). They learn to cup their tongue, to close their lips around a spoon, to use their tongue independently of their jaw, and to chew volitionally. Additionally, their vocal tract is maturing physically. It is not surprising, therefore, that protophones expand in variety.

One of the new protophones produced during this period is called **marginal babbling (MB)**. This form consists of a single consonant-vowel (CV) syllable shape without the timing constraints of adult speech. It is typically accomplished as an infant moves his articulators from a closed-mouth position to a distinct vowel (e.g., resembling /ma/).

Other vocal patterns that occur during this stage reflect experimentation with loudness (e.g., **yelling**, **whispering**), pitch (**squealing**, **growling**) and lip movements (e.g., **raspberries** or **bilabial trills**). In addition, infants learn to produce sustained vowel-like sounds resembling /a/ with the airstream directed exclusively through the oral cavity. This form is known as **a fully resonant nucleus (FRN)**. Overall, infants appear to be exploring the raw features of sound segmentation and prosody. For this reason, this period of development also may be characterized as the stage of vocal play (Menn & Stoel-Gammon, 2005). Interestingly, infants who are deaf produce consonant-like protophones that are similar to those of hearing infants but with less vari-

ety and a higher frequency of consonants that can be prolonged (e.g., /m/, /n/, /ŋ/) (Stoel-Gammon, 1988).

D. K. Oller (2006) considered this stage particularly important both from a developmental and an evolutionary perspective. He proposed that the experimentation and inherent flexibility of infant protophones is what distinguishes humans from other primates, who produce more fixed vocal patterns. This flexibility demonstrated by humans may have been favored at some point in the evolutionary process.

Stage 4 (~6–10 months)—Canonical Babbling

Canonical babbling emerges at a point in development when infants are becoming increasingly able to maneuver themselves and to manipulate objects within their environments. Crawling typically occurs for the first time during this stage, and patterns of object exploration become more sophisticated. As before, infants continue to be interested in toys and to grasp them with their hands; however, they are also learning to pick up smaller objects requiring finer degrees of coordination. They demonstrate increased control over their oral motor abilities as well. By 6 months they can pout by extending their lips, without moving their jaw. One month later, they can chew in a more rotary fashion and with lips closed. At 8 months, tongue control expands to include lateralization and elevation, independently of the jaw.

Consistent with these more general patterns of development, we see increasing sophistication in the production of protophones. For the first time, we observe **canonical babbling**, which involves the repetition of consonant-vowel (CV) syllables within the same breath-group and at a rate that is consistent with the timing of adult speech. Two canonical forms are observed. The first is **reduplicated babbling (RB)**, which consists of repeated CV-sequences containing the same consonant and the same vowel. Examples include /mamama/ and /dadada/ which are often misinterpreted as an infant's first words. However, these sequences typically are not accompanied by nonverbal behaviors that would suggest a referential semantic function. For example, an infant may say /mamama/ while looking at a toy, without any evidence of searching for his or her mother. In fact, reduplicated babbling often occurs when infants are holding an object or exploring the environment. As such it may be comparable to rhythmic hand movements which also occur in this context (e.g., Stark, Bernstein, & Demorest, 1993). As children progress in this stage, they also use reduplicated babbling when interacting with adults (Owens, 2008).

Variegated babbling (VB) is the second canonical protophone, and it emerges toward the later part of this stage. Like RB, it consists of syllable sequences that conform to the timing of adult speech. However, it is distinct from RB in that successive syllables within the same breath group may have different shapes (e.g., /magədɪbə/) and that different consonants and different vowels occur within and across syllables. Furthermore, as infants develop within this stage, their intonation patterns more closely resemble the intonation patterns of adult speech, which makes their variegated babbling patterns come ever closer to resembling the "speechiness" quality of adult utterances.

Interestingly, the babbling patterns of infants who are deaf do not demonstrate this same trajectory of growth within the canonical period. Instead, these infants produce far fewer reduplicated forms, and show a gradual decline in the frequency, variety, and quality of the babbling repertoire (Stoel-Gammon & Otomo, 1986). This is interpreted to suggest that canonical forms are reinforced in part by an infant's ability to hear him or herself and others in the production of sounds (Kuhl & Meltzoff, 1996; Menn & Stoel-Gammon, 2005).

Stage 5 (~10 months and older)—Jargon

At this stage, infants produce long strings of VB with stress and intonation patterns resembling those of the language they hear. In fact, intonation is used systematically to express meaning. Jargon is used increasingly during child-caregiver interaction to accompany intentional communicative acts, and its use overlaps with the onset of language. When caregivers hear these jargon utterances, they often feel as if the infant is trying to communicate and may even comment on it (e.g., "You don't say! Tell me more"). Infants behave as if they understand the social use of speech but that they haven't completely grasped its symbolic function. For these reasons, it is also known as conversational babble and modulated babble (Menn & Stoel-Gammon, 2005).

However, the segmental features of the protophones within this stage are continuous with the segmental features of variegated babbling. In fact, some authors do not isolate this pattern from the canonical stage per se (e.g., J. W. Oller, Oller, & Badon, 2006).

Typically developing children continue to produce jargon (increasingly mixed with speech) until about the age of 2 years. Children who are deaf and learning to talk may also eventually use jargon mixed with speech. However, they may do so for an extended period of time up to the age of 3 years.

This sequence of stages is observed in infants across languages, including American Sign Language (ASL) (Cheek, Cormier, & Meier, 1998; D. K. Oller, 2000, Pettito & Marentette, 1991). In a controlled observational study, Pettito and Marentette showed that ASL-learning infants produce repetitive hand-shape movements within the timing constraints of ASL utterances, hence resembling the format of canonical babbling. This was interpreted as an indication that the capacity for language development, while neurologically based, can be expressed in any modality. If an infant is exposed to ASL instead of speech, then the infrastructure for the acquisition of linguistic forms can be expressed in a manual format.

The specific sounds that are acquired by hearing infants during the first 12 months are also fairly consistent across cultures. During the precanonical stages, the predominant protophones consist of vowel approximations plus two consonant approximations (/g/ and /k/). In contrast, the sounds that are added during the canonical stage are predominantly consonants. Early in the canonical stage, infants produce a high frequency of front consonants such as /m/, /b/, and /d/ (Menn & Stoel-Gammon, 2005). Shortly thereafter, they begin to produce additional consonants, including groups known as stop sounds (/p, b, t, d, k, g/), nasal sounds (/m/ and /n/), and glides (/w, j/). Also observed are /s/ and /h/. Altogether, these are the consonants typically observed during the earliest stages of speech production. The consonants usually not observed are those that are normally late to be mastered when children begin to talk: /v, ð, tʃ, l, r/. For a more detailed discussion of the sound classes referenced above (e.g., stop sounds, nasals, glides), see Chapter 5 in this volume.

Cultural differences in patterns of babbling begin to emerge late in the canonical babbling stage. For example, infants will drop sounds that are not used in their native language, such as /h/ in the case of French infants. Additionally, the frequency of particular sounds within babbling will change to approximate the frequency of those sounds in an infant's native language. At this point in development, adults can sometimes guess just from listening to the babbling patterns whether an infant has been exposed to French, Chinese, Arabic, or English (e.g., de Boysson-Bardies, Sagart, & Durand, 1984).

In sum, there is a shift from universal to culture-specific patterns of vocalization produced by infants over the first year of life.

Vocal Patterns: The Contributions of Caregivers

The progression from language-universal to culture-specific babbling simply could not happen without an infant's exposure to speech models. In fact, case studies of children who have been deprived of appropriate speech and language experiences show us that language cannot develop normally without this exposure (e.g., Fromkin, Krashen, Curtiss, Rigler, & Rigler, 1974). We have already discussed the perceptual skills that infants acquire through exposure to motherese. These perceptual skills provide a store of increasingly refined acoustic templates against which infants can compare the auditory features of their own productions. The question is whether caregivers engage in behaviors that specifically scaffold the development of babbling. Surprisingly little research has addressed this question. In fact, some have observed that babbling, like other aspects of language, normally develops in an amazingly short period of time without any specific instruction (Bijou & Baer, 1965; Moerk, 1990; Owens, 2008) and that its progress largely is due to biological maturation (Lenneberg, 1976; Vygotsky, 1986/1934). However, others argue that babbling is influenced in various ways through social interaction, motherese, and imitation (e.g., Kuhl, 2004; Meltzoff, 2002; Skinner, 1957).

Reinforcement

From a behavioral perspective, infant vocalization develops in part through a process called **automatic reinforcement** (Skinner, 1957; Vaughan &

Michael, 1982). This process is set in motion when a neutral stimulus develops reinforcing properties by being paired with another stimulus that already has reinforcing properties. For example, infants typically hear their caregivers' vocalizations during routine activities such as feeding, diapering, and rocking. These vocalizations (originally neutral) are believed to acquire reinforcing properties through repeated pairings with unconditioned or conditioned reinforcers (e.g., feeding, diapering, rocking). Consequently, when infants produce sounds that approximate the sounds made by their caregivers, these approximations function as automatic reinforcers for the oral-motor movements that the infant produced to create them. In this sense, the simple pairing of positive social stimulation with vocalization (a form of **stimulus-stimulus pairing**) may enhance infant vocal development as long as the pairing of caregiver vocalizations with positive infant-caregiver interactions continues.

Five studies have examined the effects of stimulus-stimulus pairing on the vocal repertoires of very young children (Esch, Carr, & Michael, 2005; Miguel, Carr, & Michael, 2002; Smith, Michael, Sundberg, 1996; Sundberg, Michael, Partington, & Sundberg, 1996; Yoon & Bennett, 2000). Some of the children were toddlers or preschoolers with disabilities and some were developing normally. In each study, children participated in procedures that paired a vocal stimulus (e.g., "eee" or "bababa") with a reinforcing stimulus (e.g., tickling or presentation of a preferred food). The vocal stimuli consisted of sounds that were either novel, not observed in a child's repertoire, or observed at very low frequencies. The results varied somewhat across studies. In three studies, all but one child spontaneously emitted new vocal responses after the pairings (Miguel et al., 2002; Sundberg et al., 1996; Yoon & Bennett, 2000). However, the new responses returned to pre-pairing frequencies within a short time after the pairing procedure was completed. In another study, both children increased their frequency of vocalizing sounds already within repertoire, but none of the children produced new vocal responses (Smith et al., 1996), and in one last study, pairing failed to increase novel vocalizations (Esch et al., 2005).

In a follow-up to these earlier studies, Esch (2007) used a stimulus-stimulus pairing procedure with modifications. Three preschoolers with autism spectrum disorder served as participants. Their ages ranged from 2;4 (years, months) to 5;7. All communicated at a prelinguistic level. Four modifications were made to the stimulus-stimulus pairing procedures described above. The purpose of these modifications was to increase the salience of the paired stimulus and experimental control. Specifically: (1) presentations of the paired stimuli were interspersed with presentations of a neutral auditory stimulus which was never followed by the preferred stimulus; (2) a nonvocal prompt for attention was given prior to all stimulus presentations (neutral and unpaired); (3) stimulus presentations were separated from each other by a variable inter-trial interval; and (4) stimulus presentations (both neutral and unpaired) were produced using a "motherese" voice (i.e., clear articulation, exaggerated intonation, reduced rate). In combination, these procedures resulted in reliable increases of target vocalizations within sessions for all participants.

Other studies involving typical infants indicate that when even the most minimal form of social interaction is paired with speech, performance is enhanced. For example, Todd and Palmer (1968) used contingent verbal reinforcement to increase the frequency of vocalizations by two groups of 3-month-old infants. The infants in both groups received verbal reinforcement delivered through a speaker in the wall behind the crib. However, the infants in one group saw an adult near their crib whereas the infants in the other group did not. Results showed that the infants who saw the adult demonstrated significantly higher rates of vocalization. In another study, Kuhl, Tsao, and Liu (2003) compared the speech perception skills of two groups of 9-month-old English-learning infants following exposure to a Mandarin-speaking adult. Infants in both groups listened while the same adult read the same books to them and talked to them about the same toys. However, the infants in one group were in the same room with the caregiver while the infants in the other group observed the caregiver on television. Results showed that the infants who were present in the room with the adult performed significantly better on a speech perception task.

Interaction

Researchers have also examined the influence of particular types of social interaction on infant vocal-izations. Two studies demonstrated that social initiations increased the frequency of vocalizations produced by 3-month-old infants (Bloom, 1975; Bloom & Esposito, 1975). Other studies examined the effects of contingent feedback. In one, Goldstein, King, and West (2003) observed 8-month-old infants with their mothers during spontaneous play with toys. The mothers of half of the infants were asked to provide their infants with positive social feedback (e.g., smiling, moving closer to the infant) contingent on vocal behavior while the mothers of the other half of the infants were prompted to provided the same amount of positive social feedback but not contingent on vocalizations. Results indicated that the infants who received vocalized social feedback contingently produced more developmentally advanced vocalizations. Similar results were found by other researchers (e.g., Hsu, Fogel, & Messinger, 2001; Todd & Palmer, 1968).

A related study by Gross-Louis, West, Goldstein, and King (2006) assessed the amount of social feedback provided to infants spontaneously in response to their vocalizations. Ten mother-infant dyads participated, and the mean age of the infants was again 8 months. Results showed that mothers responded contingently to prelinguistic vocalizations 70% of the time, and they responded more often with verbal utterances than with nonverbal acts alone (e.g., smiling, gazing, physical contact). Furthermore, mothers acknowledged both vowel-like sounds and consonant-vowel (CV) combinations, but they responded differentially to each type. Vowel-like sounds were followed more often with play vocalizations while CV combinations were followed more often by the mother's imitations.

Imitation

Perhaps one of the most fundamental processes influencing infant vocal development is imitation. To imitate speech sounds, an infant must: (a) attend to a model, (b) translate sensory information from the model into a motor plan (cross-modal transfer), and (c) carry out the motor plan so that the acoustic (sensory) output matches the model (another level of cross-modal transfer). A carefully controlled study by Kuhl and Meltzoff (1982) demonstrated that infants as young as 4 months can recognize the relationship between specific facial movements (a visual stimulus) and acoustic features of the vowels /i/ and /a/ (an auditory vocal stimulus). In other words, infants attend to both visual and auditory information when they are exposed to speech models in a face-to-face setting.

According to Piaget (1952), imitation is challenging for newborns because of the required cross-modal transfer skills. In his view, the ability to coordinate sensory and motor information develops gradually throughout infancy. Moreover, he considered vocal imitation to be particularly challenging since an infant cannot see his or her own mouth. For example, when imitating a hand movement, an infant can see and compare the model's movement to his or her own movement. However, when imitating vocalizations, the infant can see only the model's face but not his own. Piaget argued that infants need particular kinds of experience (e.g., exposure to mirrors, tactile exploration of the caregiver's face) to learn how to imitate facial movements and that facial imitation could not be expected before 12 months. However, he did propose that infants engage in vocal contagion (the tendency to vocalize when others in the environment are vocalizing) within the first month of life.

As indicated earlier, Piaget's ideas have since been challenged by the results of experiments involving instrumentation that was not available in Piaget's time. In the case of imitation, carefully controlled laboratory studies involving sophisticated split-screen video technology have demonstrated that young infants can indeed imitate facial movements (e.g., tongue protrusion, lip protrusion, mouth opening) within days of birth (e.g., Meltzoff & Moore, 1977, 1983; Field et al., 1983). These and other related results strongly suggest that infants are born with a special capacity for **crossmodal transfer**. Meltzoff (1990) has referred to this as **active intermodal mapping (AIM)**.

To determine the age at which infants begin to imitate vocal models, Kuhl and Metzoff (1996) observed 72 infants, including 24 in each of three age groups (12, 16, and 20 weeks). In a carefully controlled laboratory environment, each infant saw and heard a woman produce one of three vowels (/a/, /i/, /u/) slowly and clearly. Each production was followed by a moment of silence. The vocalizations produced by infants within that moment were recorded and later analyzed by trained phoneticians

who were unaware of the models to which the infants were responding. Results indicated that infants as young as 12 weeks made approximations of each vowel. Moreover, when infants were later provided with the same facial cues for /a/, /i/, or /u/ but paired with nonspeech sounds, the infants produced no speech sounds. This finding indicates that infants were indeed sensitive to the vocal components of the original vowel models and that they were not simply imitating the model's facial movements. Overall, these findings indicate that infants can perform vocal imitation at least 9 months sooner than was predicted by Piaget.

In reflecting on the findings of this and previous research, Kuhl and Meltzoff (1996) proposed that infants use their vocal experiences from birth on to create an **auditory-articulatory "map."** This map relates self-produced auditory events to the motor movements that caused them. At the same time, infants are continually comparing the perceptual feedback from their own vocalizations (auditory proprioception) with perceptual feedback from speech models (auditory exteroception). Differences between the two are then used to adjust the auditory-articulatory map (Kuhl & Meltzoff, 1982).

Although Kuhl and Meltzoff (1982) provide an interesting framework for thinking about how motherese affects infant vocal development, it is unclear whether elicited imitation (i.e., imitation that is specifically requested by the adult) is a necessary component of the developmental process. In other words, infants may imitate speech sounds spontaneously without any deliberate effort on the part of caregivers to encourage it. At the same time, we see from observations of ritualized interactive games (including imitation games) that caregivers do provide infants with opportunities to hear clear, short speech segments in repetitive interactive contexts with increasing frequency as they progress from early infancy to the onset of speech. It is also true that parents imitate the acoustic features of their infants' vocalizations (e.g., Papousek & Papousek, 1989), and this may reinforce the infant's performance (Snowdon & Hausberger, 1997).

Overall, it is clear that exposure to motherese and social interaction is crucial for the development of babbling. Studies also show that pairing and contingent social interaction can influence the content of babbling and that infants must imitate features of speech in order to develop language-specific babbling patterns. What is unclear, however, is the extent to which babbling is influenced by an infant's natural motivation to engage in vocal imitation and by caregiver scaffolding patterns that influence the frequency of vocalization, vocal exploration, or vocal imitation. To determine this further studies are needed.

PRIMARY ACCOMPLISHMENTS: MORPHOLOGY AND SYNTAX

Background

To learn grammar, infants must be able to locate and distinguish linguistic units (words, phrases, sentences) in the stream of phonetic units they hear. At the broadest level, the organizing features of these units include syntax and morphology. Syntax is the system of rules that determines the sequencing of words within phrase structures such as sentences. For example, most English declarative sentences are organized in a **subject-verb-object (SVO) sequence**, as in the sentence "The cat [S] is chasing [V] a ball [O]." Note that the SVO structure is not universal; for example, Japanese uses an SOV structure. Morphology is the system of rules that determines the internal structure of words in relation to their semantic or grammatical function within an utterance. For example, the root word "swim" is used independently to represent a discrete activity (e.g., "I can swim") but it is produced with the suffix "-ing" when referring to a continuous ongoing activity (e.g., "I am swimming.") or when it functions grammatically as a noun (e.g., "Swimming is fun."). Neither morphology nor syntax is differentiated productively during the prelinguistic period; however, each contributes to the grammatic structure. For a more detailed description of morphology and syntax, see Chapter 4.

Infants identify syntactic and morphological patterns based partly on the prosodic features of speech (e.g., pauses, pitch changes, final lengthening, etc.) (e.g., Morgan, Meier, & Newport, 1987; Shi, Werker, & Morgan, 1999). Although prosody is influenced by factors other than syntax alone, there are enough prosodic features in motherese to support the identification of grammatical units (e.g., Fisher & Tokura, 1996). As we know from our discussion of speech perception, infants become sensitive to speech prosody by at least 7 months, even before they begin to comprehend words (Owens, 2008), and they produce language-specific prosodic patterns by about 9 to 10 months (e.g., de Boysson-Bardies et al., 1984). Knowledge of prosodic cues may assist infants in bootstrapping syntactic knowledge. For example, SVO languages have a systematic prosodic structure (Nespor & Vogel, 1986), and the acoustic cues associated with this structure may help infants to identify syntactic units (Werker & Tees, 1999).

Although the perception of prosody may be helpful, it alone falls short of providing all the information needed to identify the boundaries of syntactic phrase structures (Gerken, Jusczyk, & Mandel, 1994). Fortunately, it is not the only available cue. Infants also use information from the segmental features of speech to identify word-order patterns. This has been demonstrated by studies in which infants were exposed to artificial languages containing segmental patterns across nonadjacent phonetic units. For example, in one study, 12-month-olds were exposed to repeated samples of artificial "word" strings such as "vot-pel-jic-rud-tam." The boundaries of each string were always the same ("vot" and "tam"), but the "words" between the boundaries always varied. After less than 3 minutes of exposure to different word strings, infants identified the specific word order patterns that were targeted (Gomez & Gerken, 1999, 2000). In another study, 7-month-old infants were exposed to three-word sequences that followed either an ABB pattern (e.g., "ga-ti-ti") or an ABA pattern ("ga-ti-ga"). After only 2 minutes of listening to either pattern with the original word strings, the infants generalized their recognition of the ABB or ABA pattern to completely new word strings (e.g., "wo-fe-fe" and "wo-fe-wo") (Marcus, Vijayan, Bandi Rao, & Vishton, 1999).

Another clue to grammatical structure comes from information about infant perception of morphological categories. Specifically, infants are sensitive to the acoustic information that differentiates lexical words from grammatical words (Shi, Werker, & Morgan, 1999; Werker & Tees, 1999). This is supported in part by the differential phonological cues in motherese. For example, Shi, Morgan, and Allopenna (1998) found that the lexical (content) words in motherese tend to be longer, louder, and more likely to have full vowels than function (grammatical) words. Follow-up work by Shi, Werker, and Morgan (1999) suggests that the ability to discriminate the acoustic features of lexical and function words may even be present shortly after birth.

In sum, the precursors of syntax appear to emerge between about 7 to 10 months as infants become sensitive to relevant prosodic and segmental speech patterns in motherese. The precursors of morphology appear to emerge even earlier as infants demonstrate a perceptual sensitivity to differences in the acoustic features of lexical versus function words in the speech they hear. These perceptual skills are not enough to help infants decode the meanings of specific sentences or words, but they may help infants notice phonetic patterns that extend beyond individual sounds.

PRIMARY ACCOMPLISHMENTS: PRAGMATICS

Background

The rules of pragmatics determine socially appropriate communication patterns. At the most basic level, this includes the rules of turn-taking within the context of infant-caregiver interaction. As infant-caregiver interaction is also the basic context of learning, we described the development of turn-taking skills within our discussion of the semantic and lexical precursors to language (see above). To recap, we noted that behavioral turn-taking is scaffolded in two general ways. Caregivers structure interactive routines throughout the course of the infant's waking moments; and they weave their responses around the bursts and pauses of the infant's behavior. As the infant matures, he or she uses increasingly more mature behavior to take turns, and there is an increasing amount of shared control over the scripts in which infants and caregivers interact. Routine activities of daily living (e.g., feeding, dressing, play) are important contexts in which infants learn to anticipate and assume their roles, and ritualized interactive games play a particularly important role as a scaffold for learning conventional communication skills. Imitation may be the quintessential form of turn-taking, without which the cultural features of communication cannot be acquired.

In addition to turn-taking, however, the **rules of pragmatics** also determine the socially appropriate selection of form (phonology, morphology, syntax) and content (semantics) to express communicative intentions within a given context. In other words, we typically have many ways to communicate our intended messages, and the rules of pragmatics prompt us to choose the way that is most appropriate for the social occasion. Consider, for example, some different ways to request a cup of coffee: "Give me some coffee!," "Coffee please," "Is that coffee I smell?," "Man am I thirsty!," "Where's my morning Joe?," "Ich möchte Kaffee bitte," and others. What we choose to say will depend on our communicative intent, where we are, our relationship to the communicative partner, the nature of the social occasion, and other relevant features of context. In fact, mature speakers routinely consider multiple features of context in choosing their words, and in some circumstances they may choose not to express their intentions at all if other considerations take priority.

In contrast to mature speakers, infants begin with a limited repertoire of signals and have no apparent awareness of social context. At birth, much of their behavior is reflexive, and for at least the first 7 months, lacks intentionality. At this time, infants do not know that their behavior has the potential to influence others. This awareness develops gradually during the prelinguistic period together with sensitivity to social contexts.

Elizabeth Bates (1976) and her colleagues (Bates, Camaioni, & Volterra, 1975) were among the first to study the development of pragmatics from prelinguistic communication to the onset of language. Their research identified three stages in this transition. Borrowing terminology from speech act theory (Austin, 1962; Searle, 1969), they characterized these stages as perlocutionary, illocutionary, and locutionary. Below is a summary of the key features of each stage.

Perlocutionary Stage (~0 to 8 months)

This stage is characterized by pre-intentional behavior that is interpreted as meaningful by caregivers.

The behaviors include a wide range of nonverbal and vocal signals. Nonverbal signals may include gaze patterns, facial expressions, body orientation, movement, object manipulations, and others. Vocal signals may initially include reflexive and vegetative forms as well as protophones. Both types of signals are considered pre-intentional because infants do not appear to recognize the potential of these signals to affect the behavior of others.

As infants approach the next (illocutionary) stage, their signals become increasingly refined. For example, during the first month of life, caregivers interpret every salient behavior (e.g., facial expression, eye gaze, vocalization, movement patterns, burping, sneezing, yawning, etc.) as communicative signals. However, as infants develop increasingly more sophisticated behaviors (e.g., joint reference, gaze shifts, object permanence, means-ends, object play, etc.) and increasingly more speechlike babbling patterns, caregivers respond contingently to a more narrow range of signals. Through these experiences, infants gradually learn that their behaviors have the potential to influence the behavior of others.

Illocutionary Stage (~9 to 11 months)

This stage is characterized by the deliberate use of conventional gestures (e.g., pointing, showing, giving, abbreviated reaching) to express communicative intent (also known as communicative function). Sometimes infants invent their own gestures to express communicative intent. For example, Owens (2008) described a child who twisted her legs around each other to signal "potty." However, the hallmark of the illocutionary stage is the intentional use of conventional gestures, and these gestures are increasingly accompanied by canonical babbling with prosodic features that signal the infant's communicative intent. Just before the production of the first words, infants may accompany their conventional gestures with a protoword. In sum, infants now know that their signals have the potential to affect the behavior of others, and they use these signals deliberately to express their intentions with the expectation of specific responses.

How do caregivers know when an infant's signals are intentional? Sachs (2005) summarized four features typically associated with intentional communication. First, the infant accompanies his or her signals with gaze shifts between the communicative partner and the object or event to which the infant is referring. Secondly, the particular gestures are consistent, ritualized, and produced in similar ways each time they are used. Third, the infant typically pauses after his production of a gesture to wait for a response from the conversational partner, and finally, the infant will persist (and sometimes even modify his or her signals) if his or her communicative intent is not honored or misunderstood.

Bates, Camaioni, and Volterra (1975) identified two categories of communicative intentions typically expressed by infants at this stage: the **protoimperative** and the **protodeclarative**. The protoimperative involves the use of gestures for the purpose of regulating adult behavior in the service of a goal (e.g., to receive an object, participate in an activity, or engage in an action; Bruner, 1983). For example, a child may point to a cookie, look at an adult, look at the cookie, and look back at the adult to request a cookie. It is as if the child is saying, "I want that cookie and I want you to give it to me." However, protoimperatives also may be used to communicate rejection (Sachs, 2005). For example, the infant may push away an offered object or use a gesture to end an interaction. In contrast, the protodeclarative involves the use of gestures to share joint attention. For example, a child may point to a puppy, look at his or her father, and then look back at the puppy simply because he or she wishes to share the experience. It is as if the child is saying, "I see a puppy and I want you to see it too."

The protoimperative and the protodeclarative are not the only communicative intentions expressed during the illocutionary stage. For example, children also engage actively in rituals that might be classified as intentions, such as waving "bye-bye." However, the protoimperative and protodeclarative are considered major milestones in the development of pragmatic skills because they involve a deliberate coordination of object-oriented and socially-oriented acts in the service of a goal. Interestingly, Bates, Camaioni, and Volterra (1975) reported a correlation between the emergence of these skills and an infant's ability to engage in tool use (i.e., to use one object as a means of accessing another). Sachs (2005) observed that the expression of communicative intent also is correlated with an infant's emerging concept of causality (i.e., knowledge that there are causes for events). These cognitive skills (tool use, causality) typically are included in the assessment of prelinguistic communication behavior, and there may be reason for concern when a child demonstrates only one or two of these forms (e.g., tool use) in the absence of the others (e.g., protoimperative and protodeclarative). In fact, some children with disabilities (e.g., autism) may demonstrate unusually higher levels of skill in tool use and in the expression of protoimperatives but not express any protodeclaratives.

Locutionary Stage (~12 months and later)

Illocutionary communication patterns provide the communicative infrastructure to support later language use. In fact, during the locutionary stage, infants begin to use words within the same types of communicative contexts in which they previously used conventional gestures. Language is learned in the service of communication, and nowhere is the connection more direct than in the context of illocutionary communicative acts.

For mature speakers, good pragmatic skills are closely tied to an individual's theory of mind (ToM), or to the ability to appreciate the mental states, agendas, and overall perspective of others. The development of ToM during the prelinguistic period has been linked with an infant's ability to participate actively in the establishment of joint attention (Tomasello, 1995). Infants begin to share with another person the experience of attending to something at about 9 months of age (Carpenter, Nagell, & Tomasello, 1995). In the act of joint attention, each partner seeks to insure that the other partner is noticing the same reference point. To the extent that infants can perform this maneuver, they are building a path toward perspective taking. However, sharing joint attention is only the beginning. (For more information about the development of joint attention, refer to an earlier section of this chapter.)

As in every other aspect of prelinguistic development, the role of a caregiver is crucial to supporting the development of pragmatic skills. If a caregiver did not respond contingently to an infant's communication signals, then the infant would have no basis for learning that his or her signals have the power to influence others. In other words, a caregiver's

appropriate and consistent responsivity helps the infant to become aware of the communication process (Owens, 2008). Through these interactions, an infant learns that his or her behavior can have predictable consequences. However, although responsivity is important, there is normal variability among caregivers in the amount and type of responses they offer. Furthermore, it is important to note that a caregiver's behavior alone cannot account for infant communication development. What caregivers bring to the table is a responsive social environment in which the growth of intentional communication can take place.

In this section, the early development of pragmatic skills was described from a developmental linguistic perspective. We encourage readers to also consider the developmental process from a behavioral perspective in Hegde (2010) and McLaughlin (2010).

INTEGRATION OF LANGUAGE SKILLS

The development of linguistic precursors is a gradual and complex process involving a wide range of skills and systematic patterns of social support. We have divided this topic into segments for ease of discussion, although in reality, all aspects of prelinguistic development progress simultaneously and in an interdependent manner. As we have seen, all learning takes place in the context of child-caregiver interaction. Failure to adapt to an interactive turn-taking structure will severely limit an infant's opportunities to learn all of the linguistic precursors. Motherese also changes the way in which infants perceive speech sounds, and this perception is linked with changes in patterns of babbling. As speech perception and babbling develop, so do patterns of cognitive growth (e.g., object permanence, play, means-ends, imitation) and modes of communication. Altogether, we see a gradual shift from universal to culture-specific patterns of growth across all linguistic precursors.

We have described the behavior of infants and of their caregivers in separate sections, but their behaviors too are interdependent. Right from the start, infants are socially precocious, having the ability to influence their caregivers' behaviors even before they are conscious of doing so. Caregivers are drawn to their infants and their needs, and structure the environment to scaffold more advanced behaviors. As infants succeed in mastering these challenges, caregivers make further adjustments to encourage further growth. Perhaps the major integrating force behind prelinguistic communication development is the desire of infants and caregivers to communicate with each other. Neither is consciously assuming the role of teacher or learner, but each is operating in a kind of synchrony to achieve successful collaboration. Initially, caregivers assume the major responsibility for structuring successful exchanges. However, as an infant's abilities mature, there is a gradual shift toward shared control of joint activities and shared understanding of communication signals.

CONCLUSION

Language is a tool for communication, and it develops on the shoulders of previously established communication skills. In this chapter, we traced the development of this communicative infrastructure with an eye to future developments in semantics, phonology, morphology, syntax, and pragmatics. Milestones in the developmental trajectory are tied to contributions of the infant and of the social environment, since communication develops within the context of infant-caregiver interactions. The trajectory of development itself can be characterized as a shift from universal to culture-specific infant behavior with respect to precursors of each linguistic component. However, although the precursors of each component were discussed individually, their development and functions are interdependent. Taken as a whole, these skills provide an infrastructure for the onset of true linguistic content (lexicon and semantics), structure (phonology, morphology, and syntax) and function (pragmatics).

REFLECTION QUESTIONS

1. What is the difference between lexical and function words? Please provide examples of each.

2. How is the ability to participate in child-caregiver interactions related to the development of a lexicon?

3. How might object permanence, object play, means-ends development, categorization, and analogical reasoning influence the development of a lexicon?

4. What is the zone of proximal development (ZPD)? How do caregivers make use of ZPD to scaffold more advanced levels of infant behavior?

5. What is motherese? How can it help infants to learn language?

6. What is joint attention and joint reference? What are the implications of these skills for early lexical development?

7. What are the characteristics of ritualized interactive games? How are these games especially well suited for helping infants learn word meanings? What additional advantage is provided by joint book-reading?

8. Describe three methods of evaluating the comprehension of words by infants. Summarize the milestones of lexical comprehension during the first 12 months.

9. What is a protoword? How do protowords differ from real words? What is the significance of protowords?

10. What is the relationship between speech sounds and letters of the alphabet? What is the International Phonetic Alphabet (IPA) and what is the advantage of using it?

11. What is phonology, and what is the difference between the segmental versus the suprasegmental features of speech?

12. What is the difference between top-down and bottom-up processing of speech?

13. Describe the protophones associated with each stage of infant babbling development.

14. In what sense does canonical babbling resemble speech? How might social interaction and contingent feedback from a caregiver influence the development of babbling?

15. Distinguish between auditory-articulatory map, auditory proprioception, and auditory extero-

ception. How do these factors relate to the development of babbling?

16. What are syntax and morphology? How are they different and in what way are they similar?

17. What is communicative intent? Describe three stages in an infant's acquisition of communicative intent.

18. What are the criteria for deciding if an infant's nonverbal gestures are intentional?

19. Describe ways in which the development of linguistic precursors is integrated throughout the developmental process.

20. During the first year of life, infants demonstrate a shift from universal to culture-specific patterns of behavior across all linguistic components. What does this mean?

APPLICATION EXERCISES

1. Make a list of words that infants are likely to hear during feeding, dressing, and play. Interview parents of infants who are 8 to 12 months old. Ask open-ended questions (e.g., "Tell me about your child's understanding of words during feeding, bed time, and play.") Compare the items on your word list with the items reported by individual parents.

2. Interview parents about the babbling and speech of their prelinguistic infants by asking open-ended questions (e.g., "Tell me about your infant's speech sounds.") What kind of information do they give you? For example, do they tell you only about the infant's speech sounds or do they tell you about the sounds, the context, and the possible meanings?

3. Observe infants of different ages and their caregivers during routine play interactions with and without toys. If possible, videotape the observation. Describes the infant's behavior in relation to object permanence, object play, means-ends, joint attention, babbling, and language comprehension. Describe the caregiver's participation in relation to the structure of turn-taking, topics of interaction, and motherese.

4. Ask family members whether you or your siblings used made-up words. Make a list of the words and their meanings.

REFERENCES

Aslin, R. N., Saffran, J. R., Newport, E. L. (1998). Computation of conditional probability statistics by 8-month-old infants. *Psychological Science, 9,* 321–324.

Austin, J. L. (1962). *How to do things with words.* Oxford, UK: Clarendon Press.

Baillargeon, R. (1987). Object permanence in 3.5- and 4.5-mon-old infants. *Developmental Psychology, 23,* 655–664.

Baillargeon, R., & DeVos, J. (1991). Object permanence in young infants: Further evidence. *Child Development, 62,* 1227–1246.

Baillargeon, R., DeVos, J., & Graber, M. (1989). Location memory in 8-month-old infants in a nonsearch AB task: Further evidence. *Cognitive Development, 4,* 345–367.

Baillargeon, R., Graber, M., DeVos, J., & Black, J. (1990). Why do young infants fail to search for hidden objects? *Cognition, 36,* 255–284.

Bakeman, R., Adamson, L. B., Konner, N., & Barr, R. (1990). Kung infancy: The social context of object exploration. *Child Development, 61,* 794–809.

Baldwin, D., & Meyer, M. (2007). How inherently social is language? In E. Hoff & M. Schatz (Eds.), *Blackwell handbook of language development.* Malden, MA: Blackwell.

Bates, E. (1976). *Language in context: Studies in the acquisition of pragmatics.* New York, NY: Academic Press.

Bates, E. (1979). On the emergence of symbols: Ontogeny and phylogeny. In A. Collins (Ed.), *Children's language and communication: The Minnesota Symposium on Child Psychology* (Vol. 12, pp. 121–157). Hillsdale, NJ: Erlbaum Associates.

Bates, E. (1997). On the nature and nurture of language. In E. Bizzi, P. Catissano, & V. Volterra (Eds.), *Frontier de la biologica: The brain of homosapiens.* Rome, Italy: Giovanni Trecani.

Bates, E., Camaioni, L., & Volterra, V. (1975). The acquisition of performatives prior to speech. *Merrill-Palmer Quarterly, 21,* 205–216.

Bates, E., with L. Benigni, I. Bretherton, L. Camaioni, & V. Volterra. (1979). *The emergence of symbols: Cognition and communication in infancy.* New York, NY: Academic Press.

Benedict, H. (1979). Early lexical development: Comprehension and production. *Journal of Child Language, 6,* 183–200.

Berk, L. (2006). *Child development* (7th ed.). New Deli: Prentice-Hall of India.

Bijou, S. W., & Baer, D. M. (1965). *Child development: Vol 2. Universal stage of infancy.* New York, NY: Appleton-Century-Crofts.

Bloom, K. (1975). Social elicitation of infant vocal behavior. *Journal of Experimental Child Psychology, 20*(1), 51-58.

Bloom, K., & Eposito, A. (1975). Social conditioning and its proper control procedures. *Journal of Experimental Child Psychology, 19*(2), 209-222.

Bortfeld, H., Morgan, J. L., Golinkoff, R. M., & Rathbun, K. (2005). Mommy and me: Familiar names help launch babies into speech-stream segmentation. *Psychological Science, 16*(4), 298-304.

Bosch, L., & Sebastian-Galles, N. (1997). Native language recognition abilities in 4-month old infants from monolingual and bilingual environments. *Cognition, 65*, 33-69.

Bremmer, G., & Fogel, A. (2001). *Blackwell handbook of infant development.* Malden, MA: Blackwell.

Brooks, R., & Meltzoff, A. N. (2005). The development of gaze following and its relation to language. *Developmental Science, 8*, 535-543

Bruner, J. (1981). The social context of language acquisition. *Language and Communication, 1*, 155-178.

Bruner, J. (1983). *Child's talk: Learning to use language.* New York, NY: Norton.

Bruner, J., & Sherwood, V. (1976). Peekaboo and the learning of rule structures. In J. S. Bruner, A. Jolly, & K. Sylva (Eds.), *Play—Its role in development and evolution* (pp. 268-265). New York, NY: Basic Books.

Campbell, A. L., & Namy, L. L. (2003). The role of social referential context and verbal and nonverbal symbol learning. *Child Development, 74*, 549-563.

Carpenter, M., Nagell, K., & Tomasello, M. (1998). Social cognition, joint attention, and communicative competence from 9 to 15 months of age. *Monographs of the Society for Research in Child Development, 74*, 549-563.

Cheek, A., Cormier, K., & Meier, R. P. (1998). *Continuities and discontinuities between manual babbling and early signing.* Presented at the Sixth International Conference on Theoretical Issues in Sign Language Research. Gallaudet University, Washington, DC, November 12-15, 1998.

Chen, Z., Sanchez, R. P., & Campbell, T. (1997). From beyond to within their grasp: The rudiments of analogical problem solving in 10- and 13-month-olds. *Developmental Psychology, 33*(5), 790-801.

Cheour, M., Ceponiene, R., Lehtokoski, A., Luuk, A., & Allik, J. (1998). Development of language-specific phoneme representations in the infant brain. *Nature Neuroscience, 1*(5), 351-353.

Clarke-Stewart, K. A. (1973). Interactions between mothers and their young children: Characteristics and consequences. *Monographs for the Society for Research in Child Development, 38*(Serial No. 153).

Cohen, L. B. (2003). Commentary on Part I: Unresolved issues in infant categorization. In D. H. Rakison & L. M. Oakes (Eds.), *Early category and concept development: Making sense of the booming, budding confusion.* New York, NY: Oxford University Press.

Cooper, R. P., & Aslin, R. N. (1990). Preference for infant-directed speech in the first month after birth. *Child Development, 61*, 1584-1595.

Cutler, A., & Carter, D. (1987). The predominance of strong initial syllables in English vocabulary. *Computer, Speech, and Language, 2*, 133-142.

de Boysson-Bardies, B., Sagart, L., & Durand, C. (1984). Discernable differences in the babbling of infants according to target language. *Journal of Child Language, 11*, 1-5.

DeCasper, A. J., Fifer, W. P. (1980). Of human bonding: Newborns prefer their mother's voices. *Science, 208*, 1174-1176.

Dore, J., Franklin, M., Miller, R., & Ramer, A. (1976). Transitional phenomena in early language acquisition. *Journal of Child Language, 3*, 13-28.

Echols, C. H., Crowhurst, M. J., & Childers, J. B. (1997). Perception of rhythmic units in speech by infants and adults. *Journal of Memory and Language, 36*, 202-225.

Eimas, P. D. (1975). Auditory and phonetic coding of the cues for speech: Discrimination of the /r-l/ distinction by young infants. *Perception and Psychophysics, 18*, 341-347.

Eimas, P. D., Siqueland, E. R., Jusczyk, P., & Vigorito, J. (1971). Speech perception in infants. *Science, 171*, 303-306.

Esch, B. (2007). *The role of automatic reinforcement in early speech acquisition.* Unpublished dissertation, Western Michigan University, Department of Psychology.

Esch, B., Carr, J. E., & Michael, J. (2005). Evaluating stimulus-stimulus pairing and direct reinforcement in the establishment of an echoic repertoire of children diagnosed with autism. *Analysis of Verbal Behavior, 21*, 43-58.

Fenson, L., Dale, P. S., Reznick, J. S., Bates, E., Thal, D. J., & Pethick, S. J. (1994). Variability in early communicative development. *Monographs of the Society for Research in Child Development, 59*(Serial No. 242).

Fenson, L., Marchman, V. A., Thal, D. J., Dale, P. S., Reznick, J. S., & Bates, E. (2007). *MacArthur-Bates communicative development inventories* (2nd ed.). Baltimore, MD: Paul H. Brookes.

Fernald, A. (1985). Four-month-old infants prefer to listen to motherese. *Infant Behavior and Development, 8*, 181-195.

Fernald, A., & Kuhl, P. K. (1987). Acoustic determinants of infant preference for motherese speech. *Infant Behavior and Development, 10*, 279–293.

Fernald, A., & Mazzie, C. (1991). Prosody and focus in speech to infants and adults. *Developmental Psychology, 12*(2), 209–221.

Field, T. M., Woodson, R., Cohen, D., Greenberg, R., Garcia, R., & Collins, K. (1983). Discrimination and imitation of facial expressions by term and preterm neonates. *Infant Behavior and Development, 6*, 485–489.

Fisher, C., & Tokura, H. (1996). Acoustic cues to grammatical structure in infant-directed speech: Cross-linguistic evidence. *Child Development, 67*(6), 3192–3218.

Fromkin, V., Krashen, S., Curtiss, S., Rigler, D., & Rigler, M. (1974). The development of language in Genie: A case of language acquisition beyond the critical period. *Brain and Language, 1*, 81–107.

Gerken, L., Jusczyk, P. W., & Mandel, D. R. (1994). When prosody fails to cue syntactic structure: 9-month-olds' sensitivity to phonological versus syntactic phrases. *Cognition, 51*(3), 237–265.

Goldstein, M. H., King, A. P., & West, M. J. (2003). Social interaction shapes babbling: Testing parallels between birdsong and speech. *Proceedings of the National Academy of Sciences, 100*, 8030–8035.

Gomez, R. L., & Gerken, L. (1999). Artificial grammar-learning by 1-year-olds leads to specific and abstract knowledge. *Cognition, 70*, 109–135.

Gomez, R. L., & Gerken, L. (2000). Infant artificial language learning and language acquisition. *Trends in Cognitive Science, 4*, 178–186.

Goodsit, J. B., Morgan, J. L., & Kuhl, P. K. (1993). Perceptual strategies in prelingual speech segmentation. *Journal of Child Language, 20*, 229–252.

Gopnik, A., & Meltzoff, A. (1986). Relations between semantic and cognitive development in the one-word stage: The specificity hypothesis. *Child Development, 57*, 1040–1053.

Graf Este, K., Evans, J. L., Alibali, M. W., & Saffran, J. R. (2007). Can infants map meaning to newly segmented words? Statistical segmentation and word learning. *Psychological Science, 18*(3), 524–260.

Gros-Louis, J., West, M. J., Goldstein, M. H., & King, A. P. (2006). Mothers provide differential feedback to infants' prelinguistic sounds. *International Journal of Behavior Development, 30*(6), 509–516.

Gustafson, G. E., Green, J. A., & West, M. J. (1979). The infant's changing role in mother-infant games: The growth of social skills. *Infant Behavior and Development, 21*(2), 373–377.

Hauser, M. D., Newport, E. L., & Aslin, R. N. (2001). Segmentation of the speech stream in a nonhuman primate: Statistical learning in cotton-top tamarins. *Cognition, 78*, B53–B64.

Heath, S. B. (1983). *Ways with words: Language, life and work in communities and classrooms.* Cambridge, UK: Cambridge University Press.

Hegde, M. N. (2010). Language and grammar: A behavioral perspective. *Journal of Speech-Language Pathology and Applied Behavior Analysis, 5*(2), 90–113.

Hirsh-Pasek, K., & Golinkoff, R. M. (Eds.). (1996). *The origins of grammar: Evidence from early language comprehension.* Cambridge, MA: MIT Press.

Holmgren, K., Lindblom, B., Aurelius, G., Jalling, B., & Zetterstrom, R. (1986). On the phonetics of infant vocalization. In B. Lindblom & R. Zetterstrom (Eds.), *Precursors of early speech* (pp. 51–63). New York, NY: Stockton Press.

Hsu, H. C., Fogel, A., & Messinger, D. S. (2001). Infant non-stress vocalization during mother-infant, face-to-face interaction: Factors associated with quantitative and qualitative differences. *Infant Behavior and Development, 24*, 107–128.

Jusczyk, P. (1997). *The discovery of spoken language.* Cambridge, MA: MIT Press.

Jusczyk, P. W., & Hohne, E. A. (1997). Infants' memory for spoken words. *Science, 277*, 1984–1986.

Jusczyk, P. W., Houston, D. M., & Newsome, N. (1999). The beginnings of word-segmentation in English-learning infants. *Cognitive Psychology, 39*, 159–207.

Karrass, J., Braungart-Rieker, J., Mullins, J., & Lefever J. (2002). Processes in language acquisition: The roles of gender, attention, and maternal encouragement of attention over time. *Journal of Child Language, 29*, 519–543.

Kaye, K. (1979). Thickening thin data: The maternal role in developing communication and language. In M. Bullowa (Ed.), *Before speech.* New York, NY: Cambridge University Press.

Kaye, K. (1980). Why we don't talk "baby talk" to babies. *Journal of Child Language, 7*, 489–507.

Kaye, K., & Wells, A. J. (1980). Mothers' jiggling and the burst-pause pattern in neonatal feeding. *Infant Behavior and Development, 3*, 29–46.

Keller, H. (1905). *The story of my life.* New York, NY: Doubleday.

Kent, R. D. (1992). The biology of phonological development. In C. A. Ferguson, L. Menn, & C. Stoel-Gammon (Eds.), *Phonological development: Models, research, implications.* Timonium, MD: York Press.

Koopmans-van Beinum, F. K., & van der Stelt, J. M. (1986). Early stages in the development of speech movements. In B. Lindblom & R. Zetterstrom (Eds.), *Precursors of early speech* (pp. 37–50). New York, NY: Stockton Press.

Krasnegor, N. A., Rumbaugh, D. M., Schiefelbusch, R., & Studdert-Kennedy, M. (1991). *Biological and behavioral determinants of language development.* Hillsdale, NJ: L. Erlbaum.

Kuhl, P. K. (1991). Human adults and human infants show a "perceptual magnet effect" for the prototypes of speech categories, monkeys do not. *Perception and Psychophysics, 50,* 93-107.

Kuhl, P. K. (2000). A new view of language acquisition. *Proceedings of the National Academy of Sciences, 97,* 11850-11857.

Kuhl, P. K. (2004). Early language acquisition: Cracking the speech code. *Nature Reviews Neuroscience, 5,* 831-843.

Kuhl, P. K., Andruski, J. E., Chistovich, I. A., Chistovich, L. A., Kozhevnikova, A. V., Ryskina, V. L., . . . Lacerda, F. (1997). Cross-language analysis of phonetic units in language addressed to infants. *Science, 277,* 684-686.

Kuhl, P. K., & Meltzoff, A. (1982). The bimodal perception of speech in infancy. *Science, 218,* 1138-1141.

Kuhl, P. K., & Meltzoff, A. (1996). Infant vocalization in response to speech: Vocal imitation and developmental change. *Journal of the Acoustic Society of America, 100,* 2425-2438.

Kuhl, P. K., & Miller, J. D. (1975). Speech perception by the chinchilla: Voice-voiceless distinction in alveolar plosive consonants. *Science, 90,* 69-72.

Kuhl, P. K., & Miller J. D. (1978). Speech perception by the chinchilla: Identification functions for synthetic VOT stimuli. *Journal of the Acoustic Society of America, 63,* 905-917.

Kuhl, P. K., & Padden, D. M. (1983). Enhanced discriminability at the phonetic boundaries for the place feature in macaques. *Journal of the Acoustic Society of America, 73,* 1003-1010.

Kuhl, P. K., Tsao, F. M., & Liu, H.-M. (2003). Foreign language experience in infancy: Effects of short term exposure and social interaction on phonetic learning. *Proceedings of the National Academy of Sciences, 100,* 9096-9101.

Kuhl, P. K., Williams, K. A., Lacerda, F., Stevens, K. N., & Lindblom, B. (1992). *Science, 255,* 606-608.

Lamb, M. E., Bornstein, M. E., & Teti, D. B. (2002). *Development in infancy: An introduction* (4th ed.). Hillsdale, NJ: Lawrence Erlbaum.

Lenneberg, E. (1967). *The biological foundations of language.* New York, NY: Wiley.

Lieberman, P., Crelin, E. S., & Klatt, D. H. (1972). Phonetic ability and related anatomy of the newborn, adult human, Neanderthal man, and the chimpanzee. *American Anthropologist, 74,* 287-307.

Mandel, D. R., Jusczyk, P. E., & Pisoni, D. B. (1995). Infants' recognition of the sound patterns of their own names. *Psychological Science, 6,* 315-318.

Marcus, G. F., Vijayan, S., Bandi Rao, S., & Vishton, P. M. (1999). Rule learning in 7-month-old infants. *Science, 283,* 77-80.

Markus, J., Mundy, P., Morales, M., Delgado, C. E. F., & Yale, M. (2000). Individual differences in infant skills as predictors of child-caregiver joint attention and language. *Social Development, 9*(3), 302-315.

Matychuk, P. (2004). The role of child-directed speech in language acquisition: A case study. *Language Sciences, 27,* 301-379.

McClaughlin, S. (2010). Verbal behavior by BF Skinner: Contributions to analyzing early language learning. *Journal of Speech-Language Pathology and Applied Behavior Analysis, 5*(2), 114-131.

Mehler, J., Jusczyk, P., Lambertz, G., Halsted, N., Bertoncini, J., & Amiel-Tison, C. (1998). A precursor of language acquisition in young infants. *Cognition, 29,* 144-178.

Meltzoff, A. (1988). Infant imitation after a week delay: Long term memory for novel acts and multiple stimuli. *Developmental Psychology, 24,* 470-476.

Meltzoff, A. (1990). Towards a developmental cognitive science: The implications of cross-modal matching and imitation for the development of representation and memory in infancy. *Annals of the New York Academy of Sciences, 608,* 1-37.

Meltzoff, A. (2002). Elements of a developmental theory of imitation. In W. Printz & A. Meltzoff (Eds.), *The imitative mind: Development, evolution, and brain biases.* Cambridge, UK: Cambridge University Press.

Meltzoff, A., & Moore, K. (1977). Imitation of facial and manual gestures by human neonates. *Science, 198,* 75-78.

Meltzoff, A., & Moore, K. (1983). Newborn infants imitate adult facial gestures. *Child Development, 54,* 702-709.

Meltzoff, A., & Moore, K. (1999). A new foundation for cognitive development in infancy: The birth of the representational infant. In E. Scholnick, K. Nelson, P. Miller, & S. Gelman (Eds.), *Conceptual development: Piageti's legacy.* Mahwah, NJ: Erlbaum.

Menn, L., & Stoel-Gammon, C. (2005). Phonological development: Learning sounds and sound patterns. In J. Berko Gleason (Ed.), *The development of language* (6th ed., pp. 62-111). Boston, MA: Pearson, Allyn & Bacon.

Menyuk, P., Liebergott, J. W., & Schultz, M. C. (1995). *Early language development in full-term and premature infants.* Hillsdale, NJ: Erlbaum.

Mervis, C. B., & Rosch, E. (1981). *Annual Review of Psychology, 32,* 89-115.

Miguel, C. F., Carr, J. E., & Michael, J. (2002). The effects of a stimulus-stimulus pairing procedure on the vocal behavior of children diagnosd with autism. *Analysis of Verbal Behavior, 18,* 3-13.

Moerk, E. (1990). Three-term contingency patterns in mother-child verbal interactions during first language acquisition. *Journal of the Experimental Analysis of Behavior, 54,* 293-305.

Moore, K., & Meltzoff, A. (1999). New findings on object permanence: A developmental difference between two types of occlusion. *British Journal of Developmental Psychology, 17,* 563–584.

Morales, M., Mundy, P., Delgado, C., Yale, M., Messinger, D., Neal, R., & Schwartz, H. (2000). Responding to joint attention across the 6- through 24-month age period and early language acquisition. *Journal of Applied Developmental Psychology, 21*(3), 283–298.

Morales, M., Mundy, P., Rojas, J. (1998). Following the direction of gaze and language development in 6-month-olds. *Infant Behavior and Development, 21,* 373–377.

Morgan, J. L. (1994). Converging measures of speech segmentation in prelingual infants. *Infants' Behavior and Development, 17,* 387–400.

Morgan, J. L., Meier, R. P., & Newport, E. L. (1987). Structural packaging in the input to language learning. Contributions of prosodic and morphological marking of phrases to the acquisition of language. *Cognitive Psychology, 19,* 498–550.

Morgan, J. L., & Saffran, J. R. (1994). Emerging integration of sequential and suprasegmental information in preverbal speech segments. *Child Development, 66,* 911–936.

Morikawa, H., Shand, N., & Kosawa, Y. (1988). Maternal speech to prelinguistic infants in Japan and the United States: Relationships among functions, form, and referents. *Journal of Child Language, 15,* 237–256.

Nazzi, T., Bertoncini, J., & Mehler, J. (1998). Language discrimination by newborns: Towards an understanding of the role of rhythm. *Journal of Experimental Psychology: Human Perception and Performance, 24,* 756–766.

Nazzi, T., Jusczik, P. W., & Johnson, E. K. (2000). Language discrimination by English learning 5-month-olds: Effects of rhythm and familiarity. *Journal of Memory and Language, 43,* 1–19.

Nespor, M., & Vogel, I. (1986). *Prosodic phonology.* Dordrech, Netherlands: Foris.

Ninio, A., & Bruner, J. (1978). The achievement and antecedent of labeling. *Journal of Child Language, 5,* 1–15.

Oakes, L. M., & Mandole, K. L. (2003). Principles of developmental change in infants' category formation. In D. H. Rakison & L. M. Oakes (Eds.), *Early category and concept development: Making sense of the booming, budding confusion.* New York, NY: Oxford University Press.

Ochs, E., & Schieffelin, B. (1984). Language acquisition and socialization: Three developmental stories. In R. Shweder & R. LeVine (Eds.), *Culture theory: Mind, self, and emotion* (pp. 276–320). Cambridge, UK: Cambridge University Press.

Oller, D. K. (1978). Infant vocalization and the development of speech. *Allied Health and Behavioral Sciences, 1,* 523–549.

Oller, D. K. (1980). The emergence of the sounds of speech in infancy. In G. Yeni-Komshian, J. Kavanaugh, & C. Ferguson (Eds.), *Child phonology* (pp. 93–112). New York, NY: Academic Press.

Oller, D. K. (2000). *The emergence of the speech capacity.* Mahwah, NJ: Lawrence Erlbaum Associates.

Oller, D. K. (2006). Development and evolution in human vocal communication. *Biological Theory, 14,* 349–351.

Oller, J. W., Oller, S. D., & Badon, L. C. (2006). *Milestones: Normal speech and language development across the lifespan.* San Diego, CA: Plural Publishing.

Owens, R. (2008). *Language development: An introduction* (7th ed.). Boston, MA: Pearson Education.

Papousek, M., & Papousek, H. (1989). Forms and functions of vocal matching in interactions between mothers and their precanonical infants. *First Language, 9,* 137–158.

Payne, D. G., & Wenger, M. J. (1998). *Cognitive psychology.* Boston, MA: Houghton-Mifflin.

Pettito, L. A., & Marentette, P. F. (1991). Babbling in the manual mode: Evidence for the ontogeny of language. *Science, 251,* 1493–1496.

Piaget, J. (1952). *The origin of intelligence in children.* New York, NY: International Universities Press.

Platt, J., & Coggins, T. (1990). Comprehension of social-action games in prelinguistic children: Levels of participation and effect of adult structure. *Journal of Speech and Hearing Disorders, 55,* 315–326.

Ratner, N., & Bruner, J. (1978). Games, social exchange, and the acquisition of language. *Journal of Child Language, 5,* 391–401.

Rescorla, L. (1989). The Language Development Survey: A screening tool for delayed language in toddlers. *Journal of Speech and Hearing Disorders, 54,* 587–599.

Rieber, R. W. (1987). *The collected works of L. S. Vygotsky, Vol. 1.* New York, NY: Plenum.

Rollins, P. R. (2003). Caregivers' contingent comments to 9 month infants: Relationships with later language. *Journal of Applied Psycholinguistics, 24,* 221–234.

Rosch, E. (1975). Cognitive representations of semantic categories. *Journal of Experimental Psychology: General, 104,* 192–233.

Sachs, J. (2005). Communication in infancy. In J. Berko Gleason (Ed.), *The development of language* (6th ed.). Boston, MA: Pearson, Allyn & Bacon.

Saffran, J. R., Aslin, R. N., & Newport, E. (1996). Statistical learning by 8-month-old infants. *Science, 274,* 1926–1928.

Saffran, J. R., Newport, E. L., & Aslin, R. N. (1996). Word segmentation: The role of distributional cues. *Journal of Memory and Language, 35,* 606–621.

Saffran, J. R., & Thiessen, E. D. (2007). Domain-general learning capacities. In E. Hoff & M. Shatz (Eds.), *Handbook of language development* (pp. 68–86). Malden, MA: Blackwell.

Schieffelin, B. (1990). *The give and take of everyday life: Language socialization of Kaluli children.* New York, NY: Cambridge University Press.

Schliger, H. D. (2010). Behavioral vs. cognitive views of speech perception and production. *Journal of Speech-Language Pathology and Applied Behavior Analysis, 5*(2), 150–165.

Searle, J. (1969). *Speech acts: An essay in the philosophy of language.* London, UK: Cambridge University Press.

Shi, R., Morgan, J. L., & Allopenna, P. (1998). Phonological and acoustic bases for earliest grammatical category assignment. A cross-linguistic perspective. *Journal of Child Language, 25,* 169–201.

Shi, R., Werker, J. F., & Morgan, J. L. (1999). Newborn infants' sensitivity to perceptual cues to lexical and grammatical words. *Cognition,* B11–B21.

Singh, L., Morgan, J. L., & Best, C. T. (2002). Infants' listening preferences: Baby talk or happy talk? *Infancy, 3*(3), 365–394.

Skinner, B. F. (1957). *Verbal behavior.* New York, NY: Apple-Century-Crofts.

Smith, C. B., Adamson, L. B., & Bakeman, R. (1988). Interactional predictors of early language. *First Language, 8,* 143–156.

Smith, R., Michael, J., & Sundberg, M. L. (1996). Automatic reinforcement and automatic punishment in infant vocal behavior. *Analysis of Verbal Behavior, 13,* 29–48.

Snow, C. (1977). The development of conversation between mothers and babies. *Journal of Child Language, 4,* 1–22.

Snow, C. E. (1978). The conversational context of language acquisition. In R. N. Campbell & P. T. Smith (Eds.), *Recent advances in the psychology of language: Language development and mother-child interaction.* New York, NY: Plenum Press.

Snow, C., & Ferguson, C. A. (1977). *Talking to children: Language input and acquisition.* Cambridge, MA: University Press.

Snowdon, C. T., & Hausberger, M. (Eds.). (1997). *Social influences on vocal development.* Cambridge, UK: Cambridge University Press.

Stark, R. E. (1980). Prespeech segmental feature development. In G. Yeni-Komshian, J. Kavanaugh, C. Ferguson (Eds.), *Child phonology* (pp. 73–92). New York, NY: Academic Press.

Stark, R. E., Bernstein, L. E., & Demorest, M. E. (1993). Vocal communication in the first 18 months of life. *Journal of Speech and Hearing Research, 36,* 548–558.

Stoel-Gammon, C. (1988). Prelinguistic vocalizations of hearing-impaired and normally hearing subjects: A comparison of consonantal inventories. *Journal of Speech and Hearing Disorders, 53,* 302–315.

Stoel-Gammon, C., & Otomo, K. (1986). Babbling development of hearing-impaired and normally hearing subjects. *Journal of Speech and Hearing Disorders, 51,* 33–41.

Sundberg, M. L., Michael, J., Partington, J. W., & Sundberg, C. A. (1996). The role of automatic reinforcement in early language acquisition. *Analysis of Verbal Behavior, 13,* 21–37.

Thiessen, E. D., Hill, E. A., & Saffron, J. R. (2005). Infant-directed speech facilitates word segmentation. *Infancy, 7*(1), 53–71.

Tincoff, R., & Jusczyk, P. W. (1999). Some beginnings of word comprehension in 6-month-olds. *Psychological Science, 10*(2), 172–175.

Todd, G. A., & Palmer, B. (1968). Social reinforcement of infant babbling. *Child Development, 39*(2), 591–596.

Tomasello, M. (1995). Joint attention as social cognition. In C. Moore & P. J. Dunham (Eds.), *Joint attention: Its origins and role in development.* Hillsdale, NJ: Erlbaum.

Tomasello, M., Mannle, S., & Kruger, A. (1986). The linguistic environment of one to two year old twins. *Developmental Psychology, 22,* 169–176.

Tomasello, M., & Mervis, C. (1994). Commentary: The instrument is great, but measuring comprehension is still a problem. *Monographs of the Society for Research in Child Development, 59*(Serial No. 242), 174–179.

Tomasello, M., & Todd, J. (1983). Joint attention and lexical acquisition style. *First Language, 4,* 197–212.

Trehub, S. E. (1976). The discrimination of foreign speech contrasts by infants and children. *Child Development, 47,* 466–472.

Tsao, F. M., Liu, H. M., & Kuhl, P. K. (2004). Speech perception in infancy predicts language development in the second year of life: A longitudinal study. *Child Development, 75,* 1067–1084.

Uzgiris, I., & Hunt, J. (1975). *Assessment in infancy. Ordinal scales of psychological development.* Urbana, IL: University of Illinois Press.

Vaughn, M. E., & Michael, J. (1982). Automatic reinforcement: An important but ignored concept. *Behaviorism, 10,* 217–227.

Voulomanos, A., & Werker, J. F. (2004). Tuned to the signal: The privileged status of speech for young infants. *Developmental Science, 7,* 270–276.

Vygotsky, L. (1978). *Mind in society: The development of higher psychological processes.* (Eds), M. Cole, V. John-Steiner, S. Scribner, & E. Souberman (Trans.). Cambridge, MA: Harvard University Press.

Vygotsky, L. (1986/1934). *Thought and language*. Cambridge, MA: The MIT Press.

Waterson, N., & Snow, C. (1978). *The development of communication*. New York, NY: John Wiley & Sons.

Werker, J. F., & Tees, R. C. (1984). Cross-language speech perception: Evidence for perceptual reorganization during the first year of life. *Infant behavior and development, 7*, 49-64.

Werker J. F., & Tees, R. C. (1999). Influences on infant speech processing: Toward a new synthesis. *Annual Review of Psychology, 50*, 509-535.

Yoon, S., & Bennett, G. M. (2000). Effects of a stimulus-stimulus pairing procedure on conditioning vocal sounds as reinforcers. *Analysis of Verbal Behavior, 17*, 75-88.

CHAPTER 4

Language Development: Earlier Linguistic Skills

EARLIER LINGUISTIC PERIOD: PARAMETERS

In Chapter 3, we discussed the development of prelinguistic communication skills, which serve as the infrastructure on which language is built. We now turn to the development of language itself, beginning with the production of single words at about 12 months and continuing to the formulation of narratives at about 5 years.

EARLIER LINGUISTIC PERIOD: PURPOSES

The changes that take place between 12 months and 5 years are amazing as infants break the language barrier and zoom forward to a new level of communication. Initially, the meanings of their words are completely tied to the "here and now," and a listener must rely on nonlinguistic contextual cues to interpret an utterance as a statement, a request, or some other communicative intent. However, by the time children are 5 years old, listeners can understand the children's utterances without extensive reference to nonlinguistic cues, and children can use language to communicate information that transcends time and space. For example, they can describe objects that are not present, tell others about events that took place last week, plan future events, and describe the contents of their imagination. This is possible because they have learned to produce speech with increasing intelligibility and accuracy. There has been an explosion in the growth of their vocabulary. Single-word utterances have morphed into phrases, sentences, and narratives, and language has become a tool for thought. Through experience in an ever expanding social universe, children have learned to engage in extended conversations, to adjust their communication patterns in consideration of a listener's perspective, and to understand that language itself can be a topic of conversation. In this chapter, we trace these developments within and across each component of language.

PRIMARY ACCOMPLISHMENTS: LEXICON AND SEMANTICS

Children's first words mark the first directly observable indication that true linguistic communication has begun. As development continues throughout the preschool period, children's vocabularies expand to include several thousands of words. Here, we address some key issues related to this process. We review some of the concepts that mature language users know about words. We then review theories of word learning and selected features of lexical development observed during the first five years of life. We also summarize the features of social interaction and child-addressed speech that support word-learning.

Lexical Knowledge of Mature Communicators

To appreciate the scope of children's word learning, it helps to review some of what we, as experienced communicators, understand about words. Perhaps our most basic understanding is that spoken words are **sounds** used as **symbols** to **represent meaning** (e.g., *rose* is a symbol that stands for a type of flower with soft petals and a thorny stem). We also understand that word **meanings are abstract and categorical**. Independent of context, the word *rose* refers to a conceptual category rather than to a specific object in the world. However, within communicative contexts, words can be used to refer to specific real-world items (e.g., *the rose in my vase*) as well as more general categories (e.g., *There's nothing as fragrant as a rose*).

Another feature of word knowledge is that the phonetic form of a word is arbitrary but conventional. It is **arbitrary** because there is no logical relationship between a word and its meaning. Theoretically, any sound sequence could be used to represent any meaning. For example, the semantic category that we call *tree* in English is also known as *Baum, Árbol, drzew, ki, mti, pohon, δένδρο,* and *Περесо* in German, Spanish, Polish, Japanese, Swahili, Indonesian, Greek, and Russian, respectively. However, these very different words are **conventional**, because speakers of each language agree on the particular sound sequence that they will use to represent that meaning. These agreements are found in the dictionary of any language and are updated over time as word meanings evolve.

Most words can be categorized in relation to **word classes** that represent different kinds of meanings. At the broadest level, **lexical words** (e.g., nouns, verbs, adjectives) are used to represent substantive meanings and **function words** (e.g., articles, conjunctions, etc.) are used to represent grammatical meanings. Lexical words can be categorized further according to referents they typically are used to represent, including **nouns** (referring to people, places, and things), **verbs** (referring to actions and states), **adjectives** (referring to qualities of items named by nouns), and **adverbs** (referring to manners, times, and locations of actions or states named by verbs).

Some words have **unique features**. For example, in the case of some words, the relationship between sound and meaning appears less arbitrary (e.g., *meow, woof-woof, moo, hiss, clang, boom-boom, clickety-clack, choo-choo,* etc.). The sounds of these words resemble the sounds to which they refer. For this reason, they are classified as **onomatopoetic words**.

A unique feature of another set of words is that their referents shift depending on the speaker. These are known as **deictic words**. For example, the referent of the pronoun *I* shifts depending on who is using it. If I use the pronoun *I,* it refers to me, but if you use the pronoun *I,* it refers to you. Similarly, the meanings of words like *here* and *there* will shift depending on who is using them. If I say, *"bring the book over here"* I am asking someone to bring it closer to me. If someone at a distance from me says, *"Bring the book over here,"* then *here* refers to a location closer to the speaker and farther away from me.

Many words have **multiple meanings**. For example, the word *fly* can refer to an insect, a zipper, a particular kind of hit in baseball, the act of moving through the air, doing something with little preparation, and others. We understand which meaning is relevant in a particular situation by considering other information in the linguistic or nonlinguistic context (Miller, 1999). For example, in a description about the consequences of a batter's actions during a baseball game, the word *fly* points to one kind of meaning whereas in a discussion about insects the word, *fly* evokes another kind of meaning.

Sometimes words refer to **nonliteral meanings**. This may occur in the form of a **metaphor** (e.g., *She is an angel*), a **simile** (e.g., *The highway is like a parking lot*), an **idiom** (e.g., *It's raining cats and dogs*), or a **proverb** (e.g., *A stitch in time saves nine*). The ability to understand nonliteral meanings (also known as **figurative meanings**) requires us to ignore the typical meanings of words and to look for alternative meanings. The same principle underlies our ability to understand linguistic humor as well (e.g., *Metaphors be with you!*).

Words can be grouped together into **semantic networks** based on various **meaningful relationships** that exist between them. For example, words may be linked by reference to items at different **levels of categorization** (e.g., a feline house pet can be called a *tabby*, a *cat*, or an *animal*, representing **subordinate, basic,** and **superordinate** levels of categorization, respectively). Some words are associated by shared **contextual features** (e.g., *hospital, emergency, illness, nurse, doctor, medicine*, etc.) and others are **related by function** (e.g., bicycle, *car, bus, airplane*). Still others are linked because their meanings represent different or similar **points on the same continuum** (e.g., *small, medium, large*). Words at opposite ends of a continuum are **antonyms** (e.g., *hot, cold*) and words at the same end of a continuum are **synonyms** (e.g., *large, big*). Moreover, individual words can be linked with other words in multiple ways, and these linkages are believed to support the ease of word retrieval.

Finally, there is a sense in which words, by themselves, do not refer to anything at all. It is a speaker's use of words in the expression of communicative intent that activates their meanings, and it is the listener who makes an interpretation (Baldwin & Meyer, 2007). From that perspective, reference is a cognitive act (P. Bloom, 2000).

Peirce (1932) described three **levels of reference** that differ along several dimensions of interpretation. The first level is an **icon**, which is a signal that physically resembles a referent. A caricature of Albert Einstein is an icon of the man. An onomatopoetic word (e.g., *woof woof*) can be considered an icon of its referent (the barking of a dog). However, even though icons bear a physical resemblance to their referents, they are not the same as their referents, and recognition of the resemblance between the two is a cognitive act.

The second level of reference is an **index**, defined as a signal whose meaning is associated with a referent even though it bears no physical resemblance to it. For example, smoke is an index of fire; dark clouds are an index of rain; a particular smell is an index of coffee; and the beeper on an oven can indicate that cookies have finished baking. A word can be an index if its meaning is limited to a specific association. For example, a dog may understand the word *outside* because it systematically occurs prior to going for a walk. Indexes can be learned through classical or operant conditioning. For example, if a dog consistently sees his leash (signal) just before he is taken for a walk (reinforcement), he may learn to interpret the appearance of his leash as an index of going for a walk. The correlation between the index (e.g., the leash) and its referent (e.g., going for a walk) does not have to be perfect. However, the indexical relationship will weaken or fade as the correlation weakens or fades. Finally, with the exception of indexical word use, an index and its referent (e.g., smoke and fire) have a functional (rather than an arbitrary) relationship.

The third level of reference, a **symbol,** differs from an icon and an index in several important ways. First, the relationship between a signal and its referent is arbitrary but conventional (as discussed earlier). Second, listeners recognize symbols as *intentional* signals of social communication. Third, symbols are tied to other symbols within a semantic network. So, when a listener hears a word, he or she may think of other related words within the network. For example, if I point to an animal and say, "*That's my cat*" you may think about the specific cat to which I am pointing. However, your understanding of *cat* will also link with other meanings within your semantic network (e.g., *furry, allergies, sneezing*, etc.). Fourth, the memory for a word's meaning and its connections within a semantic network typically are not dependent on systematic reinforcement. For example, even though dinosaurs are extinct, the word *dinosaur* and its connection to other words remain part of your semantic network. Finally, although animals have been observed to interpret icons and indexes, the ability to interpret symbols is uniquely human. However, at the beginning of language development word meanings are likely to be indexical before they become symbolic (Cummings, 2003; Huttenlocher, 1974).

The semantic component of language is all about the content or meaning that is represented by words. We presented this information from a developmental linguistic perspective. A discussion about the representation of meaning would be presented quite differently from a behavioral perspective. Please refer to an excellent article by M. R. Hegde (2008) on meaning from a behavior analytic perspective.

For experienced language users, true linguistic knowledge of words, word meanings, and semantic networks is extensive, complex, and continues to expand throughout life. In the next section, we consider ideas about children's initial grasp of conventional word meanings.

Theories of Early Lexical Development

How do children begin to make the connection between a word and its meaning? To highlight the complexities of this puzzle, consider this vignette offered by Quine (1960): An anthropologist is in a remote location studying a tribe whose members speak an unknown language. Suddenly, he sees a rabbit scurrying by, and at precisely this moment a local tribesman points to the rabbit and says *gavagai*. How does the anthropologist interpret this word? Does he assume that it refers to the rabbit or to parts of the rabbit, such as its ears, paws, or tail? Does he assume it refers to the rabbit's hopping or perhaps to the tracks that the rabbit leaves behind? Does *gavagai* refer to the rabbit's color or to the direction in which the rabbit is running? Is *gavagai* a warning about the rabbit or simply a word to direct the linguist's attention to the rabbit? These are but a few of the possible ways to interpret *gavagai*.

During the early stages of language development, infants are in a position similar to Quine's anthropologist. Once they have learned to notice word segments, how do they solve the **gavagai problem**? How do they figure out the meaning of an unfamiliar word when the range of possible meanings is so great?

Over the decades, developmental researchers have responded to Quine's question by considering ways in which children may solve this **word mapping** problem. Four sorts of theories have evolved. These characterize word learning as **domain-specific** (i.e., based on neurologically programmed universal linguistic processes), **socially mediated** (i.e., based on scaffolding provided by caregivers during social interaction), **domain-general** (i.e., based on cognitive processes that apply across all aspects of learning), or **emergentist** (i.e., based on neurologic structures that allow for the growth of linguistic knowledge through a combination of general cognitive processes and social interaction). An in-depth discussion of these perspectives can be found in Hollich, Hirsh-Pasek, and Golinkoff (2000). A brief summary is provided below.

Domain-Specific Framework

Domain-specific views assume that the mind of a toddler is **constrained** in some way by **operating principles** that help her or him narrow down the number of possible meanings to which an unfamiliar word may refer. These principles develop gradually, so not all are available to a child at the earliest stages (Mervis & Bertrand, 1993; Waxman & Lidz, 2006). In fact, they may be acquired in a two-tier sequence (Golinkoff, Mervis, & Hirsh-Pasek, 1994; Mervis & Bertrand, 1994). Tier 1 principles are available when children first begin to talk and tier 2 principles are available later in the second year. Below is brief summary of the principles assumed to operate at each tier.

Tier 1. Three operating principles are included at tier 1. The first is called the **reference principle**, which refers a child's assumption that words stand for a person, place, or thing (Golinkoff, Mervis, & Hirsh-Pasek, 1994). The application of this principle usually leads to accurate word mapping because adults produce a higher proportion of nouns than verbs (Goldfield, 2000). However, it can lead to mapping errors if, for example, an adult points to a stove and says *hot* rather than *stove*. Also at tier 1, there is the **extendibility principle**, which refers to a child's assumption that words refer to categories of objects and not just to single instances as do proper names. This would account for a toddlers' labeling of various men as *daddy*. Third, the **object scope** principle, refers to a child's assumption that words refer to whole objects rather than to object parts or qualities For example, if someone says *teddy* while the child sees a teddy bear, the child will assume that the word refers to the teddy bear rather than to its ears, nose, paws, and so on.

Tier 2. Three additional operating principles are associated with tier 2, including the **conventionality principle**, which refers to the child's assumption that words should sound like conventional forms. Also included is the **categorical scope** principle, which refers to a child's assumption that words can be applied to other members of the same category but not to other objects that may be associated with the category. For example, the word *car* can refer to various cars, but it cannot refer to a key. The **novel name-nameless category principle** is the third tier 2 principle, which refers to a child's assumption that new words refer to categories that do not already have a name. For example, if a child sees two objects (e.g., a cat chasing a string) and knows the name for one (e.g., *cat*), the child will assume that the new word (e.g., *string*) refers to the other. As a child learns an increasing number of labels for items in the same context, the number of possible referents for new words gradually is reduced.

Social Mediation Framework

Researchers who propose social mediation frameworks note that word mapping is not really as complex as Quine (1930) originally suggested and that operating principles are not necessarily the key. Instead, they point to the supportive role of the social environment, to the emergence of children's social skills, and to the structure of language itself. They note that **caregivers serve as gatekeepers and social tutors** who protect their children from irrelevant information, structure interactive routines, simplify the language input, and scaffold word learning (e.g., Baldwin & Tomasello, 1998; L. Bloom, 1993; Nelson, 1988). Rather than leaving a child to search among a large number of potential meanings to link with unfamiliar words, caregivers follow their children's lead and name the things to which their children are already attending. As children begin to recognize the value of these social cues and to "read" the intentions of their communicative partners, they increasingly use a speaker's communicative intent to interpret word meanings (e.g., Baldwin, 1993, 1995). Finally, the style of speech typically used when talking to very young children provides children with cues about how to segment words from the speech stream and how to make inferences about word meanings.

Domain-General Framework

The domain-general framework proposes that word-learning is supported by general cognitive mechanisms, and it points to the influence of "**dumb attentional mechanisms**" in this process (Plunkett, 1997; Smith, 1995). Dumb attentional mechanisms include perceptual saliency, association, and frequency. Children are seen as information processors who pay attention only to the objects, actions, and events that are salient (i.e., noticeable, outstanding) to them in their environment, and who associate the most frequently heard label with the most salient referent. As they gain experience in the environment and begin to learn some words, different environmental conditions become salient and available for further word learning.

Aspects of all three frameworks discussed so far have been supported by research. However, none accounts for all aspects of word learning. For example, most of the proposed operating principles pertain to object labels, but children's first 10 to 20 words are not restricted to object labels (e.g., Caselli et al., 1995; Cummings, 2003;). Instead, children produce different types of words that do not fit neatly into adult grammatical categories (e.g., *bye-bye*, *up*, *boo*) as well as some that do (e.g., *mama*). Second, some of the data are not explained by any of the frameworks. For example, studies of the first 50 words show that nouns are easier to learn than verbs and words with concrete referents are easier to learn than words with abstract referents. Yet toddlers also acquire verbs (e.g., *go*) and words for abstract relationships (e.g., *uncle*). These observations suggest that word learning is a complex process involving multiple influences, including cognition, social interaction, environmental experience, and each child's unique motivations. A complete understanding cannot be limited to cognitive constraints, social features, or dumb attentional processes alone. Instead, it must be sensitive to the multiple levels of a child's participation in the complex fabric of his or her world (P. Bloom, 2000).

Emergentist Framework

As an alternative to the single-strategy frameworks described above, Hollich, Hirsh-Pasek, and Golinkoff (2000) proposed the **emergentist coalition model** (**ECM**). This theory is a hybrid of the previous frameworks, and it applies to word learning across all word classes (Hirsh-Pasek, & Golinkoff, 2006; Hirsh-Pasek, Golinkoff, Hennon, & Maguire, 2004). It is based on three assumptions. First, children are sensitive to multiple cues (e.g., perceptual, social, linguistic) in word learning. Second, word learning is developmental, and children give different weight to different sources of information at different points in development. For example, when they first begin to talk, they appear to rely more heavily on perceptual cues (e.g., shape) to map word meanings. However, with the emergence of intentional communication skills toward the end of the first year, they begin to pay more attention to social cues. Third, strategies of word learning are emergent in the sense that the strategies become more sophisticated as children become more proficient language users. For example, once they acquire grammatical skills, children can use grammatical structure as a cue to word learning. So, if they hear sentences like *Mary has a blunk* or *Mary is blunking*, they can use grammatical markers such as indefinite articles that precede nouns (e.g., *a blunk)* and verb endings (e.g., *-ing*) to identify *blunk* as a noun and *blunking* as a verb.

There is considerable support for the ECM, but it does not account for all aspects of word learning either. For example, L. Bloom (2000) noted that it does not account for the influence of a child's active participation in the world during the process of word learning. She argues that each child's own motivations and agendas will contribute to the way in which words are understood. For example, Cummings (2003) proposes that the very earliest words actually are indices, motivated by an infant's desire for social interaction. As you read the remainder of this section, think about how the evidence supports the four theories we have described.

Features of Early Lexical Development

Having considered frameworks for understanding lexical development, we now turn our attention to selected aspects of processes and products of word learning.

Emergence of Lexical Comprehension

To understand a word, an infant must be able to segment the word from a continuous stream of speech, store the word in memory, and link it with meaning. Developmentally, the word segmentation process begins first, providing a sort of envelope into which meaningful content will later be added. Initially, infants recognize wordlike phonetic forms by about 4½ months and their own names by about 5 to 6 months. By about 6 to 7 months they link a few salient words with meaning (e.g., *mommy, daddy*) and by 8 to 10 months, parents report that their infants comprehend an increasing number of words. Additional words are understood even before initial words are spoken (Fenson et al., 1994). However, word segmentation leads the way. Infants as old as 17 months map meanings more efficiently if given previous opportunities to segment a phonological form (Graf Estes, Evans, Alibali, & Saffran, 2007). Interestingly, 9- and 10-month-old infants prefer to listen to lexical words rather than function words, suggesting that they give special attention to the kinds of words that appear first in their vocabularies (Waxman & Lidz, 2006).

The words and meanings that children first understand are similar to those that they later will produce. For example, in a study of 48 infants between the ages of 10 to 21 months, Miller, Chapman, Branston, and Reichle (1980) found that single words for people and things were understood before single words that labeled actions. Moreover, words for people and things present in the environment were understood before words for people and things removed from context. Specifically, all 12-month-olds understood words for people who were present, but only half understood names for things. Words for actions were understood by most of the children older than 15 months. Slightly more than half of the 19- to 20-month-olds understood names for people and things that were not present. Unfortunately, the results of this study are limited by the fact that the children's comprehension was assessed in a structured task that included only object and action labels and not other word classes.

When infants begin to talk, there is a noticeable difference in the number of words understood and produced, and comprehension consistently leads production. Using traditional methods of assessment (e.g., parent report, direct observation in natural contexts), several researchers have found a 5- to 6-month lag between children's comprehension of 50 words at about 13 months and their production of 50 words at 18 to 19 months (Benedict, 1979; Menyuk, Liebergott, & Schultz, 1995). In Benedict's study, children learned about 22 words per month receptively and only 9 to 10 words per month expressively. A study conducted by Casselli et al. (2005) compared the comprehension and production vocabularies of American and Italian infants between 8 months and 16 months. Although they were learning different languages, the infants demonstrated surprising similarities in the sizes of their comprehension and production vocabularies. Additionally, children in both groups demonstrated an increased widening of the gap between comprehension and production between 8 and 16 months, with the widest gap appearing at 16 months.

It is important to note, however, that children's initial understandings of words are different from those of adults. For example, a toddler initially may respond to *bye-bye* only in a specific context. In fact, Huttenlocher (1974) suggested that the comprehension of children's earliest words may not even be fully linguistic. Instead, toddlers may look to co-occurring contextual cues (e.g., knowledge about event routines, the caregiver's intent) to interpret word meanings. We characterized this in Chapter 3 as **communicative comprehension**. It also may be characterized as an **indexical** (versus symbolic) form of comprehension (see the earlier discussion regarding levels of reference). However, through repeated experiences within the same routines (e.g., play, dressing, feeding, bathing, bed time, etc.) involving variations in people and objects, toddlers begin to notice categories of meaning, to represent them mentally, and to link them with appropriate phonetic forms. Once the link is established, words are understood as **symbols** and **linguistic comprehension** begins.

Differences between comprehension and production also may reflect difference between **recognition** versus **recollection** memory (Berk, 2006). Comprehension requires only that children recognize the meaning of a word that is spoken by someone else. However, production requires them to recall a word's phonetic form and meaning, to link it with a communicative intent, and to execute the oral motor movements needed to say it. So, it is easier to comprehend than to produce words.

Additional differences in comprehension and production are noted in the following discussion of word production, below. For now, one thing should be clear: We cannot draw conclusions about a child's comprehension skills based on his or her production, or vice versa. Each must be assessed separately. We now turn to a consideration of word production.

The First 25 Words

Most children begin to talk by about 12 months, with a range of from 8 to about 17 months (Reich, 1986). Most of the earliest words **resemble conventional words** in two ways: (1) they sound like the conventional word (e.g., *nana* for *banana*), and (2) they have a meaning that at least overlaps with the word's conventional meaning (e.g., *nana* may refer only to a whole banana and not to a banana slices). In addition, first words are spoken in the context to which they refer. For example, a child may say *nana* while pointing to a banana.

As in comprehension, the meanings of first words in production often are quite restricted even though they overlap with adult meanings. For example, 8-month-old Quentin Reich said *shoes* when looking at his mother's shoes in the closet but not when looking at his mother's shoes on the bedroom floor or his father's shoes in another closet (Reich, 1986). Similarly, 9-month-old Alison Bloom said *car* when looking from a window at a moving car on the street but not when in a car, when looking at a car standing still, or when looking at a picture of a car (L. Bloom, 1973). Ten-month-old Wendy said *hi* when she was in her crib and someone came into her room, but not elsewhere (Huttenlocher, 1974). These examples may reflect **indexical rather than symbolic** uses of words. At the very least, these uses of words are extremely restricted.

Cummings (2001) analyzed **the first 25 words** produced by 42 children representing three different cultures (American, British, French). Her goal was to assess the domain-specific theory, which suggests that word learning initially is influenced by operating principles that prompt infants to link new words with objects. However, the results did not support this theory. Instead, Cummings found that children's earliest vocabularies consist of at least seven different word categories, including general nouns, proper nouns, personal-social words, verbs, ritualized imitations, deictic words, and adjectives. Moreover, the combined proportion of proper nouns (including only one token) and personal-social words was greater than the proportion of object labels.

Cummings interpreted her findings as support for an emergentist framework suggesting that toddlers begin to talk by repeating frequently heard sounds that are emotionally salient and that are reinforced by the social environment. Use of these earliest words may appear referential because toddlers produce them in appropriate contexts. However, consistent with the examples of Quentin and Wendy above, they probably are indexical rather than symbolic. These initial words are context-specific and they are learned through reinforcement during social interaction.

Cummings (2003) also found that phrases like *thank you, scuse me*, and *come on* were perceived and treated by toddlers as single words. These are **segmentation errors** by adult standards, but it is easy to understand how children could arrive at incorrect conclusions about the boundaries of these words. After all, phrases like *thank you, come on*, and *excuse me* probably occur frequently in motherese during ritualized contexts of child-caregiver interaction.

The First 50+ Words

When the vocabularies of children at the 5- to 10-word stage are compared with those of children at the 11- to 25-word stage, we see a clear **increase in the proportion of object labels** (Cummings, 2003; Caselli et al., 1995). In fact, the dominance of nouns in children's early vocabularies is observed consistently across languages (Bornstein et al., 2004), and it is particularly striking at the 50-word level (Benedict, 1979; Nelson, 1973). For example, based on a longitudinal study of 18 American toddlers, Nelson found that more than half of the children's 50-word vocabularies consisted of object labels (e.g., *juice, bubbles, bottle*). Similar results were reported by others (e.g., Benedict, 1979; Caselli et al, 1995). In contrast to object labels, action labels (e.g., *go, bye-bye, up, out*) account for only about 13 to 19% of children's first 50 words; modifiers (e.g., *big, red, pretty, hot*) account for about 9% to 10% of the words; and other word categories, such as personal words (e.g., *yes, no, want, please, ouch*) and function words (e.g., *what, were, is, for*) account for 10% or fewer words (Benedict, 1979; Nelson, 11973).

Nouns continue to dominate until a child has acquired about 100 words when the proportion of verbs begins to increase slowly with a proportional

decrease in nouns. Other word classes (e.g., prepositions) do not increase proportionally until children have acquired about 400 words (Owens, 2008). Finally, although there are cross-cultural similarities in the types of words that children acquire, the specific words are based on a combination of factors such as their relevance to the child and the cultural significance of the referent (Anglin, 1995).

Rate of Early Lexical Development

The earliest words are acquired one at a time at the rate of about two per week (Carey, 1978). By the time that children have acquired their first 50 words, the rate has increased to about 9 per day (e.g., L. Bloom, 1973; Templin, 1957). Cumulatively, children typically produce about 3 to 4 words at 12 months, 90 words at 18 months, 320 words at 24 months, and 570 words at 30 months (Fenson et al., 1993). However you look at it, there is a dramatic increase in the rate of word learning, and the increase that occurs at about 18 to 19 months is often characterized as a **vocabulary spurt** (L. Bloom, 1993; Goldfield & Reznick, 1990). At this point, the largest proportion of children's words consists of object labels. The content of their vocabularies is conceptual rather than context bound, and children behave like sponges for lexical information, frequently asking *whassat?* Children appear to have gained the insight that things have names. Most researchers consider this insight to influence the rate of word learning, but others disagree. For example, P. Bloom (2000) argues that the rate of word learning increases simply because children get better at it, not because of conceptual changes.

Smith (in Reich, 1986) studied the productive vocabularies of children between the ages of 12 months and 6 years by using objects, pictures, and questions to evoke responses. Results demonstrated a gradual acquisition of words with a vocabulary spurt at about 19 months, followed by continued rapid acquisition. Children's comprehension vocabularies continue to grow in advance of their expressive vocabularies at every point along the continuum. For example, although Smith (in Reich, 1986) estimated that the productive vocabulary of 6-year-olds consist of 2,562 words, Templin (1957) estimated comprehension vocabulary at this age to include about 8,000 words.

Because word learning proceeds at a rapid rate after the initial vocabulary spurt at about 18 months, researchers have looked for factors to explain this. One is the development of **incidental learning** or the ability to learn words during spontaneous interaction without the benefit of direct instruction (Jaswal & Markman, 2001). It begins at about 24 months. A second factor is **fast mapping**, which enables children to retain a word in memory after only a few meaningful exposures, also without any direct instruction (Woodward, Markman, & Fitzimmons, 1994). It was observed in a study involving 3- and 4-year-olds who were exposed to unfamiliar words during classroom activities. Exposure occurred during requests such as, *Bring me the chromium tray, not the blue one, the chromium one.* During a probe one week later, the toddlers recalled information about the novel words. For example, they remembered the sound of the word *chromium* and that it referred to a color. Three-year-olds need more exposure to words than preschoolers, and preschoolers retain fast-mapped words for a month even though nonlinguistic information fades more rapidly (Markson & Bloom, 1997). However, the meanings of fast-mapped words are likely to be sketchy, tentative, and sometimes inaccurate. For example, Berk (2005) described the experience of Sammi, whose teacher announced that the class would go on a *field trip* (a phrase he had never heard before). When Sammy told his mother about it, she asked him where they were going. He replied *to a field, of course!* So, the capacity for fast mapping helps to ensure that new words will not be forgotten quickly even if encountered infrequently (Pan, 2005). However, once acquired, word meanings typically need further refinement (Carey, 1978).

Growth of Word Classes

Recall that object labels, verbs, and adjectives rank as the three most frequent types among the first 50 words. Below is a summary of special characteristics associated with the development of each of these word classes.

Labels for Objects. Much has been written about why object labels dominate early vocabularies, regardless of the language being learned. Researchers generally agree that objects may be easier to conceptualize (Waxman & Lidz, 2006). It is also true that caregivers name objects more often than other word categories; that object labels are more consistently accompanied by gestures (Schmidt, 1996); and that American mothers prompt their children to produce nouns more often than other word categories such as verbs (Goldfield, 2000). Object labels also may be easier to learn because their meaning is not dependent on other linguistic categories (Waxman & Lidz, 2006). For example, adjectives and verbs are predicates that require objects for their meaning, but object labels can stand alone. In fact, Waxman and Lidz consider object labels to be entry points for learning about verbs and adjectives.

Despite their importance as a reference point for verbs and adjectives, the children's early meanings of object labels are not always completely the same as those of adults'. Several explanations have been offered. Vygotsky (1934/1962) proposed that the very earliest words may be applied to new referents on the basis of **chained associations** such that the criterion for using a word varies from one referent to the next. An example involves a child who said the word *qua* (*quack*) when looking at a duck in a pond. Originally, the word referred to the entire scene. Later, she used the word in reference to a duck alone. Eventually, the word's meaning evolved in two directions. By association with the pond, its meaning was extended to include water and then milk in a baby's bottle. By association with the duck, its meaning was extended to include the image of an eagle on a round coin, then the coin itself, and eventually a round button. These chained associations in word extensions parallel the changing criteria in object sorting also observed in the performance of toddlers (Cummings, 2003).

Other researchers have identified patterns of word use known as underextension and overextension. **Underextension** is the pattern in which toddlers apply a word too narrowly. Recall 8-month-old Quentin's use of *shoes* only in reference to his mother's shoes when they were in the closet but not in reference to other shoes. This is an underextension error. It may be the result of indexical learning (as in the cases of Quentin, Alison, and Wendy) or it may reflect the content of children's early semantic categories. For example, a child may extend the word *cookie* to a variety of round cookies but never to cookies of different shapes.

In contrast to underextension, **overextension** is the pattern in which children apply a word more broadly than an adult would do, such as when a child says *kitty* in reference to a dog.

Much has been written about the possible reasons for these differences in extension patterns observed in children's use of words (e.g., Bowerman, 1978a; Clark, 1975; Mervis, 1987, 1998; Mervis & Mervis, 1988; Nelson, 1977). Three of the explanations involve theories regarding the mental processing that underlies children's extension patterns. One theory attributes overextensions to limitations in the number of semantic features in children's initial semantic concepts (Clark, 1975). Another theory (Nelson, 1977) attributes underextensions to a holistic focusing strategy that initially prevents children from differentiating the core features of a concept from the irrelevant features of a concept represented by a word. The third theory (Mervis, 1987, 1998) predicts both overextensions and underextensions based on the assumption that children, like adults, will extend a word to a referent based on their prototype for the concept represented by the word. However, children's prototypes vary from adult prototypes due to differences in experience, and therefore their word-extension patterns will differ as well.

All of these theories have been supported through research, with most of the weight supporting prototype theory. However, there may be additional reasons why children overextend words (McDonough, 2002). Several were noted by Pan (2005). For example, children may have **retrieval problems**. So, an older and more frequently used word (e.g., *cow*) might be easier to recall than the correct but less frequently used word (e.g., *moose*). Second, children may **lack the correct label**. For example, they may refer to zucchini as *cucumber* simply because they don't know its accurate name, not because they believe it to be a cucumber. Third, children may sometimes **use words analogically**. They may point to a bat and say *bird* only to indicate that the bat looks like a bird. Finally, children may sometimes **overextend words to create humor**. Pan (2005) described a two-year-old who routinely used the word *hat* while placing an overturned bowl on his head and giggling.

Labels for Actions. As indicated earlier, action labels are among the earliest words acquired, but account for a smaller proportion of first words than nouns, Moreover, they don't begin to increase in proportion until toddlers have acquired about 100 words and are beginning to produce multiword combinations.

Why are action labels more difficult to acquire? A number of explanations are summarized here, based partly on Gentner (1982) and Maguire, Hirsch-Pasek, and Golinkoff (2006). First, **actions are transient**. That is, although objects are distinct, unchanging entities that a child can examine at length, actions are dynamic and tend to disappear, making them harder to conceptualize. Second, there is a **mapping problem.** Actions typically consist of sequences of events, and it is difficult to know which part of the sequence is mapped by the verb. For example, picture a person eating an apple. They begin by holding it, bringing it to their mouth, biting into it, chewing it, and swallowing it. Which part of this sequence refers to eating? Third, there is an **extension problem.** To fully understand an action verb, a child must recognize the equivalence of actions across agents, manners, and objects (Naigles & Hoff, 2006). For example, to understand the word *throw*, the child must know that the word maps the same action performed by different agents (e.g., a child, an adult, a football player), even if it is performed in different manners (e.g., slowly, quickly) with different objects (e.g., a baseball, a pillow, a stone). Recognizing the similarities across these different contexts is challenging. Fourth, there may be a **perspective problem** (Gleitman, 1990). Specifically, the same action can be described by verbs that reflect different points of view. For example, while watching a cat chasing a dog, the labels *chasing* and *running* could both be used to describe the same event. The difference between these verbs relates to the perspective of the runner. So, the simple observation of a scene cannot provide all the information needed to interpret a verb. **Linguistic complexity** is a fifth explanation. The form of an English verb changes in at least four ways depending on tense (e.g., *walk, walks, walking, walked*), whereas nouns change only slightly in the plural form (e.g., *bike* to *bikes*). And finally, **early motherese favors nouns** (Owens, 2008). As indicated earlier, caregivers use a higher proportion of object labels just as children begin to say their first words. Object labels tend to occur at the end of caregivers' utterances, making them more salient to young listeners. Object labels more consistently are accompanied by gestures (Schmidt, 1996), and American mothers prompt their children to produce nouns more often than verbs (Goldfield, 2000).

The emergence and use of particular verbs has been studied by a number of researchers (Braunwald, 1995; Cauley & Gordon, 1987; Forbes & Poulin Dubois, 1997; Golinkoff, Hirsh-Pasek, Huttenlocher, Smiley, & Charney, 1983; Naigles, 1997; Naigles & Hoff, 2006; Smiley & Huttenlocher, 1995). Their findings confirm that verbs appear in the earliest vocabularies but that their use is limited and underextended. Huttenlocher et al. (1983) studied the verbs produced by children who had begun to produce two-word combinations and found that 90% of verb-containing utterances were produced while the children were engaged in the action they named. Smiley et al (1983) studied the use of *open*, *ride*, *sit*, and *rock* by children between 13 and 19 months, and also found that verbs were used most often when the children were engaged in the action they named, but *ride* and *rock* were also used in reference to actions produced by objects and people. So, although children do begin to use verbs at an early age, the verbs tend to refer to the children's own actions.

Studies of verb comprehension show that children understand more verbs than they use (Benedict, 1979; Goldfield, 2000; Goldin-Meadow, Seligman, & Gelman, 1976; Smith & Sachs, 1990). Using a combination of traditional methods (direction following) and the intermodal preferential looking paradigm (described in Chapter 3), Huttenlocher, Smiley, and Charney (1983) studied the comprehension of eight verbs (*wave*, *sit*, *kick*, *jump*, *put down*, *get*) by children between 20 to 40 months. They found that children comprehend these words earlier in a direction-following task than during the intermodal preferential looking (IPL) task, and this was corroborated by Golinkoff, Hirsch-Pasek, Cauley, and Gordon (1987).

Other evidence shows that the meanings of some verbs are understood before others. For example, Huttenlocher, Smiley, and Charney (1983) found that children understand **movement verbs** (e.g., *jump*, *blow*) before they understand **change verbs** (e.g., *bring*, *put down*). Comprehension also is affected by context. For example, Forbes and Poulin-Dubois (1997) observed 20-month-olds to assess their understanding of two verbs (*kick*, *pick up*). The actions corresponding to the verbs were performed by different agents, in different manners, or with new outcomes. Results showed that children could identify verbs in reference to actions performed by different agents but not when performed in different manners or with different outcomes. In summary, by adult standards, early verb comprehension appears to be restricted and underextended.

One explanation for the underextension pattern is tied to motherese (Naigles & Hoff 2006). As indicated earlier, adults label actions less often than objects, and they ask their children to name actions less often. Also, unlike object labels that are often accompanied by gestures toward the referent, action labels typically are named just before the action is performed. However, verbs that are used in motherese more frequently and in more diverse syntactic frames are acquired sooner than verbs that are used less often and in fewer syntactic frames (Naigles & Hoff-Ginsberg, 1998). A **syntactic frame** is a phrase structure. For example, *Doggie eats hamburger*, *Doggy eats noisily*, and *Doggy eats it up*, illustrate the use of *eat* in three different frames reflecting theme, manner, and outcome, respectively.

During two larger scale studies, Naigles and Hoff (2006) found several additional patterns of verb use in motherese. In one study, they observed mothers talking to their 14-month-olds during play with toys selected to encourage the use of 17 different verbs (*blow*, *bounce*, *clap*, *drink*, *eat*, *jump*, *listen*, *look*, *push*, *roll*, *sit*, *talk*, *throw*, *turn*, *walk*, and *wave*). Results showed that some were used more frequently than others (e.g., *push*, *look*, *eat*, *turn*, and *throw*) and some were not used at all (e.g., *clap*, *jump*, *roll*) during the 140 minutes of observation. In addition, some verbs were used in only one play context (e.g., *drink*, *sing*, *talk*, *throw*) whereas others were used during more than one (e.g., *eat*, *push*, *turn*).

The second study examined differences in the use of verbs types. This time, Naigles and Hoff (2006) observed 62 mothers talking to their 2-year-olds during four routine activities (mealtime, dressing, book reading, toy play). Results showed that verbs with general all-purpose meanings (**GAP verbs**) were used more often across all activities than verbs with more specialized meaning (**non-GAP verbs**). GAP words included *come*, *do*, *go*, *get*, *look*, *make*, *need*, *put*, and *want*. Non-GAP words included *drop*, *fall*, *give*, *work*, *jump*, *lay*, and others. Additionally, the authors found that both types of verbs were used significantly more often during joint book reading.

Further, GAP verbs and **internal state verbs** (e.g., *know*, *think*, *want*, *like*) were used significantly more often than non-Gap verbs and **motion verbs** (e.g., *push*, *put*, *pull*).

Labels for Object Qualities

Information about the development of adjectives is somewhat limited. We know that they occur frequently in speech addressed to toddlers and that toddlers are very sensitive to the qualities that adjectives label (e.g., color, size, texture, temperature, emotional state). Still, adjectives account for only 10% or less of toddlers' first 50 words and do not begin to emerge with any regularity until children have learned a core vocabulary of object labels, usually at about the time that they are beginning to combine words into short phrases.

Knowledge of object labels clearly supports the comprehension of adjectives. Consider this example: When toddlers as old as 3 years are presented with an unfamiliar object (e.g., a white llama) and told *it's white*, they will interpret the adjective as the object's name (Waxman & Lidz, 2006). Yet, the same toddlers will understand the word (e.g., *white*) as an adjective if it is used in combination with a familiar object label (e.g., *a white shoe*).

Based on parent reports, toddlers begin to use adjectives with some regularity by about 21 months (Fenson et al., 1994). As with object labels and verbs, their initial understanding of adjectives is somewhat restricted. For example, toddlers initially understand a new adjective only in reference to other objects within the same basic level category (Waxman & Lidz, 2006). So, if they hear someone say, *It's furry* (referring to a cat), they will understand *furry* as a label that can be applied only to other cats. However, by 24 months, if given an example, they can apply unfamiliar adjectives across appropriate basic level object categories. So, if they are shown a picture and told, *This is a blikish dog. Can you show me a blikish car?* they will understand that *blikish* is an adjective and will pick out the appropriate car (Mintz & Gleitman, 2002).

Support for Early Lexical Learning

Studies show that word learning is supported by both social and linguistic aspects of child-caregiver interaction (Gerken, 2002; Hart & Risley, 1995; Hoff, 2003; Hoff & Naigles, 2002). Below we highlight selected features of child-caregiver interaction that appear to support vocabulary development, and we summarize two studies (Hart & Risley, 1985; Hoff, 2003) that illustrate the impact of child-addressed speech on word learning.

Social Features of Interaction

The social context of word learning includes routinized interactions, child-oriented language input, and children's emerging ability to "read" their caregiver's intentions. Routinized interactions provide familiar contexts in which children can link the words they hear with the predictable focus of joint attention. In less familiar situations, caregivers help their children map meanings by following the child's lead and naming items to which the child is already attending. Towards the end of the first year, infants learn to interpret their caregiver's intentions, thus gaining additional information for making inferences about word meanings. By 18 months children's perspective-taking skills become increasingly sophisticated. They begin to understand that, if a speaker isn't paying attention to the same thing that they are, then the speaker's words probably refer to whatever the speaker is attending to (Baldwin, 1993; Hollich, Hirsh-Pasek, & Gollinkoff, 2000).

Linguistic Features of Child-Addressed Speech

The linguistic features of child-addressed speech provide crucial support for word learning. Remember that word-learning requires children to find word segments in the stream of speech, to fast-map the segments into memory, and then to flesh out the meanings of mapped words (Hoff & Naigles, 2003). In the previous chapter, we reviewed aspects of motherese that support word segmentation, including the statistical distribution of speech sounds, the prosodic features of utterances (e.g., rate, stress, pausing), and the placement of key words at the end of an utterance (e.g., Aslin, Saffran, & Newport, 1998; Morgan & Denuth, 1996). Once children have acquired a core vocabulary, they can begin to use familiar words to figure out the meanings of unfamiliar words. For example if 2- to 3-year-olds are told that *Mommy feeds the ferret*, they will understand that *ferret* refers to the animal (Goodman, McDonough, & Brown, 1998). These kinds of inferences have been shown to occur for nouns, verbs, and adjectives. In addition to the form and content of motherese, there also is a frequency effect. For example, the first words that children produce tend to include the most frequent words they hear (e.g., Hart, 1991). The number of utterances that children hear and the average length of those utterances will both influence the rate of vocabulary development (e.g., Bornstein, Haynes, & Painter, 1998; Hart & Risley, 1995).

Sharing Joint Attention

Within all interactive contexts, episodes of **joint attention** continue to be an important feature of word learning (Tomasello & Farrar, 1986; Tomasello, Mannle, & Kruger, 1986; Tomasello & Todd, 1983). Tomasello and Farrar (1986) observed 24 toddlers interacting with their mothers in a naturalistic setting at 15 months and again at 21 months. At each observation, the behaviors of a mother and her child were observed within and outside of joint attention episodes. Results showed that child behaviors were more advanced and maternal behaviors were more helpful within (versus outside of) joint attention episodes at both observation sessions. Mothers and children produced more utterances when engaged in joint attention. Mothers used shorter utterances, and they made more comments. Most importantly, mothers' references to the objects of joint attention at 15 months were positively correlated with children's vocabulary at 21 months, whereas object references that attempted to redirect the children's attention were negatively correlated.

Following Child's Lead

Caregivers not only **follow their children's focus of attention** by what they choose to label but also by what labels they choose (e.g., Anglin, 1977, 1978; Mervis & Mervis, 1982). Mervis and Mervis found that mothers of 13-month-olds used child-basic rather than adult-basic category labels when talking to their children. So, when their 13-month-old children played the same way with a toy leopard as with a toy tabby cat, mothers referred to the leopard as a *kitty-cat* (a child-basic label) even though they called it a *leopard* (adult-basic label) when talking to an adult. The authors interpreted this to mean that mothers prefer to follow their

children's lead by naming objects according to their children's level of categorization. The authors reasoned that mothers make inferences about their children's categories by watching the way in which their children play with toys. Because the children in this study played the same way with a toy tabby cat and a toy leopard, their mothers referred to each as *kitty-cat*. By the same token, mothers change their choice of words when children begin to notice critical features that link an object with the adult-basic category (Mervis & Mervis, 1988). For example, a toy dump truck initially may be labeled *car* by a mother, if her child plays with it in the same way as other toy vehicles (e.g., by rolling back and forth). However, once the child plays with the dump truck differently (e.g., by loading and unloading blocks), his or her mother is likely to begin calling it a *truck*. In summary, mothers follow their children's lead when deciding how to name the objects to which their children are attending. When children categorize objects differently than adults, mothers use child-basic object labels to fit the child's category. However, when children begin to notice critical features of an object that differentiate it from a child-basic category and link it with an adult-basic category, mothers again will follow their children's lead by using the adult-basic label.

Highlighting Linguistic Features

A recent study by Cleve and Kay-Raining Bird (2007) shows how mothers adjust their language to support children's word segmentation, fast-mapping, and elaboration. The authors observed 19 mother-child dyads including children between 20 and 36 months of age. The dyads were observed during play with a set of animal toys and a set of specially designed activity boxes. Some of the animals were known to be familiar to the children (e.g., dog, bear) and some were known to be unfamiliar (e.g., koala, raccoon). Similarly, the activity boxes were structured to invite familiar actions (e.g., push, blow) as well as unfamiliar actions (e.g., pump, scrub). Maternal utterances were recorded during play with all of the toys and later analyzed. Results showed that mothers adjusted their language depending on the child's familiarity with a word. Words that were known to be less familiar to a child were produced in the final position of utterances more often than words that were known to be familiar; and unfamiliar words were produced as single word utterances more often as well. Both of these patterns make unfamiliar words more salient, which supports the segmentation process. Evidence of support for fast-mapping also was found. Pairing of unfamiliar object labels with clear nonverbal referents occurred more often than pairing of familiar words with nonverbal referents. Finally, familiar words occurred more often in longer sentences that elaborated some aspect of the referent. This is exactly the kind of input that would help a toddler flesh out his or her understanding of previously fast-mapped words.

Providing Corrective Feedback and Direct Instruction

Sometimes word learning is influenced by **corrective feedback**, which may be either implicit or explicit. **Implicit feedback** occurs when a child simply experiences the communicative consequences of his or her word choice. For example, if a toddler who wants juice asks for *baba* (bottle), he may receive his or her bottle containing water or milk, thereby learning that *baba* is not the most efficient way to request juice. **Explicit feedback** may involve a combination of verbal instruction and demonstration. For example, if an older child mislabels an object, a caregiver may provide the correct label together with a demonstration to illustrate critical features to support the use of another word. So, if a child says *ball* in reference to a yo-yo, the adult may say, *That's a yo-yo. See?* [demonstration] *It goes up and down.* Chapman, Leonard, and Mervis (1986) found this to be the most effective way of supporting children's differentiation of adult-basic labels.

Other strategies vary depending on the level of generality, the type of target word, and the child's comprehension level (Pan, 2006). For example, when adults name objects at the basic level, they typically accompany the label with **explicit cues** for linking the word with its referent (e.g., pointing to an object and saying, *that's a ball*). However, when caregivers are asked to teach their children superordinate level category labels (e.g., *vehicle, clothing*), they use an **inclusion strategy** that links the superordinate level category with basic level examples (e.g., *An apple and a banana are kinds of fruit*). Similarly, when caregivers teach a subordinate-level object label, they link the subordinate level to the basic level (e.g., *A person is a passenger when he's riding in a car*.) If a word does not have an external referent, caregivers may link it with a child's experience. The following example is based on a study of mealtime discourse by Beals (1997, p. 682):

Mother: *You have to wait a little while so you don't get cramps.*

George: *What's cramps?*

Mother: *Cramps are when your stomach feels all tight and it hurts 'cause you have food in it.*

Participating in Joint Book Reading

Ritualized interactive games provide children with frequent opportunities to practice linguistic reference, and joint book reading stands out as a particularly important context for all sorts of language learning, including lexical development. Within these contexts, children are exposed to a wider range of words spoken within a wider range of syntactic contexts than is typical of conversational speech. Additionally, books expand the universe of topics for joint reference, and interactions during joint book reading provide children with scripts for how to talk about topics. As children demonstrate increasing skill at using words within a script, caregivers expand the script to new levels. Examples of this can be seen in successive sessions of joint book reading where the same book is used from one session to the next. Initially, caregivers may begin by encouraging toddlers to name the pictures to which they are attending and by providing the label if an object is not named. The example below is based on an interaction between a toddler and his mother while reading *Pancakes for Breakfast* (dePaola, 1978), a wordless picture book.

Toddler: (pointing at picture in book)

Mother: *What's that?*

Toddler: (still pointing at picture)

Mother: *a lady*

   It's a lady.

When the same situation recurred a few days later, the toddler recalled how to answer the question and his mother expanded the exchange:

Child: (pointing to picture in book) *lady*

Mother: *Yes, and what's she doing?*

Child: (looking at picture)

Mother: *She's cooking.*

Child: (looking back at book) cooking

Mother: *She's cooking pancakes*

A study by Snow and Goldfield (1983) examined the effects of situation-specific learning through longitudinal observations of one parent-child dyad over an 11-month period. Their results were consistent with the example above in that the child's utterances during one session of joint book-reading could be traced back to his mother's utterances during a previous session in the same context. Snow and Goldfield concluded that the routinization and the predictability of the language input helped the child to learn how to talk about the pictures in the book.

Impact of Motherese

The impact of motherese on word learning has been demonstrated by a number of studies. We have already mentioned the impact of language input during episodes of joint attention (e.g., Tomasello & Farrar, 1986). Other studies show additional important effects. For example, Hart (1991) observed that first words produced by toddlers tended to be ones that their parents frequently used in speaking to them. Below is a summary of two additional studies showing the impact of motherese on the rate of vocabulary development.

Hart and Risley (1995) used a longitudinal design to find out which features of language input affect children's vocabulary growth. Interactions between 42 individual infants and their caregivers were observed monthly over a 2½-year period beginning when the infants were 10 months old. The families represented three groups based on socioeconomic status (SES), including higher SES professional families ($n = 13$), middle to lower SES working-class families ($n = 23$), and welfare families ($n = 6$). Each group was racially and ethnically diverse.

Target behaviors included the number of different words produced by children during each observation session, and the number of utterances produced by caregivers. Caregiver utterances also were coded for three indicators of quality, including discourse features, adjacency conditions, and valence. **Discourse features** reflected the extent to which a parent encouraged a child's communication and independence. Asking the child questions (e.g., *Can you say horse?*), modeling social conventions (e.g., *thank you*), giving the child choices, and using prompt hierarchies that began with the least controlling cues were indicators of discourse quality. **Contingency features** reflected the extent to which parental responses addressed and enhanced child-initiated topics. For example, if a child said, *This soup is good*, a high quality contingent reply might be, *Yes, it's delicious.* **Valence features** reflected the emotional tone given to an interaction, such as affirmation of a child's communicative efforts. For example if a toddler said *duce* (referring to *juice*), a high quality valence response might be *that's right, juice!*

Several findings emerged from the study. First, all of the children had many similar experiences in language input. They all heard language about people, things, relationships, actions, feelings, and events, and they all engaged in interactions where their behavior was responded to, expanded on, prohibited, or affirmed. Second, by the end of the study, all the children had acquired language appropriately, including vocabularies within the normal range. However, the children in each group differed in the amount of language they heard and in the number of the quality indicators they experienced. Children of professional families heard the highest number of verbal utterances and experienced the highest number of quality of indicators. Children from welfare families heard and experienced the smallest number of each. The experiences of working class children ranked in between the other two. A third finding was that the amount of input received by the children was positively correlated with their rate of vocabulary development. Not surprisingly, then, the results showed a widening gap between the cumulative vocabularies of children across SES groups, with children from the high SES group using the largest number of different words, children from the welfare group using the lowest number of different words, and children from middle to lower SES groups ranking in between the other two. Finally, statistical analyses indicated that some factors (e.g., ethnicity/race, gender, birth order) had no affect on the rate of vocabulary growth.

Hoff (2003) replicated some of the results obtained by Hart and Risley (1995). She observed 63 mother-toddler dyads, including 33 from high SES families (i.e., parents were college-educated professionals) and 30 from mid SES families (i.e., parents had high school diplomas and unskilled or semiskilled jobs). All dyads were observed twice over a 10-week period in their homes while mothers and their toddlers were engaged in routine activities (dressing, eating, playing). At the first observation session, the mean ages of the high and mid-SES toddlers were 20.8 months and 21.6 months, respectively. The data consisted of each mother's utterances during the first session and each child's utterances during both sessions. Results showed that (a) the productive vocabulary size of the high-SES children grew more than that of mid-SES children, and (b) properties of maternal speech that differed as a function of SES fully accounted for the difference in the children's vocabularies. Mothers from the high-SES group used a larger number of words, a larger number of unique words, and longer average length of utterances.

Hoff offered two possible explanations for the differences in the style of motherese between the high and mid SES groups. One is that mid-SES families may have different beliefs about the value and appropriateness of talking to children or about the desirability of having a talkative child. This, in turn, may lead to a different communicative style (Heath, 1983; Snow de Blauw & Van Roosmalen, 1979). Another possibility is that SES may affect the amount of time available for leisurely parent-child interaction and it may affect the magnitude of other stresses on the families. Stress and time constraints, in turn, could affect both the frequency and style of child-caregiver interaction.

Of the three differences in the style of language used by the high versus mid-SES mothers, the average length maternal utterances had the strongest influence on children's vocabulary. This effect could occur for three reasons. First, longer utterances include a larger variety of words, and if children are exposed to a richer vocabulary they have more opportunities to map meanings. Second, utterances may be longer because parents are discussing word meanings rather than just labeling objects, and this would provide children with more semantic information (Gelman, Coley, Rosengren, Hartman, & Pappas, 1998). Finally, longer utterances provide more syntactic information and syntax can help children figure out word meaning. This effect was first demonstrated in an experiment by Brown (1958). He showed 3- to 5-year-olds an image of a pair of hands kneading a confettilike material in a bowl. For some of the children, the scene was accompanied by phrases like, *he likes to sib* or *he is sibbing*. These children assumed that *sib* referred to a kneading action. For other children, the picture was accompanied by phrases like *this is a sib*, and these children assumed that *sib* referred to the bowl. In other words, children made inferences about the meaning of an unfamiliar word based on the word's grammatical category within a syntactic framework.

LATER SEMANTIC DEVELOPMENT

As before, word learning continues to be influenced by a child's cognitive abilities, personal motivations, environmental experiences, social interactions, emerging language skills, and access to relevant language input. Below, we sample some of the key products of later development.

Color Terms

Some words typically are not observed in children's vocabularies until after they begin to produce multiword utterances. From our earlier discussion about adjectives, we know that a solid store of object labels and emerging syntactic skills can serve as entry points for further word learning (Waxman & Lidz, 2006). **Color terms** are a type of adjective and follow this pattern. Clearly, toddlers notice colors before they label them. For example, 2-year-olds can sort objects by color even though they use no color terms (Soja, 1994). Later, children learn to answer, *What color is this?* by providing a color term, even though their choice of the color term may be incorrect (Braisby & Dockrell, 1999). Eventually, color terms are used accurately. When talking to toddlers, caregivers tend to use primary color labels (*blue, red, green*) rather than subtler shades (e.g., *lavender, mauve*). So, it's not surprising that children's earliest color terms refer to primary colors.

Deictic Terms

Deixis comes from a Greek word meaning "to show," and deictic terms are linguistic tools for regulating joint attention (Wales, 1986). They are complex because their referents shift depending on the speaker (see discussion earlier in this chapter). Forms of deixis include pronouns (e.g., *I*, *you*), adverbs of location (e.g., *here*, *there*), verbs (e.g., *come*, *go*), and others. Here, we summarize the development of select pronouns (*I*, *you*, *this*, *that*) and adverbs (*here*, *there*) to illustrate the complexities of acquisition. Readers who are interested in further information are encouraged to consult Wales (1986), Reich (1986), and Owens (2008).

Development of **pronoun reference** involves some interesting twists and turns. Initially, many caregivers refer to their infant by name or by using the word *baby* (e.g., *Is baby hungry?*). In turn, a toddler's self-reference may begin with his or her name rather than a pronoun. Eventually, toddlers do use *I* for self-reference but may do so in combination with their names (e.g., *I Douglas pick it up*.). Redundant coding also occasionally occurs with other pronouns (e.g., *Fix it choo-choo train*) (Bloom, Lightbown, & Hood, 1975, p. 20). After toddlers begin to notice the pronoun *you*, they sometimes assume that *I* refers to the adult and *you* refers to them (e.g., saying *Hurt your elbow* to mean *I hurt my elbow*) (Tanz, 1980, p, 52). Also, certain discourse contexts are especially tricky at first. For example, when instructed by his conversational partner (a woman) to, *Ask Tom where my bike is*, the child turned to Tom and asked, *Where is your bike?* When he should have asked, *Where is her bike?* (Tanz, 1980, p. 67). By about 36 months, most toddlers have mastered the referential aspect of first person *I*. Third person pronouns (*he*, *she*, *it*) are mastered later.

The pronouns *this* and *that* and the adverbs *here* and *there* are important because they are used by caregivers while pointing out things in the environment, and they emerge early in children's vocabularies. Toddlers understand that these words are used to make reference, but their understanding of the referential targets emerges slowly. Initially, some children assume that *this* and *here* refer to new things whereas *that* and *there* refer to things they are finished playing with (Clarke & Sengul, 1978). Thereafter, each pair of terms emerges in three steps. First, the terms in each pair are used equivalently.

Later, one of the two terms is used more often than the other. Eventually, the shifting referents of each word are understood accurately in most contexts, but the distinction between *here* and *there* emerges before the distinction between *this* and *that* (Clark & Sengul, 1978; Wales, 1986). In an investigation of *this* and *that*, deVilliers and deVilliers (1974) found that 3-year-olds can understand these terms from the perspective of another person during a structured task, and 4-year-olds can adjust their use of these terms in consideration of a listener's perspective, also in a structured task. However, complete mastery is a gradual process. One experience builds on another, and mastery may not occur until early in elementary school. Also, note that even adults sometimes have difficulty interpreting these terms. For example, have you ever had difficulty understanding someone's directions when, while gesturing toward an imaginary map, they recommend that you *turn right there*?

Words for Contrasting Qualities

Some adjectives describe qualities that exist on a continuum, including *big/little*, *thick/thin*, *fat/skinny*, *more/less*, and others. According to Owens (2008), children learn the most general contrasts (e.g., *big* and *little*) before they learn the more specific contrasts (e.g., *fat/skinny*, *tall/short*). For each contrasting set, the positive label (e.g., *big*, *fat*, *tall*, *wide*) is learned before the negative label (e.g., *little*, *skinny*, *short*, *narrow*). Initially, use of these words will be restricted to contexts that resemble the ones in which they were first heard. However, as children are exposed to increasing examples involving familiar object (e.g., *tall girl*, *tall tree*, *tall building*), their understanding of the concepts expands and their use of the terms is generalized.

Invented Words

When children do not know or cannot recall the names of items they want to refer to, they sometimes invent their own words by using **derivational rules** and **rules for compounding** (e.g., Clark, 1982; Owens, 2008). Some examples are shown in Table 4–1. These examples show that, although children's invented words are not conventional, the

TABLE 4–1. Invented Words

Original Word and Word Class	Rule	Invented Word	Example
ring (Verb)	add *–er* to make a verb a noun	*ringer*	*My bike has a ringer*
jelly (Noun)	add *-ing* to make a noun a verb	*jellying*	*I'm jellying my bread* (Owens, 2008, p. 274)
dark (Adjective)	add *-ing* to make an adjective a verb	*darking*	*I'm darking the sky* (Reich, 1986)
many (N)	add *s* to make a single noun plural	*manys*	*I got manys* (Owens, 2008, p. 294)
plant (Noun)	add *man* to make a compound N	*plantman*	*The plantman is watering the flowers.*

rules used to create them certainly are. For example, it is conventional in English to refer to someone who sings as a *singer*. A person who jumps can be said to be *jumping*. More than one of something is sometimes referred to as *ones* (e.g., *These are not the ones I requested*); and the names for community workers sometimes end in *-man* (e.g., *fireman, mailman, postman*). All of the words listed in Table 4-1 reflect an **overgeneralization** of these rules. Interestingly, overgeneralization of rules is a common pattern in child language development (Slobin, 1971). Note that children's use of these rules to invent new words could not be a simple imitation of the language they hear. In fact, caregivers often respond to these utterances conversationally with comments that model the conventional word. For example, if a child says, *The plantman is here* a caregiver may say, *Yes, it's the gardener*. Hearing these models helps children learn the conventional words.

Semantic Networks

Semantic networks are groups of words that share some aspect of meaning. As children learn an increasing number of words in an increasing number of contexts, they begin to notice these meaningful relationships. They begin to notice words that occur in similar contexts (e.g., *swing, carousel, slide* are items at a *playground*), words related by taxonomic relationships (e.g., *cats, dogs, fish,* and *birds* are *animals*), words referring to qualities (e.g., *red, blue, green* are colors; *circle, square,* and *triangle* are shapes; etc.), words referring to qualities on the same continuum (e.g., *little, big, large* describe sizes); words for spatial relationships (e.g., *in, on, next to, behind*), and many others. Initially, related groups of words refer to referents that are relatively easy to sense or visualize. As children mature, they learn to recognize relationships between the meanings of words referring to concepts that are more abstract (e.g., words for mental states such as *knowing, thinking, imagining*; words for abstract categories such as *friendship, loyalty, fairness* and others).

The assumption that children organize their lexical knowledge in **semantic networks** is based on several types of evidence. One type of evidence is the observation of **within-category errors** in children's spontaneous utterances. For example, 2-year-old Christy Bowerman said, *Daddy take his pants on* when she meant . . . *pants off* (Bowerman, 1978b, p. 986). Another source of evidence is from children's performance on **word association** tasks. Nelson (1974) presented children with a target word (e.g., furniture) and asked them to name as many different words as they could that go with that word. She found that 8-year-olds can generate twice as many words as 5-year-olds, and that 5-year-olds include examples that are not categorically related (e.g., *door* in the *furniture* category). A third source of evidence comes from **free association tasks** (Brown & Berko, 1960). Here, the child is presented with one word (e.g., *dog*) and asked to say the first word that comes to mind. Brown and Berko found a **syntagmatic-paradigmatic shift** in children's responses to this task at about 7 years of age. Children younger than 7 tended to associate a given word with another word that could follow it in a sentence (e.g., *dog → barks*). Older children tended to associate a given word with a word from a related semantic category (e.g., *dog* → *cat*). This pattern may be due to changes in the semantic network. However, it also may reflect differences in the ways in which children interpret the task, differences in what children know about word meanings, or differences in conceptual organization associated with the emergence of literacy skills (Pan, 2006).

Summary of Lexical and Semantic Development During the First Five Years

Dramatic changes occur in the growth of a child's lexicon between the ages of about 12 months to five years. Comprehension typically leads production, and change in both modalities is reflected by growth in the number of words, diversity of word types, and content of lexical categories. The first 50 words in children's vocabularies tend to include a high proportion of object labels. With maturity, there is a gradual growth in other types of words as well (e.g., verbs, adjectives). The meanings of words acquired by toddlers typically are less well developed than those of adults. However, through every day experiences and interactions with others, meanings become increasingly conventional. By 5 years, children know thousands of words and recognize meaningful relationships between words based on categories (e.g., food, toys, clothing, animals, colors, etc.), associations (e.g., things in the kitchen, things outside, etc.), functions (e.g., things that cut; things that move, etc.), opposites (*wet, dry*), and synonyms (*small, little*). They also learn deictic terms and sometimes invent unconventional words by using conventional linguistic rules. Word learning is scaffolded through interactions between children and their caregivers in a variety of situations. Routine activities of daily living offer structured contexts that support the development of early vocabularies. During these predictable activity routines, caregivers communicate with their children using vocabulary that matches the topic of their joint attention. Joint book-reading is a particularly important routine for vocabulary development because it offers diverse lexical models in well-formed sentences on topics of interest to children. Frequent participation in joint book-reading is correlated with the growth of vocabulary and other skills that support children's later development of

literacy. Two studies (Hart & Risley, 1995; Hoff, 2005) demonstrate that the amount and quality of child-addressed speech has a direct impact on vocabulary development.

PRIMARY ACCOMPLISHMENTS: PHONOLOGY

Recall that the phonological component of language is the system of rules that shapes the segmental (phonetic, syllabic) and suprasegmental (prosodic) features of speech. During the prelinguistic period, infants learn to perceive and produce phonetic segments that increasingly come to resemble those that carry meaning in their linguistic community. Just prior to the production of their first words, they begin to attach meaning to some of these segments. The phonological accomplishments of the preschool language period are summarized below. These accomplishments include a qualitative shift in processing from the phonetic to the phonological level. As a background to this summary, we begin with a brief description of articulatory phonetics, which refers to speech sounds and their production.

Articulatory Phonetics

Some of the information to be considered here applies to all languages, but much of it is specific to General American English (GAE). We focus on GAE because it is the most neutral dialect with respect to accents in the United States, and we believe it is a good starting point for learning about other dialects such as Spanish-influenced English, African American vernacular, and others (e.g., Craig, Thompson, Washington, & Potter, 2003; Goldstein & Iglesias, 2004). Finally, in our discussion of articulatory phonetics, we refer readers to the Web site sponsored collaboratively by the Departments of Spanish, Portuguese, German, Speech Pathology and Audiology, and Academic Technologies at the University of Iowa: http://www.uiowa.edu/~acadtech/phonetics/#. This site contains an interactive diagram of articulatory anatomy and offers animated libraries of the phonetic sounds of English, German, and Spanish. For each consonant and vowel in each language, there is an animated articulatory diagram, a step-by-step description, and a video-audio illustration of the sound spoken in context. We encourage readers to take advantage of this Web site and to observe the features of speech sound production summarized below. For readers who wish to explore the topic of speech production in greater depth, we also recommended the following excellent sources: Bauman-Waenger (2004), Bernthal and Bankson (2004), Bleile (1995), Peña-Brooks and Hegde (2000), and Stoel-Gammon and Dunn (1985).

Speech Sounds

In all languages, speech production involves the coordinated actions of respiration, voicing, and articulation. Respiration provides the exhaled air that is used for speech production. The larynx houses vocal folds that vibrate to create voicing. The articulators (cheeks, lips, teeth, palate, tongue, and jaw) are moved to shape the vocal tract in characteristic ways to produce specific sounds.

The phonological systems of all languages include both vowels and consonants. **Vowels** generally function as the nucleus of a syllable. They are produced with vocal fold vibration and with a relatively unobstructed vocal tract configuration. For example, the production of /a/ (as in *ah*) involves voicing with an open mouth position whereas /o/ (as in *oh*) involves voicing with lip-protrusion and rounding. **Consonants**, on the other hand, are produced with greater constriction of the vocal tract. For example, the production of /m/ requires complete lip closure with voicing as the sound is directed through the nasal passages. In Chapter 3, Table 3–1 summarizes the inventory of vowels and consonants in GAE. Each sound is represented by a symbol from the International Phonetic Alphabet (IPA) and accompanied by a key word that places the sound in the context of a familiar word. Additional information pertaining to consonants and vowels is provided below.

Vowels. There are two types of vowels: pure vowels and diphthongs. Both types are produced by voicing and positioning the vocal tract in a posture allowing for the relatively unobstructed flow of air. Individual **pure vowels** are shaped by moving the tongue, jaw, lips, and cheeks into characteristic posi-

tions and by the degree of muscle tension required to achieve a particular position. Tongue position can vary from high to low. For example, during the production of [i] (as in *eat*) the tongue is relatively high up and close to the palate whereas during the production of [a] (as in *hot*) the jaw is lowered, allowing the tongue to rest on the floor of the mouth at a distance from the palate. Tongue position also can vary from front to back. For example, during the production of [i], the blade of the tongue is tensed in a more forward position below the hard palate whereas during the production of [u] (as in *two*) the back of the tongue is tensed beneath the soft palate. Lips may be rounded as in the production of [o] (e.g., *go*) or retracted as in the production of /i/. The degree of tension required to assume a posture may vary from tense (e.g., /i/, /u/, /a/) to lax as in /ə/ [in *wagon*]). Individual vowels typically are classified with respect to all three dimensions. For example, /o/ is classified as a tense, rounded, high-front vowel whereas schwa ([ə]) is classified as a lax, unrounded, mid-central vowel.

Diphthongs. Diphthongs are similar to pure vowels in that they can serve as a syllable nucleus. Also, like pure vowels, they are produced with voicing and with a relatively unobstructed vocal tract. However, unlike pure vowels, the articulatory posture shifts during the production of a diphthong, thereby creating the perception of two vowels in sequence. For example, the diphthong /aɪ/ is heard in the word *eye*. Other diphthongs can be heard in the spoken words *owl*, *boy*, *d*ay, and *sew*.

Consonants. Consonants can be cross-classified in relation to three features: voicing, place of articulation, and manner of articulation. **Voicing** is defined as the production of vocal fold vibration. Examples of voiced consonants include [m], [d], and [z]. If you position the palm of your hand on the front of your neck while producing [m], [d], or [z], you will feel the vibrations of your vocal folds while you hear them. Other consonants are produced without voicing. Examples include [p], [t], and [k].

Place of Articulation refers to the parts of the vocal tract that are constricted during the production of a sound. For example, [m], [b], [p], and [w] all involve the upper and lower lips. For this reason they are known as **bilabial** consonants. Other places of articulation are characterized as **labio-dental** (lips and teeth together, as in [f] and [v]); **interdental** (tongue between the teeth, as in [θ] and [ð]); **alveolar** (tongue and alveolar ridge, as in [d] and [t]); **palatal** (tongue moves towards palate, as in [r] and [j]); **velar** (tongue touches velum, as in [k] and [g]); and **glottal** (constriction of the space between the vocal folds, as in [h]).

Manner of Articulation refers to the way in which articulators come together. Six different manners are used in the articulation in GAE, including stops, fricatives, affricates, nasals, liquids, and glides. **Stops** are produced by completely disrupting the airflow for a period of time, as in [p], [t], and [k]. **Fricatives** require the speaker to bring articulators within close proximity but without complete closure. Examples include [f], [v], [s], [z], [θ], [ð] and [h]. **Affricates** have characteristics in common with stops and fricatives. There is brief, initial closure followed by close approximation, as in [tʃ], the initial sound in *chip*. To produce a **nasal** sound, speakers must close their oral cavity and direct the airstream through the nose. This is characteristic of [m], [n], and [ŋ]. **Liquids** ([r] and [l]) are produced by holding the tongue in characteristic positions near the palate. **Glides** ([w] and [j]) resemble vowels in that they require relatively less proximity to their points of articulation. For this reason, they are sometimes known as **semivowels**.

Phones, Phonemes, and Allophones. A **phone** is a single sound that can be produced by the vocal tract (Peña-Brooks & Hegde, 2000). For example, the isolated production of [p] represents the production of a phone. In contrast, a **phoneme** is a sound used to create meaning. This is illustrated by **minimal pairs** (i.e., words that differ by only one phoneme). For example, we recognize that that *pat* and *bat* have completely different meanings, based on a single feature (voicing) that differentiates the phonemes /p/ and /b/. On the other hand, **allophones** are different members of a phoneme category. For example, [p] can be produced with aspiration (as in the word *pin*) or without aspiration (as is normally the case in the word *cup*). However, if we produce *cup* with an aspirated /p/, the word's meaning will still remain the same.

Syllable Structures and Shapes. A syllable is defined by a vowel (V) nucleus and its surrounding consonants (C). There are two basic **syllable structures**. One is known as an **open syllable** because it ends with a vowel (e.g., *see, toy, I*). The other is known as a **closed syllable** because it ends with one or more consonants (e.g., *cup, juice, drink*). Within these basic structures, specific **syllable shapes** will differ depending on the number of consonants that precede and/or follow the vowel nucleus. GAE includes 36 different syllable shapes ranging from a single vowel (V) (e.g., *oh, I*) to the placement of consonant clusters on each side of a vowel. Examples at the low end of complexity include consonant-vowel (CV) syllables (e.g., *bee, hi*), reduplicated syllables (CVCV) involving the same consonant and the same vowel (e.g., *baby, mama, papa*), VC syllables (*up, on*), and CVC syllables (e.g., *pop, ball*). At the high end of complexity there are shapes such as CCCVCCC (e.g., *sprints*) and CCCVCCCC (e.g., *strengths*).

Coarticulation. As you can see, the phonetic repertoire is complex. The production of individual sounds involves many exquisite adjustments of the oral mechanism. Additionally, variations in these adjustments are required to accommodate surrounding phonemes. Notice the difference in the movement of your tongue when you produce /r/ in the word *ring* and in the word *green*. When all of these issues are considered it is not surprising that children find ways to simplify the system during the early acquisition process.

Developmental Patterns

As discussed in Chapter 3, prelinguistic infants are sensitive to a complex array of speech sounds and speech sound patterns. This has been demonstrated by a wide range of studies on infant speech perception (e.g., Kuhl, 2004). However, sensitivity to sound patterns is not the same as sensitivity to meanings represented by sound patterns. In other word, speech sound perception does not automatically imply phonemic perception. The two skills involve different levels of processing.

Speech Perception During Early Word Learning

Toward the second half of the prelinguistic period, infants pay more attention to the sounds within their own language communities. There also is evidence that they associate specific syllables with their referents (e.g., *mama*) and that the number of these associations increases as infants move toward the transition to spoken language. However, it is not clear whether infants perceive words holistically as a single unit or whether they recognize the phonetic details within each word. In a sense, this is analogous to the difference between sight reading and phonetic decoding. So, when an infant consistently orients to his or her mother after hearing "mama," we do not know whether the infant processes the word as a single acoustic shape or whether he or she perceives the phonetic details ([mamə]) within the sound segment.

An interesting paradox about language development is that the very building blocks that allow children to move from one level of information processing to the next sometimes become challenging at the next higher level. Perhaps the demands of early word learning do not leave early word learners with enough processing space to notice all of the phonetic detail of novel words. This type of explanation was suggested by Werker, Fennel, Corcoran, and Stager's (2002) research on early word learning. Using a habituation paradigm, they compared 14-, 17-, and 20-month-olds on their ability to discriminate between two similar sounding words (i.e., *dih* and *pih*) when systematically paired with two very different objects. All of the children discriminated between the words in the habituation phase of the experiments. However, during the test phase, when the pairing of words with objects was sometimes switched, only the 20-month-olds and some of the 17-month-olds noticed the switch. Based on the results of this study, these researchers concluded that, at the earliest stage of word learning, children appear to process words as whole units rather than paying attention to phonetic details.

Speech Production During Early Lexical Learning

During the canonical and jargon stages of babbling, infants simply are playing with the raw phonetic materials of their language. Their patterns of reduplicated babbling and jargon suggest that they perceive these raw materials at the syllable level and that their productions increasingly resemble the syllable structure of their language community, albeit in the absence of referential meaning.

Children typically produce their first word by about 12 months and their first 50 words by about 18 to 20 months. Within this span of time, their repertoire of sounds and syllable structures resembles the repertoire of sounds and syllable structures used during the later stages of babbling (Leonard, Newhoff, & Meselam, 1980; Stoel-Gammon, 1998; Stoel-Gammon & Cooper, 1984). The term **phonetic inventory** often is used to refer to the variety of sounds produced in words, regardless of whether those sounds match the conventional forms to which they refer. Within the first 50 words, such inventories typically include stops (/p,b,t,d,k,g/), nasals (/m,n,ŋ/), and glides (/w,j/). Typically, they do not include sounds that occur infrequently in the language (e.g., /v/) or sounds that require higher degrees of articulatory precision such as /ʃ/ (e.g., *ship*), /tʃ/ (*chip*), /dʒ/ (e.g., *juice*), /θ/ (e.g., *thumb*), /ð/ (e.g., *this*), and /r/ (e.g., *red*). The most frequent syllable shapes include consonant-vowel (CV) as in *go*, CVC (e.g., *pop*), and CVCV (e.g., *mama*). These patterns are consistent cross-linguistically. However, because 90% of the multisyllabic words in GAE follow a trochaic pattern (i.e., stress on the first syllable), infants exposed to GAE tend to adopt a trochaic stress pattern in their early vocabularies. Different developmental patterns are observed in other languages (e.g., French) that follow an iambic pattern (stress on the second syllable).

Phonological Development After the First 50 Words

One way to track improvements in phonological ability is to track changes in overall **intelligibility**. Intelligibility is estimated by noting the percentage of a speaker's utterances that a listener can recognize, even if the speaker's articulation is not completely accurate. For example, a child who says *wed wabbit* may be understood to mean *red rabbit* even though the form of his or her utterance is unconventional. Intelligibility estimates typically are based on the judgment of an unfamiliar listener. Using this strategy, Coplan and Gleason (1988) estimated 50%, 75%, and 100% intelligibility rates at 24, 36, and 48 months, respectively.

Although there are considerable individual variations between children with respect to the trajectory of specific phonological accomplishments, the steady increase of intelligibility represents a common ground. Children who do not meet these milestones should be referred for a speech-language evaluation.

The fact that intelligibility ratings increase even before the phonological system is mastered suggests that developmental production errors are relatively easy for listeners to decode. Indeed, when children's productions are compared to conventional forms, we typically find that the difference between the children's forms and the conventional forms reflect systematic phonological simplification processes (Stampe, 1969). Some of these processes affect the syllable structure of whole words; others affect smaller speech segments. Table 4–2 provides exam-

ples based on Vihman (2004). In consideration of these examples, note that the segment change processes apply to all of the phonemes within a class rather than to isolated phonetic forms. For example, stopping of fricatives generally applies to all fricatives, not just to /s/. Second, the list of examples is incomplete. For a more complete listing of processes, please see Bleile (1995). Third, there is considerable individual variation in the specific processes used by children. Some children may use many processes and others may use only a few. Fourth, children demonstrate varying degrees of intraword variability (Stoel-Gammon, 2007). They may pronounce the same word differently at the same point in developmental time. Specific productions may be influenced by the production demands of the utterance as a whole. Fifth, the use of simplification processes does not imply the inability to produce a particular phoneme. For example, the same child who says *poon* when referring to a spoon may produce /s/ correctly when saying *soap*. That is because the production of *poon* was based on a

TABLE 4–2. Systematic Phonological Simplification Processes

Examples of Whole Word Processes	Simplification	Target Word
Unstressed syllable deletion (the unstressed syllable is deleted from a word)	/nænə/	*banana*
Final consonant deletion(the final consonant is deleted from the final syllable)	/kʌ/	*cup*
Reduplication (two or more syllables are produced based on the sound of one or more syllables in the target word)	/bʌbʌ/	*bottle*
Consonant cluster simplification (a sequence of two or more consonants is reduced to one)	/pun/	*spoon*
Examples of Segment Change Processes		
Velar fronting (a velar consonant is replaced by an alveolar or interdental consonant)	/tɪdɪ/	*kitty*
Stopping (a fricative is replaced by a stop)	/dop/	*soap*
Gliding (replacing a liquid (/r,l/) with a glide (/w,j/)	/jʌv/	*love*
Assimilation (changing one segment of a word to resemble another)	/gɔgɪ/	*doggy*
Voicing alteration (a voiceless sound becomes voiced or a voiced sound becomes devoiced)	/gʌʊ/	*cow*

constraint against consonant clusters and not on limitations in the articulatory movements needed to produce /s/. Finally, notice that children sometimes use more than one phonological process at a time. For example, a child who says /dʌ/ to mean "cup" is using velar fronting (velar /k/ → alveolar /d/), voicing alterations (voiceless /k/ → voiced /d/), and final consonant deletion (CVC → CV). Note that the more processes involved in the production of a given word, the greater the impact on the word's intelligibility.

The use and suppression of specific phonological processes by children between 24 months and 5 years has been studied by a number of researchers. Bankson and Bernthal (2004) summarized some of these data based on observations of children between 2;0 (years; months) and 6;0. Their summary indicates that some processes (reduplication; stopping of fricatives /f/, /s/, and /tʃ/; and voicing alterations) begin to fade from use by children between 24 to 30 months. Most others seem to fade by 30 to 42 months. Similarly, Vihman (2004) observed that whole-word processes typically are the first to be suppressed and segmental change processes follow shortly thereafter. Readers who are interested in a more in-depth summary of the phonological, articulatory, and oral motor skills demonstrated by children between birth and 6 years should see McLeod and Bleile (2003).

The question yet to be answered is how children's use of simplification processes relates to their underlying representations of words. Do children's underlying representations lack the details of the adult phonological system? Alternatively, are children's underlying representations similar to those of adults but become simplified in the output? Or do both of these explanations pertain to different aspects of children's phonological repertoires? There are some reasons to believe that children's representations are more detailed than their productions. One is based on the **"fis" phenomenon**, which refers to children's rejection of simplified productions that are consistent with their own production patterns (Berko & Brown, 1960; Hoff, 2005). For example, I remember a 3-year-old named Amanda who used a number of phonological simplification processes including cluster reduction. One day when she asked me for a "poon," I replied, "I don't have a

poon." She then raised her voice and clarified her request by saying, "Not a <u>poon</u>, I need a <u>poon</u>!" Yet, there are children who seem blissfully unaware of a difference between their own production and a model. Further research is needed to sort this out. What we do know is that children's productive phonological rules becomes increasingly more conventional with opportunities to hear good speech models, with experience in speech production, and with attention to their own internal feedback (Menn & Stoel-Gammon, 2005).

It is important to note that there is much **individual variation** with respect to the specific trajectory of phonological growth, including the use of phonological simplification processes. Menn and Stoel-Gammon (2005) suggest that general statements about the order of acquisition of particular segments can be made only in probabilistic terms. Some children initially show preferences for certain sounds and avoid words that don't contain those sounds (e.g., Stoel-Gammon & Cooper, 1984). Others appear to begin by developing small sets of words with similar features (canonical forms) and reconfigure other words to fit those features (e.g., Waterson. 1971). Most children seem to progress according to their own system of phonological rules even though a few of their productions may not fit those rules. **Phonological idioms** illustrate this point. These are words that are produced accurately even though they require the use of phonological patterns that are simplified by the child in other contexts. For example, if a child produces the word *pretty* accurately while reducing clusters during the production of other words, then the word *pretty* would be considered a phonological idiom. This very example was documented in an extensive diary study by Leopold (1939-1949). One explanation for it is that phonological idioms represent memorized forms that are acquired before a child begins to process speech as a rule-based system. This explanation applies to developmental patterns in other areas of language as well. For example, in the acquisition of irregular past tense verbs, children begin by using memorized forms (e.g., *went*). However, when they learn the rule for regular past tense *-ed*, they begin to apply it to most irregular forms as well (e.g., *wented*). Still, there may be irregular forms that continue to be used correctly, even though the child is over-generalizing the regular past-tense rule.

As a final consideration, researchers have found an important relationship between phonological development and the size of a child's expressive vocabulary. Specifically, it appears that same-age children with larger productive vocabularies tend to have more conventional phonetic inventories and syllable structures (Stoel-Gammon, 1998). In other words, although toddlers initially may limit their acquisition of words to those that include preferred sounds, at some later point the motivation to learn new words seems to override this constraint and motivate the development of more conventional phonological skills (Stoel-Gammon, 2007).

Traditional Measures

To this point, our focus has been on children's development of rule-based phonological skills that pertain to categories of phonemes and syllables. Traditionally, development of the phonological repertoire was measured by observing children's productions of individual phonemes during highly structured speaking tasks. Specifically, children named pictured items that were preselected to evoke the production of each individual phoneme in the initial, medial, and final positions of single words. The results of two such studies summarized by Sander (1972) showed a developmental sequence representing the **ages of customary production** (i.e., when 50% of the observed children produced the sound correctly in at least two word positions) and a sequence of representing the **ages of mastery** (when 90% of the observed children produced the sound conventionally in all three word positions) with considerable variability across phonemes and between children in the times at which phoneme production became stable during a structured speaking task. A summary of the patterns for each phoneme follows.

Phoneme	[1]ACP	[2]AOM
/p/	1;0	3;0
/m/	1;0	3;0
/h/	1;0	3;0
/n/	1;0	3;0
/w/	1;0	3;0
/b/	1;0	3;0
/k/	2;0	4;0
/g/	2;0	4;0
/d/	2;0	4;0
/t/	2;0	6;0
/ŋ/	2;0	6;0
/f/	3;0	4;0
/j/	3;0	4;0
/r/	3;6	6;0
/l/	3;6	6;0
/s/	3;6	8;0
/tʃ/	4;0	7;0
/ʃ/	4;0	7;0
/z/	4;0	8;0
/dʒ/	4;6	7;0
/v/	4;6	8;0
/θ/	5;0	7;0
/ð/	5;6	8;0
/ʒ/	6;6	>8;0

[1]ACP = age of customary production represented in years;months (based on Sanders, 1972). [2]AOM = age of mastery represented in years;months (based on Sanders, 1972).

Note that this information is limited in certain ways. First, because the data are based on structured productions of single words, they do not reflect children's productions during spontaneous speech, which involves more complex processing demands. Second, because each phoneme was tested in only three word positions, the data do not reflect coarticulation effects (i.e., the extent to which a sound's production varies, depending on the sounds that precede and follow it). So, although these data provide a good snapshot of information about children's productions of individual phonemes, they do not represent the dynamics of children's phonological systems.

Phonological Awareness

Phonological awareness refers to a conscious understanding of the phonological structure of language. It involves the ability to use language to talk about speech as a topic of conversation. It requires a person to look beyond the referential meanings of language to the structure of the sound system itself. It accounts for the correct answer to the question requiring children to make judgments about words (e.g., Which word is longer, *automobile* or *train*?). Children under the age of 4 years have difficulty with this. Phonological awareness emerges gradually during the early language period. We see this, for example, in children's enjoyment of many Dr. Seuss books that emphasize this aspect of language (e.g., *There's a Wocket in my Pocket*). We hear it in presleep monologues of some children, who play with rhyming words (e.g., Weir, 1962), and we understand it as the basis of some children's enjoyment in learning artificial languages like Pig Latin, which involve awareness and manipulation of syllables within words (e.g., Cowan, 1989). Phonological awareness is an important basis for the development of reading, which is discussed in the next chapter.

Theoretical Frameworks

Four theories of phonological development were described by Stoel-Gammon (2007). The first is **prosodic theory** (Waterson, 1971), which proposes that children's underlying phonological representations are different from those of adults. They are determined by features of language input and by children's developing perceptual abilities. Initially, prosodic features (stress, intonation, melodic contour) provide an acoustic framework for segmental patterns, allowing children to develop a number of schemas or categories of word types (canonical forms) to use as templates for their own productions. An example from Waterson's data includes one child's development of a "sibilant" schema based on words like *fish, fetch, brush*, and *dish*. Children typically develop several schemas, each based on a different set of features, and each being shaped by a combination of the child's perceptual system, output abilities, and salient features of the language

input. With increasing exposure to language input, maturation of perceptual skills, and internal production feedback, early schemas gradually expand, become integrated, and approximate conventional representations.

Cognitive theory is associated with the work of Ferguson and Farwell (1975). In their view, children participate actively in the development of their phonological systems. They choose words based on their own communicative needs, articulatory abilities, and perceptual preferences. They formulate hypotheses about phonological forms and test them through production and feedback mechanisms. Their hypotheses may be based on phonological features or on individual word shapes. This accounts for individual variability as well as exceptions to rule-based patterns. Developmental changes are thought to be motivated by children's desire to approximate the adult model.

Biological theories emphasize the fundamental role of anatomic and motor development in the acquisition of phonological skills (Kent, 1992). Development is seen as ". . . a process in which the child progressively applies available resources in attempting to emulate the mature behavior" (Kent, 1992, p. 85). Similar to prosodic theory and cognitive theory, biological theories stand in contrast to earlier theories, which proposed that children simplify fully comprehended versions of the adult system. In biological theories, early words are assumed to be holistic "motor scores" that become more reliable as coordination improves. Phonemic organization emerges through "global mapping between sensory and motor routines" (Stoel-Gammon, 2007, p. 251).

Usage-based phonology (Kemmer & Barlow, 2000) emphasizes the role of language (input and use) in shaping children's production and in modifying their phonological systems. Phonology is seen as part of the overall development of language in context, and not as a system that is developmentally independent of the other language components. Two issues associated with usage-based phonological theory are: (1) the frequency of particular forms in the child's language input, and (2) neighborhood density of individual words (i.e., the phonological relationships between words in an individual's lexicon). It is assumed that the frequency of production will enhance the growth of the phonological skills required. It is also assumed that words in dense neighborhoods (e.g., *bat, mat, pit, pet, past, spat, at*) may need more detailed phonological representations than words whose phonological structures are more different from others. There is some evidence to support both assumptions.

The **behaviorist model** is not included in Stoel-Gammon's (2007) review of developmental theories. We include it here because behavioral procedures (e.g., modeling, imitation, differential reinforcement) are routinely included in successful treatment programs for children with atypical phonological development. In a nutshell, behavioral models propose that patterns of babbling and speech are developed through exposure to models and differential reinforcement of successive approximations to the target language (Mowrer, 1960; Skinner, 1957). Support for this position comes, in part, from various studies which confirm that a responsive vocal environment supports the development of speech and language (e.g., Goldstein, King, & West, 2003; Hart & Risley, 1995; Vellman, Mangipudi, & Locke, 1989). However, opponents of this model point out that some sounds are acquired later than others, even though they would be reinforced with equal consistency. Second, caregivers do not selectively reinforce every speech sound. Third, and perhaps most importantly, the development of phonology is seen, from a psycholinguistic perspective, as the development of an abstract rule-based system. However, because traditional behavioral models address only the development of observable behavior, they cannot account for the acquisition of abstract linguistic rules. In consideration of these issues, Hoff (2005) concludes that "the problem with behaviorism is not that it is wrong but that it is insufficient" (Hoff, 2005, p. 131). See Cerutti (1989) for an explanation of how rule-governed behavior is handled by behavioral models. Further research is needed.

Summary of Early Phonological Development

In this section, we described articulatory phonetics, milestones in phonological development, and theories about how this process evolves. We hope that these perspectives enhanced your understanding of children's typical phonological performance and that considerations of these dimensions will be helpful as you reflect on the performance of children in your care.

PRIMARY ACCOMPLISHMENTS: MORPHOLOGY AND SYNTAX

We now consider the development of grammar. Recall that language has form (phonology, morphology, syntax), content (semantics), and function (pragmatics). **Grammar** refers to two aspects of its form: syntax and morphology. The rules of **syntax** determine the order of words in a sentence. For example, English typically uses a subject-verb-object (SVO) word order. The rules of **morphology** specify changes in the forms of words depending on their syntactic or semantic functions. For example, the word *talk* will be changed to *talking* or *talked*, depending on whether we want to comment on an ongoing action (e.g., *John is talking*) or an action that has ended (*John talked*). Altogether, these are the kinds of rules that children learn in the course of grammatical development. Following a short summary of theoretical frameworks for the development of grammar, we describe five stages of grammatical development.

Theoretical Frameworks

About 90% of grammatical rules are acquired by children between the ages of 18 and 48 months without much specific instruction at a time when they are not even able to tie their own shoes. Most adults learning a second language don't do nearly as well. Clearly, neurological factors and some kind of a bootstrapping process are in play, but researchers disagree on just what these factors are and how they interact. Some think that infants are born with domain-specific learning capabilities (e.g., A. N. Chomsky, 1984). Others assume that semantic knowledge or pragmatic abilities are key to cracking the code (Pinker, 1984; Tomasello, 2002). Still others consider behavioral principles to be at work (e.g., Hegde, 1980, in press; McLaughlin & Cullinan, 1981; Moerk, 1992; Skinner, 1974). All agree that neurology, language input, and social interaction play a role in the process.

MLU and Stages of Grammatical Development

Grammatical skills obviously become more complex as children mature. Yet, like every other aspect of development, children learn grammatical skills at different rates. In fact, the **mean length of utterance** (MLU) is a better predictor of grammatical complexity than age (Brown, 1973), and it is frequently used by researchers, speech-language pathologists, and educators as a gross estimate of syntactic growth.

MLU is measured by counting morphemes rather than words. **Morphemes** are the smallest units of meaning in a language. They may appear as single words (e.g., *jump*) or in the form of affixes such as prefixes and suffixes that are added to root words. For example, the word *jumping* contains two morphemes: *jump* and *-ing*. Table 4–3 lists the specific rules described by Brown (1973) for counting morphemes in young children's utterances.

The calculation of MLU is done according to procedures defined by Brown (1973). The first step is to record and transcribe a sample of spontaneous

TABLE 4–3. Brown's (1973) Rules for Counting Morphemes

Count as 1 morpheme	Count as 2 morphemes
• Object labels (e.g., "house" counts as 1)	• Possessive nouns (e.g., "Daddy's counts as 2)
• Dysfluencies (1 point for the full word) (e.g., "c-c-c-candy" = 1)	• Plural nouns (e.g., crayons counts as 2)
• Reoccurrence of a word for emphasis (1 point for each word) (e.g., "big, big house" = 3)	• 3rd person singular of present tense verbs (e.g., "jumps" counts as 2)
• Compound words (e.g., "birthday" = 1)	• Regular past tense verbs (e.g., "jumped" counts as 2)
• Proper names (e.g., "Big Bird" = 1)	• Present progressive verbs (e.g., "jumping" counts as 2)
• Ritualized reduplications (e.g., "night-night" = 1)	• Negative contractions (if parts of contraction are used independently in the transcript) (e.g., "isn't" = 2)
• Irregular past tense vs (e.g., "ate" = 1)	**Count as 0 morphemes**
• Diminutives (e.g., "doggie" = 1)	• Fillers (e.g., "um," "ah," "uh")
• Auxiliary Verbs (e.g., "is," "have," "do" each count as 1)	• As indicated in the first column, the dysfluent parts of utterances receive a count of zero. Only the final word is counted.
• Catenatives (e.g., "gonna," "hafta," "wanna" each count as 1)	
• Indefinite pronouns (e.g., "anybody," "somebody" each count as 1)	

Source: Based on R. Brown (1973). *A first language: The early stages.* Cambridge, MA: Harvard University Press, p. 54.

language produced by a child during interactive play with a nondirective conversational partner and a set of developmentally-appropriate toys. Next, the utterances are segmented and numbered. Then, each utterance is analyzed for length in morphemes according to Brown's rules. Here is an example of how these rules would be applied:

Utterances	# Morphemes
1 Mommy is play-ing	4
2 Oscar is tickl-ing Elmo	5
3 Today is my birthday	4
4 We went to the store	5
5 No, no, no, no, don't do it.	8
Total # Morphemes	**26**

After the morphemes in each utterance are counted, they are added to determine the total number of morphemes in the language sample. This result is divided by the total number of utterances to arrive at the MLU value. For example, if the total number of morphemes found in a language sample of 100 utterances is 250, then the MLU value would be 250 divided by 100 or 2.5 morphemes.

Similar to Jean Piaget's investigations of children's cognitive development, Roger Brown (1973) studied language development through in-depth, longitudinal observations of three children (Adam, Eve, and Sarah) during their transition from single-word utterances to grammatical speech. He frequently measured each child's MLU, and compared MLU values with the kinds of syntactic patterns that the children were using. Based on these procedures, he found that MLU increased dramatically once the children began to combine words. However, there were differences between the children in the ages at which word combinations first emerged. For Eve, this occurred at 18 months, but for Adam and Sarah, it began at 26 months. Therefore, MLU was a better index of grammatical complexity than chronologic age.

The grammatical achievements associated with different MLU values were characterized by Brown (1973) in relation to five developmental stages. Table 4-4 summarizes each stage with respect to MLU values, approximate ages, and emerging grammatical skills. The table shows that the entry into syntax begins with children's production of telegraphic speech. These utterances enable children to comment on semantic relationships that extend beyond the lexical meanings of words. Next, they develop grammatical morphemes that code semantic relationships into linguistic structures. Later, children begin to produce complete sentences for making statements (declarative) asking questions (interrogative), disagreeing, negating, or rejecting ideas (negative), and issuing commands (imperative). Once basic sentences are established, children begin to embed phrases and clauses within them, thus creating complex sentences. As a final step, they learn to connect sentences with conjunctions, thereby

TABLE 4–4. Stages of Grammatical Development Based on MLU Measured in Morphemes

[1]Stage	[1]MLU	[2]Approximate Age in Mos.	[1]Emerging Forms
I	1.00–1.99	19.1 to 26.9	Formulating semantic relations—telegraphic speech
II	2.00–2.50	27.7 to 30.8	Modulating meanings—grammatical morphemes
III	2.50–3.00	31.6 to 34.8	Formulating basic sentence modalities
IV	3.00–3.75	35.6 to 39.5	Embedding phrases and clauses
V	3.75–4.50	40.3 to 46.6	Conjoining clauses

[1]Stages, MLU values, and emerging forms are based on R. Brown (1973). *A first language: The early stages.* Cambridge, MA: Harvard University Press, pp. 54–59.

[2]Age ranges correlated with MLU values are based on J. Miller (1981). *Assessing language production in children.* Baltimore, MD: University Park Press, p. 26.

creating compound sentences, including some that embed phrases and clauses. Estimates of the age ranges correlated with MLU values are based on a study by Miller and Chapman (in Miller, 1981) involving 123 children from Madison, Wisconsin. Note the individual variation between children with respect to patterns of growth, and the overlap that exists between the stages.

After children have learned to embed clauses into compound sentences, MLU ceases to be a useful measure of grammatical complexity. That is because sentences can be lengthened by conjoining clauses without necessarily adding any new grammatical features. We now consider some of the developmental products associated with these stages.

Development at Brown's Stage I

Comprehension of Word Order

What patterns would infants need to notice in order to crack the syntactic code? Recall that English syntax generally follows an SVO (subject-verb-object) word order. Knowledge of this pattern helps us to recognize the semantic functions or roles of the words in an utterance. Consider two sentences:

Big Bird is tickling Cookie Monster.

Cookie Monster is tickling Big Bird.

Each sentence contains exactly the same words, but we recognize different meanings because of the word order. In the first sentence, we recognize Big Bird as the **agent** of the action "tickle" and in the second sentence we recognize Cookie Monster as the agent. In the first sentence Cookie Monster is the **object** acted upon, but in the second sentence Big Bird is the object. Agent and object are semantic roles marked in English by word order.

Considering the importance of word order, a number of researchers have studied children to find out just when they become sensitive to the semantic roles marked in this way. The earliest studies utilized naturalistic procedures by asking toddlers to manipulate toys according to verbal instructions (e.g., Chapman & Miller, 1975; deVilliers & deVilliers,

1973; Wetstone & Friedlander, 1973). Sometimes the verbal instructions referred to likely actions (e.g., *Make the boy push the boat*) and sometimes they referred to less likely actions (e.g., *Make the boat push the shoe*). Instructions for the less likely actions were necessary to rule out the possibility that children would use their world knowledge (rather than their knowledge of language structure) to interpret the semantic roles of words. By using these methods, the researchers found that children begin to combine words in their own speech before they can make sense of word order receptively.

More recently, studies utilizing innovative observational techniques have offered surprising new insights into children's word-order comprehension. In a sequence of two studies utilizing the Intermodal Preferential Looking Paradigm (IPLP), Hirsh-Pasek and Golinkoff (1996) demonstrated that toddlers at the single-word stage, including some with as few as three words in their expressive vocabularies, make use of word order to identify the agents and objects in the utterances they hear. Forty-eight toddlers from 16 to 19 months of age participated in both studies. The average number of words in their expressive vocabularies was 67.6 with a wide range of from 2 to 255. More than half the children did not produce any two-word combinations; 9 were just beginning to combine words; and 13 used word combinations regularly.

In the first study, children were presented with two video screens at equal distances from them. Each screen illustrated an interaction between Big Bird (BB) and the Cookie Monster (CM). Sometimes BB was the agent of an action (tickling, feeding, washing, hugging), and sometimes CM served in that role. With each simultaneous presentation of two video segments, the toddlers heard verbal instructions coming from a speaker located midway between the two video screens. The instructions were stated in a consistent manner during each trial. For example: *Look, Cookie Monster is tickling Big Bird. Where is Cookie Monster tickling Big Bird?* In this case, one video segment showed BB tickling CM and the other showed CM tickling BB. As soon as the toddlers heard an instruction, the researchers recorded the length of time that the toddlers spent looking at each of the two video segments. If toddlers systematically spent more time looking at the video segments corresponding to the verbal instructions they heard, it was assumed that they understood the semantic roles of the words in the utterance. This is exactly what happened. Furthermore, toddlers who produced only single words in their spontaneous speech showed the same preferences as toddlers who were already using word combinations.

The second study was conducted with the same toddlers also using the IPLP procedure. The toddlers were shown the same sets of video segments and provided with the same opening statement (e.g., *Look! Big Bird is tickling Cookie Monster*.) However, this time the follow-up question was shortened. For example, instead of being asked, *Where is Big Bird Tickling Cookie Monster?* children were simply asked *Where is Big Bird?*

The purpose of the second study was to determine whether the results of the first study occurred simply because the toddlers paid attention to the first character named rather than processing the entire question. If they only paid attention to the first character named, then the results for the second study should be the same as the results for the first. However, if toddlers are truly sensitive to word order information, then the shorter question (e.g., *"Where's Big Bird?"*) should result in roughly equal amounts of time spent looking at each screen. As expected, no preferential looking was observed. Therefore, the alternate explanation for the children's performance during the first study could be ruled out, thereby confirming the interpretation that infants comprehend word order information even before they are able to combine words in their expressive language.

Relational Use of Single Words

Do children use their knowledge of semantic roles in their single-word utterances? L. Bloom and Lahey (1978) observed that toddlers often use single words to acknowledge their attention to a particular referent (e.g., saying *ball* while looking at a ball). However, they also use single words to comment on relationships between objects. For example, when asked, *"Where's the ball?"* a child may point to a chair and say *"chair"* to indicate a location relationship between the ball and the chair. Similarly, a

child may point to an empty chair and say *"Daddy,"* to mean that this is Daddy's chair (a possessor-possession relationship). These comments about the relationships between objects indicate that knowledge of semantic roles influences children's use of words even at the single-word level. Furthermore, when caregivers hear toddlers making these comments, they often expand their utterance within a conversational framework as in the following example:

Adult: *Where's your ball?*

Child: *Chair* (pointing to a location under the chair)

Adult: *Oh, it's under the chair*.

As a by-product of such communicative exchanges, children have the opportunity to notice how their relational meanings are expressed in the adult language system.

Two-Word Combinations

Armed with the ability to interpret word order and with the emerging ability to comment on semantic roles, children typically begin to produce connected utterances when their vocabulary has increased to about 50 words. The average age of children at this time is about 18 months, with a range from 15 to 24 months (Bates, Dale, & Thal, 1995). Just as Brown (1973) discovered through his observations of Adam, Eve, and Sarah, there is wide variability among children.

For some children, the earliest of these utterance types includes two-word combinations that comment on different manifestations of a single object, such as existence (e.g., *"there kitty"*), non-existence (e.g., *"no cookie"*), disappearance (*"allgone bubble"*), or recurrence (*"more bubble"*) (Bloom, 1973). Because these utterances refer to relationships of an object to itself, they are classified as **reflexive object relations**. That toddlers frequently comment on different states of an object during the second year of life is not surprising, as this is the time when their concept of object permanence is being fully developed.

Shortly after the emergence of reflexive object relations (and sometimes at the same time), children begin to comment on relationships between agents, actions, and other referents. These are called **semantic relations**. Table 4–5 provides examples of some common semantic relations expressed with two-word utterances (Brown, 1973). These same relationships are expressed by children learning a variety of different languages (Tager-Flusberg, 2005).

As with reflexive object relations, semantic relations are vehicles for commenting about objects, what they do, what is being done to them, where they are located, who has them, and what qualities they have. However, what is so remarkable about the emergence of two-word combinations is that they show that children are separating the lexical meaning of a word from its semantic role. For example, in the utterance *Doggy bark*, the lexical meaning of *doggy* is now paired with a higher-level semantic role (agent). Furthermore, when caregivers interact with their children, they often respond to these utterances by expanding them (just as they did with the single-word utterances):

Child: *Doggy bark*

Adult: *Yes, he's barking*

Again, these interactions provide children with opportunities to hear how their own meanings are expressed in more advanced grammatical forms. Note, however, that most researchers interpret these exchanges as conversational. For example, based on an analysis of language addressed to Adam, Eve, and Sarah, Brown and Hanlon (1970) reported that caregivers were more likely to comment on the value of a child's utterance than on its grammatical accuracy. However, not all researchers agree. For example, in a reanalysis of utterances addressed to Eve, Moerk (1994) found considerable evidence of corrective feedback contingent on errors in syntactic

TABLE 4–5. Semantic Relations Frequently Occurring in Brown's Stage I

	Semantic Relations	Child's Utterance	Interpretation (based on context)
Frequent at Brown's Stage II	Agent + Action	Doggy bark	The dog is barking
	Action + Object	Put block	Put block (into a can)
	Agent + Object	Mommy baby	Mommy's washing the baby
	Action + Location	Go store	Go to the store
	Entity + Location	Ball chair	The ball is by the chair
	Possessor + Possession	Daddy chair	That's daddy's chair
	Entity + Attribute	Diaper dirty	The diaper is dirty
	Demonstrative + Entity	That kitty	That's a kitty
Less frequent at Brown's Stage II	Instrumental (Action + Tool)	Color crayon	Color with a crayon
	Benefactive (For + Benfactor)	For Mommy	That's for Mommy
	Dative	Give me	Give me that
	Experiencer	Daddy sick	Daddy is sick
	Comitative	Go you	Go with you
	Conjunction	Cookies, milk	Cookies and milk
	Classificatory	Pookie dog	Pookie is a dog.

Source: Based on R. Brown (1973). *A first language: The early stages.* Cambridge, MA: Harvard University Press, pp. 173, 179.

production. Further research could help to identify factors that may favor corrective feedback from those that do not.

Telegraphic Speech

Brown and Fraser (1963) characterized all of children's early word combinations as **telegraphic speech** because they include mostly content words (nouns, verbs, adjectives) and few if any grammatical function words (e.g., articles, conjunctions, etc.). This continues to be true as children begin to expand their semantic relations into three-word utterances. Table 4–6 provides examples.

Once again, it is interesting to note the discourse patterns that appear to support the transition from two- to three-term telegraphic utterances. Here is an example:

Child: *Daddy go*

Mother: *Yes, and where's he going?*

Child: *outside*

Mother: *Mm hm, Daddy's going outside*

Child: *Daddy go outside*

This example illustrates the tendency of caregivers to acknowledge their children's comments and to connect them with semantic relations of interest to the child. In this case, the child comments on an agent + action relationship (*Daddy go*). Her mother acknowledges the comment (*Yes*) and connects it to the larger framework (agent + action + location) by asking a question (*and where is he going?*). When children have the vocabulary to answer these questions (e.g., *outside*), their caregivers often respond by affirming the complete thought (e.g., *Daddy's going outside*). Interestingly, young children often repeat utterances that are slightly beyond the range of their spontaneous repertoires but within their zone of proximal development. So, in conversations such as the one illustrated above, they are likely to repeat a three-term semantic relation (*Daddy go outside*). Once again, the emphasis of these exchanges is conversational but the effect is instructive.

Limitations of Telegraphic Speech. Although telegraphic speech enables children to comment on relationships that extend beyond the lexical meanings of words, the interpretation of telegraphic utterance often requires heavy reliance on nonlinguistic contextual cues. This is called **rich interpretation**, and it is especially obvious in the case of two-term semantic relations. Consider the utterance *baby crib*. A toddler producing this utterance might be expressing any of the relationships shown in Table 4–7 (and maybe others). The only way for a listener to be sure about the toddler's intended meaning is to listen for prosodic cues, to observe the child's gestures, and to consider features of the physical environment that would suggest a particular meaning. Fortunately, some of the ambiguity in telegraphic

TABLE 4–6. Examples of Three- and Four-Term Telegraphic Utterances

Semantic Roles	Examples	Interpretation (Based on Context)
Agent + Action + Object	*I kick ball.*	I am kicking the ball
Agent + Action + Locative	*Daddy sit chair.*	Daddy is sitting in the chair
Action + Dative + Object	*Give baby bottle.*	Give the baby a bottle
Action + Object + Locative	*Put ring box.*	Put the ring in the box
Agent + Action + Object + Locative	*Mommy put baby bed.*	Mommy pub the baby in the bed

Source: Based on R. Brown (1973). *A first language: The early stages.* Cambridge, MA: Harvard University Press, p. 205.

TABLE 4–7. Multiple Interpretations of the Same Two-Word Combination

Utterance	Semantic Relation	Interpretation
Baby crib =	Entity + Location	The baby is in the crib
Baby crib =	Action + Location	The baby is going into the crib
Baby crib =	Possessor + Possession	This is the baby's crib

utterances begins to decline as children acquire grammatical morphemes in the next stage of grammatical development.

Development at Brown's Stage II

Proficient language users can communicate about a wide range of ideas without any dependence on context, partly owing to the use of **grammatical morphemes**. Grammatical morphemes are suffixes and individual words that serve grammatical rather than lexical functions. Some specify semantic roles. For example, in the phrase *Baby's bed*, the possessive morpheme *-s* signals the semantic role of possessor. Others specify aspects of verb tense. For example, we add the grammatical morpheme *-ing* to a verb to represent an ongoing action (e.g., *James is playing Nintendo*). The emerging ability to use grammatical morphemes is the central feature of Brown's Stage II.

Brown (1973) identified **14 morphemes** that occur frequently in speech and are essential for the production of grammatical sentences. Table 4–8 shows the average order of emergence of these morphemes and it provides an example of each. It also shows that not all of these morphemes are mastered at once.

Brown's (1973) **mastery criterion** required children to produce the correct form of a morpheme in 9 of 10 linguistic contexts during spontaneous speech. Using this criterion, only the first four or five morphemes (*-ing, in, on*, plural *-s*, and irregular past tense) typically are mastered at Brown's stage II. Acquisition of the rest is protracted over the remaining MLU stages. The last ones to be acquired are the contractible copula and the auxiliary at some point

late in stage V. Although the three participants in Brown's study (Adam, Eve, Sarah) were quite variable in their rate of language development, it is interesting to note that the order in which they acquired the 14 grammatical morphemes was remarkably similar.

Researchers have wondered why the 14 morphemes typically are acquired in this order. An analysis of Brown's (1973) data suggests that the complexity of the morphemes determines the developmental sequence. Complexity is defined by the number of semantic meanings that are encoded by a morpheme and by the number of syntactic rules needed to use it. For example, a morpheme like plural "-s", which encodes only number (e.g., *crayon* vs. *crayons*), would be easier to acquire than the copula, which encodes both number and tense (e.g., *I am* vs. *She is* vs. *They are*).

Finally, there are some interesting patterns in the development of **irregular forms**, such as irregular noun plurals (e.g., *mice, deer*, etc.) and irregular past tense verbs (e.g., *ate, went*). These forms are acquired in a three-step sequence. First, children appear to memorize individual forms and use them appropriately. Later, when children are beginning to acquire the regular plural morpheme (*-s*) and the regular past tense morpheme (*-ed*), they begin to apply these regular endings to the irregular forms (e.g., *mouses* and *goed*). This is known as an **overregularization error**. These errors are interesting because they suggest that children are learning grammatical rules and not simply imitating the speech they hear. Finally, when children have become fluent in the application of the regular forms, they begin to recognize the exceptions, and return to using the appropriate irregular forms (*mice*, and *went*).

TABLE 4–8. The Average Ages and Stages of Mastery[1] of 14 Grammatical Morphemes

	[2]Stages	[3]Average Ages (in mos.)	[2]Morphemes	Examples
1.	II	27.7 to 30.8	Present progressive *-ing*	*jump**ing**, tickl**ing***
2.	II		Preposition *in*	*block **in** can*
3.	II		Preposition *on*	*dolly **on** chair*
4.	II		Plural *-s*	*cup**s**, key**s***
5.	II		Irregular past tense	*went, ate*
6.	III	31.6 to 34.8	Possessive *-s*	*baby's shoe*
7.	III		Uncontractible copula *is*	*This **is** dirty.*
8.	III–IV	31.6 to 39.5	Articles *a* and *the*	*the kitty, a baby*
9.	V	40.3 to 46.6	Regular past tense *-ed*	*jump**ed**, tickl**ed***
10.	V		Regular 3rd person verb agreement *-s*	*She jump**s***
11.	V		Irregular 3rd person verb agreement	*Mom **has** cookies*
12.	V		Uncontractible auxiliary *is*	*Kitty **is** purring*
13.	V		Contractible copula *-s*	*Daddy's here.*
14.	V		Contractible auxiliary *-s*	*John's hitting the ball.*

[1]Mastery is defined as correct use in 90% of contexts where it is required.

[2]Stages, selection of morphemes, and order of acquisition is based on R. Brown (1973), *A First Language.* MA: Harvard University Press.

[3]Average ages are based on J. Miller (1981), *Assessing Langage Production in Children: Experimental Procedures.* Baltimore, MD: University Park Press.

Development at Brown's Stage III

The major achievement of Brown's Stage III is the ability to form complete sentences in all of the basic modalities (statements, negations, questions, and commands). The use of language for commenting, questioning, negating, and commanding is not new to children at this stage. During previous stages, they used phrases to accomplish these communicative tasks. What is different at this stage is that they now can do so by using complete sentences. Note that this developmental relationship between function and form is a theme in language development. Children often learn new forms to represent previously acquired semantic functions, and they learn new semantic functions by using

previously acquired forms (Slobin, 1973). We saw this at stage II as children learned to code semantic functions (e.g., possessor-possession) into morphological forms (e.g., -'s), and now at stage III we see it as children are learning to combine topics and comments (another level of semantic function) into complete sentences. For example, instead of saying "*baby bed*" (which is ambiguous without the benefit of contextual cues), they can now say, "*That's the baby's bed*" (which clearly specifies the semantic relationships through linguistic forms).

A thorough developmental description of all sentence types is far beyond the scope of this chapter. Please refer to the following excellent sources which provide this information in greater detail: Avrutin (1999), Kuczaj (1982), McLaughlin (2006),

Owens (2008), and Reich (1986). However, we will illustrate the achievements of this stage by summarizing highlights in the emergence of declarative, interrogative, and negative sentences.

Declarative Sentences

To appreciate just what develops, we begin with a sampling of the structures involved in sentence production. First, at the broadest level, every **sentence (S)** must have a **noun phrase (NP)** and a **verb phrase (VP)**. The NP serves as the sentence subject and the VP serves as the predicate. This is often designated as

$$S \rightarrow NP + VP.$$

The components of each phrase range from single words to multiword sequences. Consider the following examples illustrating six variations in NP structure:

1. *He*

2. *Dinosaur*

3. *the dinosaur*

4. *the purple dinosaur*

5. *the first purple dinosaur*

6. *the first purple dinosaur on TV*

Notice that examples 1 and 2 consists of single words (1 is the pronoun *he*, and 2 is the object label, *dinosaur*). Examples 3 to 6 become increasingly complex as items are added to expand the NP. Specifically, example 3 includes a **determiner** (*the*); 4 includes an **adjective** (*purple*); 5 includes an **ordinal term** (*first*), and 6 includes a **post-noun modifier** (*on TV*).

VPs also range in complexity. Eleven examples are provided in Table 4–9. Each example shows the same verb phrase in a sentence following a subject pronoun, and pronouns are varied to show that the form of a verb must sometimes be adjusted depending on whether the subject represents first, second, or third person voice.

Several features of verbs are illustrated by the examples in Table 4–9. First, some verbs (e.g., *play* in example 1 and *have* in example 2) must be followed by a NP that names the object of the verb. These are known as **transitive verbs**. Other verbs (e.g., *am*, *are*, *is*) must be followed by an adjective

TABLE 4–9. Variations in Verb Phrase Structure Depending on Noun Phrase and Verb Tense

	First Person	Second Person	Third Person
1.	I *play* Nintendo.	You *play* Nintendo.	She *plays Nintendo*.
2.	I *have* ice cream.	You *have* ice cream.	She *has* ice cream.
3.	I *am happy*.	You *are* happy.	She *is happy*.
4.	I *am* at school.	You *are* at school.	She *is at school*.
5.	I *am* watching.	You *are watching*.	She *is watching*.
6.	I *jogged*.	You *jogged*.	She *jogged*.
7.	I *will paint*.	You *will paint*.	She *will paint*.
8.	I *might do* it.	You *might do* it.	She *might do* it.
9.	I *should do* it quickly.	You *should do* it quickly.	She *should do* it quickly.
10.	I *may do* it later.	You *may do* it later.	She *may do* it later.
11.	I can play *outside*.	You *can play* outside.	She *can play* outside.

(as in example 3), or a statement of location (as in example 4). These are known as **copula verbs**. Most verbs represent tense and must be marked accordingly. Example 5 illustrates present progressive tense as marked by an auxiliary verb (*am*, *are*, or *is*) and the suffix *-ing* (e.g., *is watching*). Example 6 illustrates past tense and requires the suffix *-ed* (e.g., *jogged*). Example 7 illustrates future tense, which is marked by auxiliary *will* (e.g., *will paint*). Notice that the copula verbs look just like the auxiliary verbs *is*, *am*, and *are*. However, they function differently. Each copula verb functions as the main verb in a sentence whereas each auxiliary verb functions to support a main verb. Also notice that some auxiliary verbs simply support the main verb (e.g., *is*, *am*, *are* in example 5) whereas others (e.g., *might*, *should*, *can*, and *may* in examples 8 to 11) modulate the meaning of the verb. Finally, examples 9 to 11 show that verbs can be qualified by adverbs, which specify the manner, time, and place of an action.

These examples represent only some of the features involved in sentence construction, but they offer enough information to indicate the complexity involved. As you know from our discussion of developments at Brown's stages I and II, children enter stage III with some important skills for tackling this challenge. They know how to create utterances containing various semantic relations that are expressed by declarative sentences (e.g., agent + action + object; possessor-possession; etc.); and they have begun to master grammatical morphemes. Some of these morphemes mark semantic roles (e.g., possessor) and some mark verb tense (e.g., present progressive). Throughout stage III, they learn to expand the NP in the subject and object positions by using adjectives and articles (*a*, *the*). They also learn to elaborate the VP by using the copula and some auxiliary verbs (e.g., *can*, *do*, *have*, *will*, *be*) with increasing frequency. So, by the end of stage III, they combine NP and VP to create the following types of declarative sentences:

That's a pretty kitty.

I have some cookies.

Me fell down.

Mommy is eating strawberry ice cream.

Brown bear is riding the big bike.

He works at the night time.

I didn't see something.

Daddy will be here.

I can make it go.

Interrogative Sentence Development

Two interrogative forms are used frequently by young children: yes/no-questions and wh-questions. **Yes/no-questions** require only a "yes" or "no" answer from the conversational partner. Both are spoken with a rising intonation, but their syntax can take two forms. One form involves the basic structure of any noninterrogative sentence type, for example, *You play Space Invaders?* Also see examples 1, 2, and 3 in Table 4–10. The second option requires a speaker to make structural changes in the underlying sentence components. However, the changes will vary somewhat, depending on the verb structure of a particular sentence. If a copula (*is*, *am*, or *are*) appears in the basic sentence, or if the verb structure of the basic sentence includes an auxiliary (e.g., *is*, *am*, *are*, *can*, *will*, etc.), then the copula or the auxiliary is moved to the front of the sentence and the subject is inverted (moved to second place). See examples 4, 5, 6, and 7 in Table 4–10. If the basic sentence includes neither a copula nor an auxiliary verb, then a form of *do* is added to the front of the sentence and the main verb is adjusted (if necessary) to coordinate with *do*. Examples 8, 9, and 10 in Table 4–10 illustrate this scenario. Note that this is a simplistic description of the grammatical process. For a more thorough review, see Santelmann, Berk, Austin, and Lust (2002). Also note that children who are just acquiring basic sentence forms may not have access to the same underlying structures as adults. However, our description does provide insight into the complexity involved when something as seemingly simple as a yes/no-question is produced.

Developmentally, children begin at Brown's stage I by using rising intonation with single words, then phrases, and then (at stage II) phrases with grammatical morphemes. By stage III, they learn to use rising intonation with basic sentence forms as illustrated by examples 1, 2, and 3 in Table 4–10.

TABLE 4–10. Formulation of Yes/No-Questions

Options	Basic Sentence	Examples of Corresponding Yes/No-Questions
Option 1 Use rising intonation with any noninterrogative sentence form.	Scott likes video games. James isn't here. Sit down.	1. Scott likes video games? 2. James isn't here? 3. Sit down?
Option 2a If the basic sentence includes a copula or an auxiliary verb, place it in the initial position of the sentence.	I am supposed to see it. Philip can speak French. Tim isn't a swimmer. We're coming over.	4. Am I supposed to see it? 5. Can Philip speak French? 6. Isn't Tim a swimmer? 7. Are you coming over?
Option 2b If the basic sentence does not include a copula or an auxiliary verb, then add the appropriate form of "do" to the front of the sentence and adjust the main verb if needed.	Teresa dances. They don't enjoy skiing. They sit together at lunch.	8. Does Teresa dance? 9. Don't they enjoy skiing? 10. Do they sit together at lunch?

Also at stage III, they begin to front the copula or the auxiliary when these are present in the basic sentence. However, there will be a period of instability before mastery. If a sentence does not have an auxiliary, children will begin to use *do* support (inconsistently at first), and there are likely to be errors in the form of the main verb. For example, they may say sentences like, *Does this goes here?* So, although the beginning of yes/no-sentence construction can clearly be seen in stage III, its complete development often extends into stage IV.

Wh-questions differ from yes/no-questions in that they invite the conversational partner to provide specific categories of information. All wh-questions begin with one of the following wh-words: *what, where, who, which, whose, when, why,* or *how.* Like yes/no-questions, the syntactic structure of wh-questions requires the inversion of subject and auxiliary or copula; and if there isn't a copula or auxiliary in the basic sentence, then do-support must be added. Table 4–11 provides examples.

When adults produce interrogative sentences, they have the advantage of knowing the components of the basic sentence from which the interrogative form is derived. However, children may not. So, they make approximations to the conventional

TABLE 4–11. Examples of Wh-Question Formation

Examples of Basic Sentences	Examples of Yes/No-Questions
That's [something].	1. What's that?
You're doing [something].	2. What are you doing?
The ball is [somewhere].	3. Where's the ball?
[Someone] is on TV.	4. Who is on TV?
Mary has [someone's] book.	5. Whose book is that?
He eats lunch [some time].	6. When does he eat lunch?
I ate [some] dessert.	7. Which dessert did you eat?
I fell [for some reason].	8. Why did you fall?
She bakes cookies [somehow].	9. How does she bake cookies?

interrogative form in small steps. At first, they use an interrogative form without a copula or auxiliary (e.g., *What that?* or *Where kitty go?*). Next, they include a copula or auxiliary verb but do not consistently move it next to the wh-word (e.g., *Where kitty is going?*). However, by the end of stage III, children are beginning to produce wh-questions using the conventional sequence (e.g., *Where is the kitty going?*). Still, inconsistencies in productions continue even at stage 4, when children begin to embed phrases and clauses.

Some researchers have suggested that the pattern of wh-question development may be repeated at different times for each different wh-question form (de Villiers, Roeper, & Vainikka, 1990). However, this needs to be confirmed. What is clear is that the question words themselves emerge in a developmental sequence. *What, where,* and *who* are used first, and *when, how,* and *why* are used later (Wootten, Merkin, Hood, & Bloom, 1979). A similar sequence is observed in comprehension (Winzemer in Valian, 1981). Two processes influence this sequence. One is cognitive. It is easier to conceptualize objects, locations, and people than it is to conceptualize time, manner, and causality. Second, answers to questions about what, where, and who generally are shorter than answers to questions about when, how, or why. Because very young children have limitations in attention and processing space, questions requiring longer responses will be acquired later (Tager-Flusberg, 2005). Finally, when children are asked questions that they do not comprehend, they tend to interpret the questions according to the wh-words that they do comprehend (McLaughlin, 2006). For example, if asked, "*How do you play ball?*" a toddler might say, "*outside.*"

Negative Sentences

Negative sentence development was studied first by Bellugi (in Brown, 1973). She analyzed the utterances produced by Adam, Eve, and Sarah in Brown's (1973) transcripts and identified a three-part developmental sequence. Initially (at Brown's stage I), the children used just a few negative markers (e.g., *no* or *not*) and placed them in the first position of an utterance (e.g., *No go nap*). Sometime later (late in Brown's Stage I), the children began to insert a negative word within the phrase itself (e.g., *I **no** go*). At about the same time, children occasionally also included a contracted auxiliary verb within the phrase (e.g., *Don't go*). Finally, by the end of stage

III, the children began to use a variety of auxiliaries and did so consistently (e.g., *I'm not sad now; You can't have this one*).

Wode (1977) studied the development of negative sentences by considering function as well as structure. The participants in his study were toddlers learning English, German, and Swedish. Like Bellugi (in Brown, 1973), Wode found that children acquired these sentences in a three-step sequence. Initially (during Brown's stage I), they used a negative morpheme (e.g., *no*) alone, and it was typically the one that occurred most often in their parents' speech. Next (also during Brown's stage I), they combined the negative morpheme with another word. At first, this was done anaphorically (i.e., to deny content in the previous utterance made by their conversational partner). For example:

Adult: *Do you want some milk?* (holding a glass of milk)

Child: *No milk.* (= I don't want that milk.)

Later, this was done nonanaphorically (i.e., to negate information in the rest of their own utterance, as in *no eat peas,* meaning "*I don't want to eat peas.*" Finally (late in Brown's stage II and early in stage III), negative elements were inserted inside of the child's utterance, and a larger variety of negative morphemes began to emerge (e.g., *not*), as in *Kathryn not quite through.* Other researchers have confirmed and extended the findings of Bellugi and of Wode (e.g., deVilliers & deVilliers, 1979).

Development at Brown's Stage IV

During Brown's Stage III, children learn to express complete thoughts by using sentences. Throughout Stage IV, their awareness of cognitive, social, and linguistic concepts continues to expand, and they learn to package more information into a single utterance. This is accomplished by **embedding** phrases and clauses within the major grammatical constituents (NP, VP) of sentences.

Phrases

A **phrase** is a group of words with either a subject or a predicate. We noted earlier that a basic sentence consists of two primary phrases: the NP and the VP. However, three other types of phrases can be embedded within these sentence constituents. Each type of phrases is built around grammatical forms, known as prepositions, participles, and gerunds, respectively.

Prepositions include words like *in*, *on*, *under*, *beside* and others. Children begin to use *in* and *on* during Brown's stage II. Other prepositions develop throughout the preschool period. A **prepositional phrase** consists of a preposition and a noun phrase (e.g., *in the box*, *on the table*), and it can function as an adjectival phrase to modify a noun (e.g., *The man in the car looked familiar*) or as an adverbial phrase to specify the time, place, or manner of an action (e.g., *I'm going swimming in the morning*).

A **gerund** is the *-ing* form of a verb used as a noun. For example, in the sentence *Diving is fun*, the word *diving* is a gerund because it is used as a noun. A **gerund phrase** may include only the gerund (e.g., *diving*) or the gerund with modifiers (e.g., *Deep-sea diving can be fun*). As can be seen in the previous example, a gerund phrase functions in the same way as a noun phrase.

A **participle** is a form of a verb used as an adjective. For example, in the sentence *Slithering snakes make me nervous*, the word *slithering* functions as an adjective to modify the word *snakes*. Notice that some participles (e.g., *slithering*) utilize the *-ing* form of a verb. In that sense, they look just like a gerund. However, they differ from gerunds in that they function like an adjective and not like a noun. Other participles utilize past participle verb forms (e.g., *frozen food*, *glazed doughnuts*). **Participial phrases** may include only a participle and a noun (e.g., *smiling children*) or they may be expanded by modifiers. Because preschoolers do not use expanded participial phrases, we do not address them here. Table 4–12 provides a range of examples showing sentences with all forms of phrases described so far.

Sometimes infinitives are included in a discussion of phrases (Justice & Ezell, 2002; Owens, 2008). An **infinitive** is the "*to* + V" form of a verb (e.g., *to jump*, *to run*). An infinitive phrase may include only an infinitive (e.g., *I like to jog*) or an infinitive with modifiers (e.g., *I like to jog in the evening*). However, infinitives are sometimes accompanied by a subject (e.g., *Mom wants **you** to clean your room*). For this reason, they are also classified as clauses, and we discuss them with other clauses, below.

Clauses

A **clause** is a group of words with both a subject and a predicate. When a clause is embedded within sentences, the result is a **complex sentence**. Like embedded phrases, embedded clauses serve grammatical functions. Note that a sentence itself is an **independent clause** because it can stand alone as

TABLE 4–12. Examples of Phrasal Embedding

Phrase Type	Example	Grammatical Function
Prepositional Phrase	The book **on the top shelf** fell down.	Adjectival phrase (postnoun modifier)
Prepositional Phrase	James is hiding **under the desk**.	Adverbial—specifying where
Prepositional Phrase	You may go swimming **after lunch**.	Adverbial—specifying when
Prepositional Phrase	Jamie came back **with the dog**	Adverbial—specifying how
Gerund phrase	**Swinging** is fun.	Subject Noun Phrase
Gerund phrase	Teresa likes **drawing pictures**.	Object Noun Phrase
Participial phrase	**Dancing clowns** make me laugh.	Subject Noun Phrase
Participial phrase	Tim enjoys **text messaging**.	Object Noun Phrase

a complete thought. However, it also can be embedded into another sentence. For example:

I guess you have your own bike

Nancy knows James is home from school

In both of these examples, the embedded clauses function as the object NP of the main verb and are therefore classified as **object NP complements**.

Some word sequences are classified as **dependent clauses**, because they do not express a complete thought even though they include both a subject and a predicate. Here, we summarize five types of dependent clauses that are used by young children. As in the example above, one is classified as an **object NP complement**. It is introduced by a pronoun (*that*) and functions as the object of the main verb (e.g., *Scott saw that you hid the ball*). A second type of dependent clause is known as a **wh-question clause**. It is introduced by a wh-word (e.g., "what," *where, when, why, how*) and also functions as the object of a verb (e.g., *I wonder what it is*). A third type of clause, known as a **relative clause**, is introduced by a relative pronoun (e.g., *who, whose, which, that*) and refers back to the noun that it follows (e.g., *The boy who sits next to me plays baseball*). The fourth type is an **infinitive clause**, which consists of the infinitive form of a

verb (e.g., *to jump, to run, to listen*), an object, and sometimes other modifiers. It can function as the object in an SVO sentence (e.g., *Roger wants Candice to play*.) and it can function as an adjective complement (e.g., *John is easy to please*). Notice that the object of an infinitive phrase is sometimes understood (e.g., *I like to play with my cat*.). Finally, **wh-adverbial clauses** specify the time that an action takes place (e.g., *We stopped playing outside when it rained*). For ease of comparison and review, Table 4–13 provides examples of all forms of clausal embedding discussed so far.

The development of embedding progresses gradually. Brown (1973) reported that the ability to embed a complete sentence in the object position (e.g., *I think you did it*.) and the ability to produce embedded wh-questions (e.g., *I wonder what it is*.) emerge at stage IV. However, embedded wh-questions may be produced without the required inversion of subject and verb (e.g., *Show me where can I get one*). Infinitive clauses emerge late in stage IV. Initially, the subject is understood and relates back to the sentence subject (e.g., *Mom wants to see you*). Later, children also learn to produce infinitive clauses that include an explicit subject different from the sentence subject (e.g., *Katrina wants Philip to play with her*). Relative clauses do not emerge until Brown's Stage V. The earliest forms are used to modify

TABLE 4–13. Examples of Clausal Embedding (Complex Sentences)

Type of Clause	Example	Grammatical Function
Independent clause	Kim says *you should come inside*.	Object complement
Dependent clauses		
Object complement	Kathy thinks *that Scott is cute*.	Object complement
Wh-question clause	Fabi wonders *what Teresa painted*.	Object complement
Wh-adverbial clause	I'll go *when it stops raining*.	Modifies main verb
Relative clause (modifying object)	Mark has a cat *that always purrs*.	Postnoun modifier
Relative clause (modifying subject)	The boy *who sits next to me* sings.	Postnoun modifier
Infinitive clause (explicit subject)	Roger wants *Candice to dance*.	Object complement
Infinitive clause (implied subject)	I like *to walk in the woods*.	Object complement
Infinitive clause (implied subject)	Sabine is *easy to please*.	Adjective complement

nouns in the object position of a sentence (e.g., *He's the one who left*). The ability to embed relative clauses in the post-subject position does not begin until after stage V (e.g., *The car that was speeding hit a truck.*). Other forms (e.g., *wh*-adverbial clauses) are also acquired later.

Development at Brown's Stage V

The major achievement of Stage V is the ability to produce compound sentences. A **compound sentence** is a complete sentence that consists of two independent clauses joined by a coordinating conjunction (e.g., *and, but, or*). Throughout stage V, children prefer to use *and* for this purpose. The first use of *and* makes its appearance during Brown's stage I when children are commenting on things that go together (e.g., *milk and cookies*). At stage III, they may use *and* to introduce a clause within the context of a conversation, as in the following example:

Adult: *Trina is running*

Child: *and her shoe is untied*

They also may name compound subjects within the context of a dialogue:

Adult: *Who is wearing a yellow shirt?*

Child: *Patty and Katy*

However, at stage V *and* emerges as a tool for connecting two independent clauses. Some compound sentences are used to comment on the relationship between two different observations (e.g., *Gia has a yellow crayon and I have a blue one.*). Some are used to comment on an identical event involving two different subjects, as in *Terri and Patti have a cat named Zuzo.* (The underlying structure in this example is presumed to be *Terri has a cat named Zuzo* and *Patti has a cat named Zuzo*). Similar compounding can occur with predicates (e.g., *We giggled and laughed*) and objects (e.g., *Michael saw lions and tigers.*). Table 4–14 summarizes the patterns of conjoining that may occur by using the conjunction "and."

The value of compound sentences is that they permit a speaker to comment on relationships be-

TABLE 4–14. Patterns of Sentence Coordination

Compound sentence	Gia has a yellow crayon and I have a blue one.
Compound subject	Terri and Patti have a cat name Zuzo.
Compound predicates	Tippy barked and ran away.
Compound objects	Paul built a castle and a fort.

tween semantic relations. For example, L. Bloom, Lahey, Hood, and Lifter (1980) studied the compound sentences used by preschoolers and found that *and* is used to express four different types of relationships. The first, **additive**, involves the combining of sentences simply to list two events with no particular connection (e.g., *I ate some ice cream and I picked some flowers*). The second relationship is **temporal**, specifying the order in which events occur (e.g., *I found a cookie and I ate it.*). Third, children comment on **causal relationships** (e.g., *Cara hurt her knee and she cried.*). A fourth use of *and* is to comment on **adversative** or contrasting relationships (e.g., *This one is old and this one is new.*). Notice that adults would use different conjunctions (coordinating or subordinating) to express some of these relationships. For example, to express an adversative relationship, an adult might use the coordinating conjunction *but* (e.g., *This one is old, but this one is new*). However, children do not begin to expand their use of coordinating or subordinating conjunctions to comment on relationships between relations until after stage V. This is yet another example of Slobin's (1973) **form and function rule** (i.e., children express new functions by using previously learned forms, and they learn new forms to express previously learned functions).

Soon after children begin to conjoin sentences, they begin to form sentences that include conjoining and embedding (e.g., *I'm going home and then I'll play with the Legos that I got for my birthday.*). At this point, MLU is no longer a good index of syntactic complexity. Until now, sentences became longer as children learned to use new grammatical structures. However, the process of conjoining results in the creation of longer sentences without adding complexity. Therefore, other methods are used to assess children's grammatical complexity at this point.

Sentence Comprehension at Stages III to V

The comprehension of sentences is aided in the natural environment by contextual cues that support the interpretation of language. In addition, children also sometimes use linguistic strategies to understand sentences including structures they cannot yet process. One strategy was already mentioned in our review of *wh*-question development. Recall that when children do not understand a wh-word, they are likely to respond to the question by **treating the unfamiliar wh-word as a familiar one**. So, if asked, "Why is there mud on your shoes?" a child might say, "Mud is dirty." Based on McLaughlin's (2006) description, we present a summary of other strategies used by children to comprehend syntactic forms that are not yet established in their repertoires.

Compound and Complex Sentence Comprehension

The ability to understand compound and complex sentences may be influenced by sentence length, complexity, or a combination. For example, it often is easier for preschoolers to understand a sentence with compound predicates than a sentence with two independent clauses as in the following examples:

Compound predicate: *Colleen kissed and hugged the baby*.

Compound sentence: *Colleen kissed the baby and then she hugged the baby*.

Similarly, it may be easier to understand a sentence with only one embedded clause than a sentence with more than one embedded clause as in the following examples:

One embedded clause: *Margaret has some video games that she borrowed from a friend*.

Multiple embeddings: *Margaret has some video games that she borrowed from a friend who got them from his dad when they went on vacation*.

Sentences with relative clauses are especially difficulty for preschoolers to understand, particularly if the clauses are center embedded to modify the subject as in the following examples:

One center-embedded clause: *The bike that I got for my birthday is red*.

Two center-embedded clauses: *The girl that the boy that had racing stripes met won the contest*.

A preschooler who hears the second sentence above may interpret it by using a **compounding strategy**. This strategy assumes that all actions named in a sentence are performed by the first noun mentioned. If, after hearing the second sentence, the preschooler was asked, "Who has racing stripes?" he or she might say, "The girl." On the other hand, sentences with only one relative clause following the grammatical object are easier to understand, as in the following example:

My Mom has a phone that rings like a wind chime.

Some sentences with **infinitive clauses** also are difficult to understand, depending on the verb (C. S. Chomsky, 1969) and on the way the clause functions in the sentence (Reich, 1986). Consider the following examples:

1. The teacher told <u>Alice to draw a picture</u>

2. Mom asked <u>Betsy to clean her room</u>.

3. Doug promised <u>Heather to feed the cat</u>.

4. Tom asked <u>Julie what to fix</u>.

5. Jim is <u>easy [for someone] to please</u>.

In most dependent clauses, the subject of the infinitive is the closest preceding noun. This rule of thumb is known as the **minimal distance principle (MDP)** (Rosenbaum, 1967). In the examples above, it applies to sentence 1 (involving the verb *tell*) and to sentence 2 (involving the verb *ask*). In sentence 1, *Alice* is the closest noun preceding the infinitive (*to draw*), and Alice is the intended agent of the action (*to draw*). In sentence 2, *Betsy* is the closest noun preceding the infinitive (*to clean*), and Betsy is the intended agent of the action (*to clean*). However, the MDP never applies when an infinitive clause follows *promise* (as in sentence 3), and it sometimes does not apply when an infinitive clause follows *ask* (as in sentence 4). In sentence 3, *Heather* is the closest noun preceding the infinitive (*to feed*), but Mom is the intended agent of the action. In sentence 4, *Julie* is the closest noun preceding the infinitive (*to fix*) but Tom is the intended agent of the action. MDP also is not applicable in some clauses that function as predicate adjectives and in which the subject is implied (e.g., sentence 5). No wonder this is difficult for preschoolers to sort out!

Developmentally, infinitive clauses are not understood until late in the preschool period. According to C. S. Chomsky's (1969) research, sentences with *tell* (which always follow the MDP) and with *ask* (where *ask* functions as a polite form of *tell*) are understood first at about 5 years. Sentences with *promise* (which never follow the MDP) are understood next (at about 7 years), and sentences with *ask* (where *ask* functions to introduce a wh-question) are understood last (at about 9 years). Other studies have reported similar results (e.g., Kessel, 1970).

Passive Sentence Comprehension

We have already noted that: (a) most sentences heard in conversational speech by English-learning preschoolers are spoken in the **active voice,** which follows the grammatical SVO sequence, and (b) for these sentences, children use the grammatical SVO sequence to identify the semantic agent, action, and object, respectively. However, in the case of **passive sentences**, the grammatical SVO sequence does not represent the semantic agent, action, and object. Consider two sets of examples in Table 4-15. Note that both sentences in each example have the same meaning, and both present the same grammatical SVO sequence. However, because the semantic object of the passive sentence is the object of the preposition *by*, the sequence of seman-

tic roles is reversed (i.e., object-action-agent). In other words, *Jack chased Jill* means the same thing as *Jill was chased by Jack*, even though the sequence of nouns is reversed in the surface structure. This is confusing for preschoolers, particularly when the incorrect interpretation is plausible (i.e., It is just as possible for Jack to be chasing Jill as it is for Jill to be chasing Jack.) When such plausibility exists, the sentence is classified as a **reversible passive**. In other passive sentences, the reversibility of roles is less plausible (e.g., *The cheese was eaten by the mouse*). These sentences are classified as **nonreversible passives**.

Developmentally, children begin to understand passive sentences at about the age of 4 years by using **nonsyntactic strategies**. However, these strategies are helpful only some of the time. For example, children use the **order-of-mention strategy** to process reversible passives, assuming that the grammatical SVO sequence refers to the semantic agent, action, and object, respectively (Maratsos, 1974). This obviously leads them to incorrect interpretations. At the same time, they use a **plausible event strategy** to interpret nonreversible passives (McLaughlin, 2006). So, if they hear a sentence like, *The cheese was eaten by the mouse*, they assume that the mouse is the agent of the action because it wouldn't make sense otherwise. This obviously is more helpful, but it is based on cognitive knowledge and not linguistic comprehension. The ability to use linguistic strategies for comprehending passive sentences does not emerge until after stage V and is not mastered until school age.

The production of passive sentences begins in the context of dialogue by use of **truncated forms**. Consider the following example:

Adult: *What happened to the vase?*

Child: *It got broken*

TABLE 4–15. Examples of Active and Passive Sentence Structures

Sentence Type	Example	Sequence of Semantic Roles
Active	*Jack chased Jill*	Agent-Action-Object
Passive	*Jill was chased by Jack*	Object-Action-Agent

The child's utterance is a truncated because the agent of the action is not named explicitly as it would be in a **full passive** sentence (e.g., *It got broken by me*). Pragmatically, truncated passives offer the option to deemphasize the agent of the action. Full passives emerge after stage V and are not mastered until school age.

Motherese and Syntactic Development

As noted previously, speech addressed to toddlers and preschoolers is different on almost every dimension when compared with speech addressed to adults. However, certain features are especially likely to support children's grammatical development. For example, it is helpful for caregivers to use a **reduced speech rate** and that their utterances are remarkably **well formed**. In fact, error rates in motherese have been reported to be as low as one in 15,000 utterances (Newport, 1976). Caregivers also produce utterances that are **highly repetitive**, probably to accompany their child's attempts at following directions. For example:

Put the blocks in the can . . . the blocks . . . in the can . . . put them in . . . Good, put the blocks in the can . . .

From a linguistic perspective, this redundancy provides toddlers with opportunities to hear complete sentences and parts of sentences in reference to meaningful ongoing activity. Finally, caregivers **adjust their MLU** in sync with the growth of grammatical complexity in their children's utterances (Philips, 1973; Snow, 1972). This probably reflects the caregiver's perception that, as their child uses longer utterances, he or she probably understands longer utterances as well.

Throughout this discussion, we have mentioned **discourse patterns** that appear to support grammatical growth. Generally, it is assumed that caregivers use these patterns in the service of communication rather than for the purpose of direct instruction (e.g., Brown & Hanlon, 1970). However, the form, content, and contingent nature of these patterns do appear to support children's grammatical development (e.g., Moerk, 1992). The following is a summary of three such discourse patterns described by

Reich (1986). The first is **expansion**, the repetition of content from a child's utterances within a grammatically more advanced form. This strategy provides a grammatical model that exactly matches the child's intended meaning, and it has been associated with syntactic growth. For example,

Child: *That doggy*

Caregiver: *Yes, that's a dog.*

Child: *Daddy go work.*

Caregiver. *Mm hm, Daddy is going to work.*

The second is **extension**, defined as the repetition of a child's utterance with the addition of semantically related information. For example:

Child: *Doggy barking*

Caregiver: *Yes, and he's running too.*

Child: *Car*

Caregiver: *A big red car*

The last strategy is known as **recasting,** which involves restating the content of a child's utterance in a different syntactic form. For example:

Child: *Doggy barking*

Caregiver: *Is he barking?*
　Bark, Dog!
　He is barking.

These utterances serve a number of functions. Communicatively, they keep the conversation going on a topic of the child's interest. Linguistically, they provide a child with examples of different grammatical frames for the same information.

Summary of Early Morphological and Syntactic Development

Our review of early syntactic development showed that grammar develops gradually as children learn to code an increasing amount of information in linguistic form. Throughout most of the preschool period, mean length of utterance (MLU) is a sensitive index of grammatical complexity. Brown's five stages of grammatical development are associated with characteristic elements of growth, including the production of telegraphic speech, the emergence of grammatical morphemes, the formulation of complete sentences, embedding, and conjoining, respectively. Changes in grammatical development are supported by patterns of child-addressed speech including expansion, extension, and recasting. These strategies appear to be particularly supportive of grammatical development. Children's initial use of new structures often occurs in the context of discourse where established semantic functions are modeled by caregivers in new forms, and new forms are used by children to express established semantic functions. We move now to a consideration of children's development of pragmatic skills.

PRIMARY ACCOMPLISHMENTS: PRAGMATICS

Although the development of pragmatics is mentioned last in this chapter, it is one of the most important motivating and integrating factors behind language acquisition. Because communication develops before speech, some researchers consider the pragmatic functions of language to play a role in bootstrapping other linguistic knowledge such that semantics, grammar, and phonology develop in the service of communication (e.g., L. Bloom, 1993; Snow, 1999). When toddlers begin to use words in addition to gestures for communicating their intentions, they experience the power of language as a tool for connecting with others, for learning about their world, and for self-regulation. Recall that the rules of pragmatics influence the selection of content (semantics) and form (grammar, phonology) relative to context. Hence, the growth of content and form may be motivated at least in part by the desire of children to communicate more effectively across an increasing range of situations and conversational partners.

The contexts to which children are sensitive expand throughout the developmental period. This section describes development in reference to the intentional context (**pragmatic functions**), the social interactive context (**discourse functions**), and the cultural context (**sociolinguistic functions**).

The Intentional Context (Communicative Functions)

Like all contexts, the **intentional context** influences our choice of linguistic content and form. In the previous chapter, we introduced the concept of the speech act (Austin, 1962; Searle, 1969). Recall that every speech act can be analyzed at three levels: (a) its locutionary form, the language signal itself (e.g., speech); (b) its illocutionary force, the function that the speaker intends his or her utterance to serve; and (c) its perlocutionary effect, the listener's interpretation of the speaker's utterance. Consistent with this framework, the intentional context refers to the illocutionary force or the speaker's intended function. For example, a person may speak to make a request, to offer advice, to give directions, to share experience, to tell a story, or for other reasons. Such goals are referred to as **communicative intentions** or **communicative functions**. Each constitutes the core around which the content and form of an utterance are built.

Recall that children begin to express communicative functions intentionally at the end of the first year during the illocutionary (intentional) period of communication development (Bates, Camaioni, & Volterra, 1975). They do so by using gestures and vocalizations deliberately to regulate joint attention (protodeclarative) and to regulate the behavior of others (proto-imperative). With the emergence of language, toddlers begin to use words plus gestures to regulate behavior, joint attention, and social interaction. Later, with the development of more advanced vocabulary, grammatical, cognitive, and social skills, we see a comparable expansion of communicative functions.

Early Communicative Functions

Communicative functions have been studied by researchers in developmental and behavioral psychology. Although there is some degree of overlap between the two, conceptually, they are different so we present them separately. Both frameworks have added value to strategies of assessment and intervention in the education of children with disabilities.

The Developmental Framework

Several developmental researchers have classified the communicative functions expressed by children during prelinguistic (illocutionary) and emerging language (locutionary) periods (e.g., Bates, Camaioni, & Volterra, 1975; Coggins & Carpenter, 1981; Dore, 1975; Halliday, 1975). Although categories overlap in the classification systems developed by individual researchers, the systems are not exactly the same. This is due to variations in the degree to which discourse features, aspects of context, and aspects of linguistic form are embedded in the coding systems (Chapman, 1981; Westby, 1994). Table 4–16 offers an integration of these categories to characterize the range of functions expressed during the first two years of life.

Table 4–16 shows that 11 of the 15 communicative functions expressed with emerging language are the same as those expressed with intentional gestures during the prelinguistic period (Westby, 1994a). For example, during the prelinguistic period, an infant may point to an object and look at his caregiver to initiate joint attention with the caregiver to the object, but during the emergent language period, a child may name an object to accomplish the same communicative goal.

Table 4–16 also shows that the range of communicative functions expands by at least four as children enter the emergent language period. For example, children learn to request linguistic information (e.g., *What's that?*) and to relabel items in the service of pretend play (e.g., referring to a shoe box as the *baby's bed*). These new functions develop as children acquire more mature cognitive and social skills (e.g., Chapman, 1984; Westby, 1994b; Wetherby, Crain, Yonclas, & Walker, 1988).

All of the communicative functions listed in Table 4–16 become increasingly differentiated as children develop more sophisticated linguistic skills throughout the emerging and later language periods. For example, initial requests for information may refer to individual objects in the present context (e.g., "*What's that?*"), although later requests may refer to nonpresent items (e.g., "*Where ball?*"), semantic relationships (e.g., "*How do you blow a bubble?*"), and many other possible referents. Additionally, intentions may combine to reflect emerging discourse skills. For example, during the emerging language period, a child may acknowledge a partner's communicative act by repeating part or all of an utterance, or a child may request an item. However, with increasing linguistic skill, a child may respond to a communicative partner's previous utterance by both acknowledging and requesting as in Table 4–17.

The relationship between linguistic competence and communicative competence is complex (Ninio & Snow, 1999). For example, children with specific language impairments use a wider range of communicative functions than younger children at the same level of syntactic maturity (Rollins, Pan, Conti-Ramsden, & Snow, 1994). Moreover, some children with an abnormally restricted range of pragmatic functions use age-appropriate semantic and syntactic skills. Furthermore, first-born children typically outperform same-age second-born children on linguistic tasks, whereas second-born children typically outperform same age first-born children on measures of pragmatic ability (Hoff, 2005). Observations of this sort have led some researchers to question the pragmatic bootstrapping theory. Specifically, if communicative competence is the gateway to semantic and grammatical development, they question how it is possible for a child with poor pragmatic skills to be advanced in semantics and grammar. Similarly, they question how it is possible for first-born children (who outperform same-age second-born children on linguistic measures) to perform more poorly on measures of pragmatics. Further research is needed to address these questions. We raise them here to highlight the complexity of the relationship between communicative functions and linguistic forms.

Other findings related to the expression of communicative functions during the first two years of life indicate that toddlers initiate communication more frequently as they mature (e.g., Snow, Pan, Imbens-Bailey, & Herman 1996). They express a wider range of intentions per unit of time (Ninio, 1995), and they begin to learn how to express the same communicative function in more than one way (Ninio, 1995). In addition, as toddlers reach the age of about 24 months, their utterance-level intentions increasingly are produced within a discourse structure, resulting in a new level of conversational competence. Conversational skills are discussed in more detail under discourse development, below.

TABLE 4–16. Social-Communicative Functions First Expressed During the Prelinguistic (PL), Emerging Language (EL), and Preschool Language (PSL) Periods

	PL[1]	EL[2]	PSL[3]
Regulation of Behavior (aka "protoimperatives" during prelinguistic period)			
1. Requesting objects or action	X	→	→
2. Rejecting objects or actions	X	→	→
3. Negotiating (and later clarifying) failed messages	X	→	→
Regulation of Social Interaction			
4. Greetings	X	→	→
5. Participating in ritualized interactive games	X	→	→
6. Showing off	X	→	→
7. Calling for attention	X	→	→
8. Acknowledging someone's communicative act	X	→	→
9. Expressing moods or feelings	X	→	→
Regulation of joint attention (aka "protodeclaratives" during prelinguistic period)			
10. Transferring objects from self to another person	X	→	→
11. Directing someone's attention to an object or event (joint referencing)	X	→	→
Functions that are more efficiently communicated in language			
12. Requesting linguistic information (e.g., Asking "What's X?")		X	→
13. Responding to a caregiver's request for verbal information (e.g., Labeling an item when asked, "what's X?")		X	→
14. Sharing information about non-present items (e.g., objects or events) (e.g., Sharing a recent zoo experience such as, "See a giraffe")		X*	→
15. Using language to structure symbolic play (e.g., Referring to a shoe box as a "doll's bed")		X*	→

[1]PL = prelinguistic period of development (~9 to 12 mos.). [2]EL = emergent language period (~12 to 24 mos.). [3]PR = preschool period (~2 years to 5 years). X = function first observed. X* = function first observed at about 24 months (late in the early language period). → = function continues to be expressed and differentiated.

Based on E. Bates, L. Camaioni, and V. Volterra (1975), The acquisition of performatives prior to speech. *Merrill-Palmer Quarterly, 21*, 205–216; R. Chapman (1981). Exploring children's communicative intents, In J. Miller (Ed.), *Assessing language production in children: Experimental procedures*, pp. 111–136; J. Dore (1975), Holophrases, speech acts, and language universals. *Journal of Child Language, 2*, 21–40; R. Golinkoff (1983), The preverbal negotiations of failed messages: Insights into the transition period. In R. M. Olinkoff (Ed.), *The transition from prelinguistic to linguistic communication.* Hillside, NJ: Erlbaum; M. K. Halliday (1975), *Learning how to mean: Explorations in the development of language.* New York, NY: Arnold; C. Westby (1994a), Sociocommunicative bases of communication development (pp. 199–229), in W. O. Haynes and B. B. Shulman (Eds.), *Communication development: Foundations, processes, and clinical applications.* Englewood Cliffs, NJ: Prentice-Hall; C. Westby (1994b), Communicative refinement in school-age and adolescence (pp. 341–383), in W. O. Haynes and B. B. Shulman (Eds.), *Communication development: Foundations, processes, and clinical applications.* Englewood Cliffs, NJ:

TABLE 4–17. Emerging Complexity in the Expression of Communicative Intentions

	Acknowledging	Requesting
Emergent Language	Mother: *There's a bunny.*	Mother: *Time for bed*
	Child: *Bunny!*	Child: *Brown Bear* (requesting a book)
	Acknowledging and Requesting	
Later Language	Mother: *Let's read <u>Pancakes for Breakfast</u>*	
	Child: *Ok, where the book is?*	

Verbal Behavior Functions

So far, we have summarized the development of communicative functions from within a developmental psycholinguistic framework. However, some evidence-based educational strategies for language instruction are derived from a framework based on applied behavior analysis (e.g., Frost & Bondy, 2006; Greer & Ross, 2008; Sundberg & Partington, 1998). This framework evolved from the work of B. F. Skinner (1957), whose research and ideas constitute the foundation of modern behavior analysis.

Skinner differentiated between two types of behavior: respondent and operant. **Respondent behavior** is reflexive. Examples include the knee jerk reflex, and the eye-blink reflex. These behaviors are hard-wired into human neurology. They are elicited by a stimulus and performed in just about the same way each time the stimulus is presented. In contrast, **operant behaviors** are voluntary behaviors that may be evoked by a particular stimulus but are shaped by their consequences. For example, I used to answer my phone when I heard it ring, because the caller was usually someone with whom I wanted to speak. However, when telemarketers began calling, I quickly learned to ignore the phone's ring altogether. Both of these behavior patterns were shaped by different sets of consequences for responding to the phone's ring.

As in the example of my phone-answering behavior, every operant behavior is embedded in a **three-term contingency**, which includes an antecedent (A), a behavior (B), and a consequence (C). This **ABC** contingency often is represented as follows:

Antecedent → Behavior → Consequence

The **antecedent** may be an event in the physical environment (e.g., a ringing phone, an object, a picture, printed matter, a previous verbal utterance, etc.) or it may be a **motivational operation (MO)** such as deprivation or an annoyance of some sort. For example, if I am thirsty (deprivation), I am likely to engage in behaviors that result in getting a drink. If I am at the movie theatre and people behind me are speaking loudly (annoyance), I may ask them to be quiet. **Consequences** may include reinforcement or punishment. **Reinforcement** is a consequence that will increase the frequency of the behavior that it follows, and **punishment** has the opposite effect (i.e., it decreases the frequency of the behavior it follows). In my example above, telephone answering was reinforced initially by opportunities to speak with friends but it was punished by the intrusion of telemarketers. These principles of reinforcement and punishment are just the tip of the iceberg of the behavioral model. For thorough descriptions of behavioral principles, please refer to the following excellent resources: Cooper, Heron, and Heward (2007); Mallott, Whaley, and Mallott (1997); and Miller (1997).

Skinner (1957) considered language to be a set of operant behaviors whose reinforcement is mediated by the social enviornment. He used the term **verbal behavior** (VB) to differentiate his functional conceptualization from the structural conceptualizations of the prevailing linguistics models (e.g., A. N. Chomsky, 1965). Unlike the structuralist views, which emphasized linguistic units such as syntax, Skinner's analysis of VB consisted of functional units. Seven of these functional units (or types of verbal behavior) are summarized in Table 4-18.

TABLE 4–18. Elementary Verbal Behavior (VB) Functions Within the Three-Term Contingency

Antecedent	VB	Consequence	Example
Verbal Behavior	Echoic	General Social Reinforcement	Mother: *There's daddy* Toddler: *Daddy* Daddy: (Gives toddler attention and hugs)
Motivating Operation	Mand	Direct reinforcement by receiving requested item	Mary: (feels thirsty) *Juice please* Mother: (Provides Mary with juice) Tara: (unable to tie shoe) *Help!* Mother: (helps Tara tie her shoe)
Environmental Stimulus	Tact	General Social Reinforcement	Martin: (sees a hot air balloon) *Look, a balloon!* Mother: (Looks at the hot air baloon) *Yes! A big one!*
Verbal Behavior	Intraverbal/ Sequelic	General Social reinforcement	Adult: *How old are you?* Carson: *Four years.* *This many* (holds up four fingers) Adult: *You are a smart kid!*
Environmental Stimulus or Verbal Behavior	Autoclitic	Direct Reinforcement	Mike: (sees two cars) <u>*May*</u> *I* <u>*please*</u> *have the red car?* Dad: (gives Mike the red car) Dad: *Look at that car!* Mike: *I see <u>five</u> cars.* Dad: *The one turning the corner.*
Environmental Stimulus	Textual Responding	General social reinforcement	Scott: (looking at a stop sign) *stop* Mom: *You're a good reader!*

Echoic—Repeating what is heard. It is a hear-say response reflecting point-to-point correspondence with the antecedent VB.

Mand—Asking for a specific reinforcement when deprived (e.g., being hungry) or when annoyed (e.g., trying to listen in a noisy environment)

Tact—Naming or identifying objects, actions, events, etc. that are seen. This is a see-say response.

Intraverbal/Sequelics—An utterance is controlled by words in a previous utterance. This is a hear-say response with no point-to-point correspondence to the previous utterance. It can occur in a conversation in as a response to another speaker or as a response to one's own previous utterance.

Autoclitic—A primary verbal behavior (mand, tact, echoic, intraverbal) containing qualifying information that further specifies a listener's interpretation. For example, tacting with qualifiers ("Look at the <u>blue</u> car on the road) or manding with politeness markers ("Pass the cookies <u>please</u>"). This can be a see-say or hear-say type of response.

Textual Responding—Verbal behavior under the control of print. This is a see (print)-say response.

Source: Adapted from L. Frost and A. Bondy (2006). A common language: Using B.F. Skinner's *Verbal Behavior* for assessment and treatment of communication disabilities in SLP-ABA. *Journal of Speech-Language Pathology and Applied Behavior Analysis, 2–3,* 103–110. http://www.behavior-analyst-today.com/SLP-ABA-VOL-1/SLP-ABA-1-2.pdf; R. D. Greer and D. E. Ross (2008). *Verbal behavior analysis: Inducing and expanding new verbal capabilities in children with language delays.* New York, NY: Pearson, Allyn & Bacon.

These units are known as **echoic**, **mand**, **tact**, **intra-verbal/sequelic**, **autoclitic**, and **textual**, respectively. Each is defined by its controlling variables within the three-term contingency.

Looking at Table 4–18, you may notice that a number of the VB functions are similar to functions included in the developmental psycholinguistic framework. For example, "echoic," "mand," and "tact" are comparable to "imitation," "requesting," and "naming." Skinner chose to use words that were different from those used in casual English, because he wanted to define each VB function precisely in relation to its unique pattern of controlling variables (antecedents and consequences). In fact, it is important to note that the term "function" has a different meaning in the developmental and the behavioral literature. Developmentally, a communicative function refers to the goal that a communicator seeks to meet by producing a signal. In the behavioral literature, the term "function" refers to the verbal behavior and its controlling variables (antecedents, consequences).

All the VB functions in Table 4–16 are expected in the repertoires of preschool children, including textual responding. Although most preschoolers are not fluent readers, many can recognize their names and the names of a few words that are routinely embedded in their environmental experiences (e.g., *stop*, *McDonald's*, *Toys-R-Us*, *Exit*, etc.).

In summary, we presented two frameworks for conceptualizing the development of communicative functions expressed by young children. The developmental framework is helpful for conceptualizing the continuity between prelinguistic communication and subsequent language development. The behavioral framework is helpful for analyzing developmental obstacles experienced by children who do not follow the normal pattern (e.g., Frost & Bondy, 2006; Greer & Ross, 2007). For some of these children, a word that is learned as a tact (e.g., saying *juice* to label juice) may not generalize spontaneously to function as a mand (e.g., saying *juice* to request juice). A developmental analysis that simply notes the words in a child's vocabulary and the range of communicative functions expressed by the child would miss this deficit. Therefore, an analysis of VB functions can be a helpful tool for pinpointing learning deficits and for suggesting possible solutions.

The Social Context (Discourse Development)

In contrast to utterance-level communicative functions, **discourse** refers to a sequence of utterances that are related to the same topic. Discourse can occur in the form of a **dialogue** when conversational partners are discussing the same topic. It also can occur in the form of a **monologue** when one person is producing a string of related utterances to share an experience, tell a story, or even to think outloud. Depending on their functions, monologues can be further classified as **narratives** (when they function to share experiences or stories) or **expository forms** (e.g., when they function to inform or instruct). Additionally, young children produce monologues that function as **language play** and **private speech** (i.e., thinking outloud). In this section, we look more closely at dialogue discourse, narrative discourse, and private speech.

Dialogue Discourse

The philosopher Paul Grice (1975) described five **conversational maxims** (i.e., rules of conduct) to which mature conversational partners adhere. These are summarized in Table 4–19. Included are maxims pertaining to quantity (say enough, but not too much), quality (be truthful), relevance (stay on topic), and manner (be clear, organized, and brief). During the preschool period, children's demonstrate emerging abilities to follow the rules of relevance.

Initially, toddlers produce single utterances while interacting with their conversational partners. As during the prelinguistic period, caregivers continue to scaffold their children's responses during the emerging and early language period. They do so by following their child's focus of attention, offering verbal commentary, and using conversational devices (e.g., questioning, modeling) to maintain the dialogue. Consider the following interaction between 20-month-old Kyle and his mother during play:

1. Kyle: (looking at blocks in his hand)

2. Mother: *What do you have?*

3. Kyle: (Puts blocks on floor)

4. Mother: *Blocks.*
   Are you going to build?

TABLE 4–19. Grice's (1975) Conversational Maxims

Maxim of Quantity:

1. Make your contribution to the conversation as informative as necessary.

2. Do not make your contribution to the conversation more informative than necessary.

Maxim of Quality:

1. Do not say what you believe to be false.

2. Do not say that for which you lack adequate evidence.

Maxim of Relevance:

Be relevant (i.e., say things related to the current topic of the conversation).

Maxim of Manner:

1. Avoid obscurity of expression.

2. Avoid ambiguity.

3. Be brief (avoid unnecessary wordiness).

4. Be orderly.

Source: Based on H. P. Grice (1975). Logic and conversation. In P. Cole & J. L. Morgan (Eds.), *Syntax and semantics, Vol. 3: Speech acts.* New York, NY: Academic Press.

5. Kyle: *Make tower*

6. Mother: (stabilizing a block) *Make a big tower!*

7. Kyle: (trying to stack blocks)

8. Mother: (helping) *put it on.*

9. Kyle: *up, up, up*

10. Mother: *Yes, build it up high*!

11. Kyle: *Boom!* (bashes the tower)

The exchange begins within a play interaction where Kyle picks up some wooden blocks (line 1). Notice how his mother scaffolds Kyle's continued participation in dialogue over six consecutive turns. First, she responds (line 2) by asking a question about the objects to which Kyle is attending. When he fails to respond (line 3), she models an answer for him (line 4) and asks another question. When Kyle replies (line 5), his mother expands the answer (line 6). In the absence of a follow-up verbal response by Kyle (line 7), she labels his ongoing action (line 8). When

Kyle responds to this (line 9), his mother again expands his comments. Clearly, the play activity serves as the shared topic to which all of the utterances refer, and Kyle's mother structures comments and questions to invite and maintain the dialogue.

Toddlers are effective at **initiating topics** of interest to them, particularly when there are contextual cues to help a listener understand the utterance. However, they need support for maintaining and extending the conversational topic. With support, and experience, they gradually become more responsive to conversational partners. By the age of 3 years, children demonstrate an overall increase in the amount of talkativeness, and they become capable of sustaining conversational topics over a larger number of volleys. (A **volley** is a conversational turn that maintains the topic of the conversational partner's previous utterance.) By this time, they also are able to engage in conversational turn taking with peers (Ervin-Tripp, 1979; Keenan & Kline, 1975).

A number of studies have demonstrated improvements in children's **topic maintenance** during the emerging language to preschool period (e.g., L. Bloom, Rocissano, & Hood, 1976; Wanska & Bedrosian, 1985). For example, L. Bloom et al. studied the topic maintenance patterns of four children ages 21 to 36 months and varying in grammatical maturity (Brown's stages I, II, and V). All children were observed during child-mother play interactions. Individual child utterances were transcribed and coded according to whether they occurred **adjacent** to or **nonadjacent** to (i.e., independent of) an adult utterance. Additionally, all adjacent utterances were coded as to whether they were **noncontingent** (i.e., unrelated to the topic of the adjacent utterance), **imitative** (i.e., repeating information in the adjacent utterance), or **contingent** (expanding the topic of the adjacent utterance). Not surprisingly, the authors found that nonadjacent utterances accounted for the highest proportion of utterances produced by the children at stages I and II, whereas contingent utterances accounted for the highest proportion of utterances by children at stage V. Additionally, the proportion of noncontingent and imitative utterances decreased as the proportion of contingent utterances increased at stage V. Wanska and Bedrosian (1985) also noted that children between about 3 years and 6 years used topic shading increasingly often. **Topic shading** is a type of contingent utterance in which some aspect of the topic is preserved while a new feature of the topic is introduced. The following is an example:

Mother: *Let's make a tall building* (referring to blocks)

Child: *Daddy work in big building.*

It is easier to describe the general increase in contingent utterances as children mature than it is to predict even the average number of topically related utterances that might be expected at particular ages or levels of grammatical maturity, because reports have varied. For example, Bloom, Rocissano, and Hood, (1976) reported that the 3-year-olds in their study maintained conversational topics for more than two volleys. Byrne and Hayden (1980) observed that children between 3 to 5 years old produced from five to seven topic-related utterances in conversation with their mothers; and Owens (2008) reported that 50% of 3-year-olds can sustain a topic for up to 12 or more consecutive volleys. The variations between these estimates reflect (among other things) differences in the contexts of the observations on which the estimates are based. Similar to adults, children are likely to sustain a topic over a longer number of volleys if they are interested in the topic, if they are motivated to interact with their conversational partner, if their conversational partner is willing to support them, and if the environment is free of other events to compete for the child's attention. So, a 3-year-old in conversation with a caregiver who follows the child's lead and supports the child's participation is likely to sustain a topic over a larger number of volleys than a 3-year-old who is conversing about a more neutral topic with a less familiar conversational partner.

Conversations between preschool peers are interesting to consider, as peers lack the maturity and the range of shared experiences that enable mothers to scaffold topic maintenance when interacting with their young children. A classic study by Garvey and Hogan (1973) described conversations between dyads involving 3- to 5-year-olds during a free play activity. These children exchanged between 4 to 12 utterances around the same topic. Schober-Peterson and Johnson (1989) found similar patterns among dyads involving 4-year-olds. Seventy-five percent of the topics discussed by these children involved fewer than 12 consecutive utterances. However, some topics were maintained over 13 to 91 consecutive utterances. These results indicate that there is considerable variability in the number of utterances exchanged by peers around a single topic.

Although maintenance is a key feature of dialogue discourse, other features are also important. For example, successful **topic initiation** improves as children are better able to judge how much information a listener needs to understand the reference to a topic removed from the here and now. Improvements also occur in **conversational repair**. This requires a speaker to revise an utterance to resolve a misunderstanding that occurred within the dialogue. Repair strategies have been studied by a number of researchers (e.g., Anselmi, Tomasello, & Acunzo, 1986; Brinton, Fujuki, Loab, & Winkler, 1986; Furrow & Lewis, 1987; Gallagher, 1977; Tomasello, Farrar, & Dines, 1984; Wilcox & Webster, 1980). In one of the first studies, Gallagher (1977) observed children varying in age (from 20 to 30 months) and in linguistic maturity (Brown's stages I, II, and III) during conversation with an adult. Clarification was requested by the adult who asked, "*What?*" following 20 child utterances in a 60-minute period. All of the children revised the majority of the utterances that were followed by a clarification request. Their strategies included phonological revisions (i.e., saying the same word again with clearer articulation); elaboration (i.e., providing more information about the topic), substitutions (i.e., using a word with similar meaning to state the idea in another way), or reduction (i.e., repeating the same idea in fewer words). However, the older children's repairs were more sophisticated. Table 4–20 provides examples of these repair strategies.

By the age of 5 years, verbal turn-taking abilities continue to improve within a dialog context. Children can initiate and end topics appropriately and sustain topics for extended periods. At this age, children also are willing to give up their own conversational turn to avoid simultaneous talking and to preserve the topic. Moreover, they can predict the direction in which a topic may move, and may help a conversational partner finish a statement if it appears that the partner is having difficulty (Hulit & Howard, 2006).

TABLE 4–20. Examples of Conversational Repair Strategies

Type of Repair	Example
Phonological Revision	C: I see a poon A: What? C: I see a spoon
Deletion	C: There's a red car? A: What? C: The red car
Substitution	C: She's drinking milk A: What? C: Mommy's drinking milk
Linguistic Revision	C: Mine is little A: What? C: I have a mall one

Source: Based on T. Gallagher (1977), Revision behaviors in the speech of normal children developing language. *Journal of Speech and Hearing Research, 20,* 303–318.

Despite these considerable advances in children's verbal turn taking, limitations remain. Specifically, preschoolers may have difficulty taking turns in the context of triadic or small-group interactions. In these contexts, children may revert to less mature patterns of turn taking (Hulit & Howard, 2006). They also have difficulty using appropriate ways to gain a listener's attention and are likely to interrupt others inappropriately. Children who attend preschool or other group-based child-care arrangements have the opportunity to learn patterns of turn taking required in small group contexts and to learn appropriate ways to gain someone's attention.

Narrative Discourse

Discourse development includes not only conversational turn taking (**dialogue discourse**) but also the ability to formulate narratives. In the simplest terms, **narrative discourse** consists of utterances used to retell a past experience (Hughes, McGillivray, & Schmidek, 1997; Liles, 1993; McCabe & Rollins, 1994). The experience may be real (e.g., telling about a trip to the zoo) or fictional (e.g., retelling a story one has read or heard). Narrative language serves as an important means of connecting with others and as a bridge to the development of literacy skills.

Although all narratives have an event sequence at their core, 14 different subtypes have been identified (e.g., Engel, 1995; Heath, 1986; Hughes, McGillivray, & Schmidek, 1997; Peterson & McCabe, 1983; Preece, 1987). The five noted most frequently are described here. The first, known as a **recount**, is prompted by others and used to share an experience. For example, a child might be prompted by his or her mother to, "*Tell Daddy what we did at the store.*" Similarly, a teacher might ask a student to, "*Tell us about your summer vacation*" as part of a show-and-tell event. When a child, in response to a request, describes an experience that happened to someone else, this is also considered to be a recount. Recounts characteristically describe an atypical event (e.g., a trip to an amusement park) rather than a predictable and routine activity of daily living (e.g., brushing one's teeth).

A second narrative subtype is known as an **account.** Accounts are produced spontaneously to describe an experience. They differ from recounts primarily by the fact that they are generated spontaneously rather than being prompted by a listener. Accounts typically are used to share information that the listener did not experience with the speaker. Accounts sometimes are known as **personal narratives** or **personal event narratives**.

A third narrative subtype is known as an **event cast**. This involves a description of ongoing activity. For example, the speaker may describe a game that he or she is observing (e.g., *It's Gillian's turn. She's rolling the dice. She rolled a six. It looks like she will win.*). Event cast narratives also may be used to structure an ongoing pretend play activity (e.g., "*We're riding on a train. Here comes our stop. Now we're getting off . . .* ").

A fourth narrative subtype is a **story** consisting of a fictional account of animate beings who are engaged in goal-oriented behavior. Stories typically have an overall organization (macrostructure) that can include a beginning, middle, and end. Stein and Glenn (1979) conceptualized the beginning as the setting (e.g., time and place, main characters, protagonist, and one or more goals), and the middle as an episode structure involving one or more episodes. Each episode includes an initiating event that interferes with the protagonist's goal, reactions, plans, an attempt to resolve the problem, and a result. A story's end may be marked by the protagonist's final reaction, a conclusion, a lesson, or just by the words "the end."

A fifth narrative subtype is known as the **verbal script**, and it includes a verbal account of what typically happens in a situation. Scripts are based on a child's routine experiences and usually are told in the present tense. They may be produced in response to a prompt (e.g., "*Tell Grandpa how we work the DVD player*"). They differ from recounts in that they are used to describe typical or routine experiences, and they sometimes are known as **procedural discourse**. As such, they come closest of all narrative types to a type of **expository discourse**.

The **development of narrative discourse** involves a complex intertwining of influences from cultural, social, cognitive, and linguistic domains. Many children begin to produce narratives by the time they are about 27 months old (McCabe & Peterson, 1991). At first, their narratives tend to include only one past event. By 36 months, they may include two events. By the age of 4 years, narratives are expanded to include an increasing amount of information. At this time, some children initially use a "**leapfrogging**" pattern where events are not described in the order of occurrence; important events may be skipped; and some events may seem contradictory (McCabe & Peterson, 1983). Below is an example of leapfrogging produced by a 4-year-old in a study by Peterson (1994, p. 265)

R [Researcher]: *Tell me what happened to your arm.*

C [Child]: *He picked me up last morning. I was gone to the doctor.*

R: *He picked you up when you went to the doctor?*

C: *Yep*

R: *What happened to your arm?*

C: *I fell down.*

(discussion about present activity)

R: *Tell me about when you fell down and hurt your arm. Tell me what happened.*

C: *The cops picked me up. That fell down.*

R: *The cops picked you up?*

C: *I was gone school.*

R: *You were gone to school.*

C: *And the bus picked me up.*

R: *The bus picked you up.*

C: *And I was (..?..). And Robert comed with me. And Robert comed with me.*

R: *Robert came with you. Uh huh?*

C: *He came with my school.*

R: *Yeah?*

C: *And he dressed me up.*

Eisenberg (1985) described the changes she observed in the development of event sharing (recounting, accounting) by two young, Spanish-speaking girls while interacting with their caregivers. Based on these data, she identified three phases in the emergence of event sharing. In Phase I, caregivers prompt the narratives and supply a rich amount of scaffolding. Below is an example of this pattern based on my own experience with an English-speaking 36-month-old:

Mother: *Tell Grandpa where we went today.*

Child: *Hershey Park*

Mother: *What did we do there?*

Child: *ride a train*

Mother: *We rode the Chocolate train. What else?*

Child: *ride a bump car*

Mother: *You and Dad rode a bumper car. Was it fun?*

Child: (silent)

Mother: *Did you have fun?*

Child: *have fun*

In Phase II, children gradually learn to rely less on the questions asked by adults and include more information spontaneously. However, when recounting a specific event, they sometimes combine general information from their script knowledge with specific information about the event. For example, if asked to tell about a specific trip to the zoo, they may include common details about zoos that were not a part of the specific event they are sharing. During Phase III, children produce accounts that are independent of prompting and free of script information.

Changes in narrative language are also observed when young children interact with their peers. Umiker-Sebeok (1979) observed 3-, 4-, and 5-year-olds in preschool during peer interactions. Changes were observed in the percentage of conversations that included narratives (23% at 3 years vs. 35% at 5 years), in the average length of narratives (1.7 clauses at 3 years vs. 2.8 clauses at 5 years), and in the complexity of the narratives (e.g., at 4 years children began to include more elements of story structure).

All types of narratives involve past or fictional event sequences. However, the **macrostructure** (i.e., the manner in which event sequences are introduced, organized, and ended) may differ somewhat across narrative types. We noted this earlier in the case of fictional narratives for which the macrostructure (also known as **story grammar**) typically includes a setting and an episode sequence (Stein & Glenn, 1979) beginning with an initiating event, followed by a reaction, a plan, an attempt, and an outcome. The number of episodes in an episode sequence may very from one to many. Table 4–21 provides an example based on a story by Paola (1978) called *Pancakes for Breakfast*. Notice that the episode sequence in this example includes three related episodes. At the end of a story, typically,

TABLE 4–21. Examples of Narrative Structure Elements

Macrostructure Elements		Example (based on *Pancakes for Breakfast* by de Paola, 1978)
Setting (introduction of characters, location, time)		A lady wakes up one morning thinking about making delicious pancakes for breakfast in her kitchen.
Episode Structure (may include one or more initiating events, reactions, plans, attempts, and outcomes and a reaction)	**Initiating Event #1**	When she goes to her kitchen, she sees that there are no eggs, milk, or butter
	Reaction	She's disappointed
	Plan	She decides to buy the items
	Attempt	She goes to the store
	Outcome	She buys the items, brings them home, and makes pancakes
	Initiating Event #2	After making the pancakes she discovers she has no syrup
	Reaction	She's disappointed because pancakes need syrup
	Plan	She decides to buy some syrup at the syrup store.
	Attempt	She purchases the syrup
	Outcome	She takes the syrup home
	Initiating Event #3	She discovers that her dog and cat have eaten the pancakes
	Reaction	She's angry and disappointed
	Plan	She decides to visit her neighbors and see what they have for breakfast
	Attempt	The neighbors invite her in for pancakes
	Outcome	The pancakes are delicious
Final Reaction (may include lessons learned)		She's happy. Lesson: If at first you don't succeed, try, try again

there is a final reaction and sometimes a lesson to be learned, as in the example on Table 4–21.

Narratives also have a **microstructure** that consists of the words and sentences used to represent specific elements of the macrostructure. These linguistic features allow a listener who is unfamiliar with the story to reconstruct it accurately from the words alone. Important ingredients of the microstructure include the **cohesion markers** (i.e., words and grammatical structures) that enable a speaker to introduce new story elements, refer back to previous story elements, and connect information across successive clauses and sentences in a manner that is clear and logically coherent (e.g., Halliday & Hassan, 1976). The following example illustrates the use of a pronoun (*she*) in the first position of the second sentence for establishing a cohesive intersentential tie with a referent (*a cat named Katrina*) in the first sentence.

Once upon a time a <u>cat named Katrina</u> wandered into a strange house. <u>She</u> sniffed the ground and looked around to see what she could find . . .

The skillful use of microstructure elements requires a level of cognitive maturity, social perspective taking, and linguistic sophistication that continues to emerge throughout elementary school.

Clearly, the formulation of narratives is a complex undertaking. In fact, the ability to share stories and events only begins to develop during the preschool period. Refinement and expansion of narrative forms continues from elementary school through high school. Opportunities to engage in oral narrative formulation and to participate with others in shared storybook reading support this process and provide a bridge for the later development of reading comprehension and written language formulation.

Finally, it is important to note that there are **cultural variations** in children's development of narratives. One source of variation pertains to the amount of detail that children include in their narratives. For example, middle-class American English-speaking children typically are encouraged to produce narratives that are long, detailed, and explicit. In contrast, Japanese children are encouraged to produce narratives that, like Haiku poetry, are succinct and implicit (Minami & McCabe, 1995). This narrative style is accomplished by omitting pronouns and other information that can be inferred in context by a listener. Japanese mothers encourage this succinct style of narration by asking fewer questions, requesting less information, and providing more frequent acknowledgments, which actually interrupt their children's speech. Below is an example of a narrative produced by a 4-year-old Japanese girl to describe an injury that she experienced. The example was transcribed by Masahiko Minami (in McCabe & Bliss, 2003). Omissions in the narrative are shown in parentheses: "(I) bled. (I) had (it) cleaned. That was good. (I) was alright," (p. 92).

Another source of variation pertains to the topic structure of narratives. For example, the narratives of middle-class American children often are characterized as **topic centered**, whereas the narratives of some African American children have been described **as topic associating** (Heath, 1986; Michaels, 1983). In other words, instead of elaborating ideas around one central topic, some African American children tend to structure their narratives by describing loosely connected sequences of personal anecdotes. This style is also known as **performative narration**, because each of the associated topics is unified by tempo and/or tone (Champion, 1998). Not all African American children use a topic associating style, and some use other features of narration that differ from the narratives of mainstream American children in other ways. Excellent descriptions and examples of these and other variations can be found in McCabe and Bliss (2003). It is important for teachers and speech-language pathologists to be aware of these variations so that they are not misinterpreted as aberrant patterns.

Theory of Mind (ToM)

Both dialogue and narrative discourse require a speaker to make adjustments in consideration of a listener's perspective. The ability to do this requires a child to take the listener's perspective. Perspective taking is associated with **theory of mind (ToM)**, an aspect of social-cognitive knowledge defined as the understanding that (1) each individual has a unique set of perspectives and agendas and (2) the behavior of others can be predicted and explained on the basis of these unique mental states (Baron-Cohen, 2000; Baron-Cohen, Tager-Flusberg, & Cohen, 1993, 2003). ToM is basic to all aspects of successful communication (oral and written). For example, ToM skills prompt us to choose topics of interest or relevance to our conversational partners, to provide the right amount of information, to select words and sentences that match the partner's comprehension level, to avoid boring them with too much information, and to refrain from confusing them or hurting their feelings.

Development of ToM Skills

Development of Attention and Perspective Taking. Like other aspects of cognition and language, ToM skills develop gradually and become evident in an increasing range of contexts. The earliest manifestation of ToM may be seen in the emergence of **joint attention** during the prelinguistic period (e.g., Carpenter, Nagell, & Tomasello, 1998; Tomasello, 1995). It also is evident in children's initial comprehension of lexical forms (Tomasello, 1995). Recall that infants initially look to their caregivers for cues regarding the referents of the words they hear.

By about 18 months, children begin to demonstrate greater sensitivity to the perspective of others. They begin to use words such as *want*, *wish*, and *hope* to refer to their own and their partner's mental states (Repacholi & Gopnik, 1997). They also begin to talk and act as if different persons may have different desires. For example, children can acknowledge that they prefer one kind of food (e.g., crackers) but that another person wants a different kind of food (e.g., broccoli) (Repacholi & Gopnik, 1997). By about 30 months, toddlers begin to use words like *think*, and *know* in a truly mentalistic sense to refer to the beliefs held by different agents (Bartsch & Wellman, 1995; Wellman, 1991). Also by the age of about 30 months, toddlers begin to engage in pretend play that includes acting out social roles that differ from their own (Youngblade & Dunn, 1995). Still, at this age, children think that people always behave in ways consistent with their desires and they do not understand that beliefs affect their actions (Bartsch & Wellman, 1995).

Between 3 and 4 years old, children's beliefs about how the mind works become increasingly differentiated. By 3 years, they begin to appreciate simple causal relations among desires, outcomes, emotions, and actions. For example, they seem to understand that people will feel good if they get what they want and that they will feel bad if they do not (Bartsch & Wellman in Flavell, 2004). Similarly, they begin to understand that desires and beliefs can influence actions. For example, by the time they are 4 years old, children understand that people may have **false beliefs** that combine with desire to influence their behavior (Perner, 1991). This has been demonstrated in various ways (Baron-Cohen, Tager-Flusberg, & Cohen, 2000; Miller, 2006). In a study by Perner, Leekam, and Wimmer (1987), 3- and 4-year-olds were shown a closed box with a label depicting Smarties Candy Rolls. When the experimenter asked the children what they thought was inside the box, they said Smarties candy, but when the box was opened, the children saw that it actually contained a pencil. Next, they were told to close the box (with the pencil still inside) and to predict what an adult (not yet present in the room) would say was inside if he or she were shown the same box now. Four-year-olds (but not 3-year-olds) reliably predicted that the adult would say there were Smarties in the box. This pattern of responding suggests that the 4-year-olds can subordinate their own knowledge about an event to consider what another person thinks.

In a study by Sodian (1991), children ages 2½ to 4 years were invited to drive a toy truck to the other side of a small sandbox and then to hide the truck driver under one of five cups lined up on a shelf along the edge of the sandbox. The experimenter instructed the children to hide the man so that an adult (who was currently out of the room) would not be able to find him when the adult came into the room. The experimenter pointed out to all of the children that the truck left telltale tracks in the sand, showing where it had been. In the end, 4-year-olds (but not 2- or 3-year-olds) smoothed the sand so that the adult would not see the truck's tracks. Some children even laid false tracks to mislead the adult into thinking that the driver was under a different cup. Sensitivity to false beliefs and their impact on behavior strengthens throughout the preschool period and beyond (Flavell, 1999; Flavell & Miller, 1998; Wellman, Cross, & Watson, 2001). Mastery of this concept is an important developmental milestone, because it indicates that a child recognizes beliefs as a basis for interpretations (Berk, 2006).

Development of Visual Perspective Taking. So far, we have reviewed the sequence of developments pertaining to children's understanding of other people's thoughts. A closely related series of developments pertains to the emerging appreciation of the **visual perspective of others**. Toddlers begin using vision-related words (e.g., *see*) correctly as early as 18 months. Soon thereafter, they learn that a person will see an object if and only if the person's eyes are open and aimed in its direction and if there are no vision-blocking objects between the person and the target object (Flavell, 1992). With this information, they can infer that others may see something that they (the child) cannot see, or that they (the child) can see something that another person cannot see. This type of inference is known as **Level I knowledge** about visual perception (Flavell, 1992). Later in the preschool period, children come to recognize that two people may look at the same object and see different parts of it if they are standing in different positions in relation to the object. This is known as **Level II knowledge** (Flavell, 1992). Awareness of both levels can help a child make decisions about how to describe objects to a conversational partner and how to understand another person's descriptions.

Linguistic Forms That Encode Perspective. Because all aspects of social communication are influenced by a speaker's sensitivity to a listener's perspective, it is somewhat artificial to highlight specific forms. However, several forms do directly encode assumptions about the perspective of a conversational partner, and they are summarized briefly here. **Deictic terms** fit this criterion. Recall that deictic terns are words whose referent shifts depending on the speaker. For example, the referent of pronouns (*I, you*) and certain adverbs (e.g., *here, there*) extend to different referents depending on the speaker. The ability to acquire these terms involves an understanding of speaker listener perspective.

Ellipsis, which also requires ToM skills, is a discourse cohesion device that enables a speaker to connect two separate utterances by deleting the topic from the second utterance. Consider, for example, the following exchange between a server and a customer in a restaurant:

Server: *How do you like your steak?*

Customer: [I like my steak] *Well done*

Notice that the customer's reply depends on a **presupposition** that the server understands the unspoken words (provided here in brackets). Ellipsis reduces redundancy and extends the meaning from one utterance to another.

Other patterns of discourse must be finely tuned to a listener's perspective for communication to occur successfully. Included here are **responses to clarification requests.** Responses to clarification requests can be successful only if the speaker provides the listener with the information that he or she needs to resolve a misunderstanding or ambiguity. To do this, the speaker needs to know why a misunderstanding occurred. We often make such assumptions accurately without explicitly asking the conversational partner, but sometimes it is necessary to ask. Please refer to the discussion of clarification patterns under discourse functions above. For an example of how referential communication can become hopelessly confused when conversational partners fail to consider each other's perspectives, we invite you to review the hilarious and celebrated example of Abbot and Costello's comedic portrayal of a dialogue between Sebation Dinwiddle (peanut salesman) and Dexter Broadhurt (manager of a baseball team) called, "*Who's on First.*" This dialogue can be accessed at the following Web sites in print and on video: http://www.baseball-almanac .com/humor4.shtml, http://www.youtube.com/ watch?v=sShMA85pv8M

Like dialogue discourse, **narrative discourse** requires multiple adjustments to a conversational partner's perspective. This becomes increasingly true as children learn to share fictional stories about imaginary characters, places, and events. Storytelling involves the verbal formulation of an event sequence so that a listener who did not read the story can recreate the images in his or her imagination. It becomes crucial for the storyteller to represent the characters, settings, and events in a way that is clear from the perspective of the listener.

Finally, **speech registers** also involve a collection of adjustments to meet the needs of the conversational partner's overall perspective. These are discussed later in this chapter under the topic of sociolinguistic functions.

In summary, in this section we provided a thumbnail sketch of selected issues pertaining to ToM. Further information about ToM development is available in many excellent references on this topic (Baron-Cohen, Tager-Flusberg, & Cohen, 2000; Farrar & Maag; 2002; Hale & Tager-Flussberg, 2003; Miller, 2006; Tomasello, 1999). Issues of perspective taking become increasingly important as children transition from preschool to kindergarten and elementary school. In these contexts, they will encounter an increasing number of conversational partners with whom they have less shared experience. To share experiences with a larger number of peers, they will be required to formulate narratives. Throughout the school years, they will be asked to formulate oral and written narratives using an oral literate style of language, requiring them to consider the perspectives of readers who are not even present in the environment. Some of the issues are considered in the next chapter.

Private Speech

A type of discourse that on the surface seems to require little ToM knowledge is **private speech:** speech that is spoken either to oneself or to no particular listener (Zivin, 1979). Piaget characterized such utterances as **egocentric speech** because he believed that children were speaking to others but were failing to adjust their language to a listener's perspective (Ginsberg & Opper, 1969). However, a preponderance of evidence over 40 years of research has supported the interpretation of this behavior as private speech (Berk, 1992).

Vygotsky (1934/1962) regarded private speech as a tool for self-guidance and self-direction. Consistent with this view, the frequency of private speech has been found to increases when children are engaged in challenging tasks, when they make errors, or when they are confused about how to proceed (Berk, 1994). For example, one of the authors (MK) observed young preschoolers who, while attempting to place geometric shapes into matching spaces

on a puzzle grid, say things like, "*That goes here. Uh oh! Not there! That's ok. Try again. Put it here.*" In a sense, these utterances sound like an event cast, but they are not addressed to anyone in particular.

Studies have shown that private speech follows a developmental progression (Bivens & Berk, 1990; Duncan & Pratt, 1997). During the preschool period, most private speech is completely audible. As children mature, its production occurs in whispers and sometimes can be seen only as small lip movements. Eventually, it becomes inaudible. Children who use task-related private speech in challenging situations are more attentive, more involved, and show greater improvement in their performance than children who use private speech less often (Behrend, Rosengren, & Perlmutter, 1992; Berk & Spuhl, 1995). Moreover, children with learning problems tend to engage in higher rates of audible private speech over a longer period of time (Berk & Landau, 1993; Diaz & Berk, 1992), and this is considered a positive accommodation to their learning challenges.

Vygotsky proposed that private speech, like all aspects of discourse, originates in the context of child-caregiver interaction. As discussed in the previous chapter, caregivers tend to structure activities with their children within the **zone of proximal development (ZPD)**. The ZPD is a level of task difficulty just above a child's independent capabilities but in which a child can succeed if provided with a small amount of scaffolding. Within such contexts, caregivers encourage their children to succeed by providing a small amount of prompting and verbal encouragement. For example, while working on a geometric puzzle, a caregiver might say, "*Try the circle. Does it fit? Uh oh. Maybe not. That's ok. Try another one. Good job, you did it!*" Children internalize these models and repeat variations of them when confronted with a challenging task to complete independently.

As children learn to regulate their behavior in this way, private speech becomes a tool for thinking. It also provides one basis for the later developments of metacognitive awareness and executive function. **Metacognitive awareness** is the ability to reflect on the products and processes of one's own thoughts. For example, it includes knowing how much information you can store in memory and at what point you will need to take notes. Another example is to know what strategies you may need to use to understand new information. If you are reading a textbook, do you need to make an outline? Keep track of key words? Draw pictures?

We began our discussion of private speech by suggesting that, on the surface, private speech seems to require little ToM knowledge. However, private speech is not entirely unrelated to ToM. Fernyhough and Meins (2009) proposed three possible relationships between the two. First, recognizing that one's behavior can be regulated through private speech involves some of the same social awareness as the recognition that mental states can be influenced by information. Second, the process of using private speech provides children with opportunities to experience themselves as thinking agents. Third, the content of private speech may include internalized dialogues between the child and his or her social partners. This process requires the child to take on the "voice" as well as the perspective of the other. Preliminary data reported by Fernyhough and Meins indicates that 3- and 4-year-olds who are more advanced in the use of self-regulatory private speech also tend to score higher on measures of ToM. However, by the age of 5 to 6 years, the overt use of self-regulatory private speech appears to decrease whereas the performance on ToM tasks tends to increase.

Private speech is also closely related to **executive function**, which is "an umbrella term for all of the complex set of cognitive processes that underlie flexible goal-directed responses to novel or difficult situations" (Hughes & Graham, 2002, p. 131). According to Müller, Jacques, Brocki, and Zelazo (2009), executive function begins when language acquired in the service of social communication begins to function as a tool for goal-oriented self-regulation. Vygotsky (1962/1934) considered every newly acquired word to be a "microcosm of human consciousness" (p. 153), and as language leads to consciousness, it is the conscious use of self-directed language that leads to purposeful, goal-directed behavior (Müller et al., 2009). As children mature, executive function includes **metacognition** as a basis for planning, monitoring, and adjusting strategies for task completion. For example, assume you need to study for a test. After reflecting on your own learning style, you may plan a preparation strategy that includes reviewing five pages of notes

each day for two weeks. As you follow your plan, you will monitor your progress. If you find that the task takes longer than you thought, you may adjust your plan in some way to become more efficient. Maybe you will pick a place to study where there are fewer distractions. Maybe you will study at a time of day when you are more alert. And if you are less successful than you had hoped, you will consider the strengths and limitations of your strategy when planning for the next test. Private speech is only the beginning of higher level thinking skills. Executive function and metacognitive awareness develop extensively during the school years and into adulthood.

Sociolinguistic Functions

Dialects

The sociolinguistic skills of a competent language user include knowledge of dialects and registers. **Dialects** are variations in language that are influenced by the geographical, cultural, and even gender identification of a speaker. Our discussion is limited to geographical and cultural variations. For example, individuals who acquire language in New Orleans, Louisiana use a distinctly different dialect than individuals who acquire language in Brooklyn, New York or Peoria, IL. Cultural differences can be appreciated by comparing the speech and language of individuals who have learned Spanish-influenced English with the speech and language of those who have learned General American English (GAE).

Geographic and cultural dialects differ from the dominant form of a language in all components of language (form, content, and use). For example, when compared to speakers of GAE, individuals who acquire English in the Philadelphia area tend to demonstrate subtle differences in phonology. Their vocabulary choices tend to differ in some respects (e.g., "hoagie" vs. "submarine"; "pocketbook" vs. "purse"). They tend to use some different syntactic patterns (e.g., "I'm done the dishes" vs. "I'm done with the dishes") and there may be differences in language use.

Because we all acquire the language of our local social communities, we all acquire a dialect. No dialect is superior to another on linguistic grounds, and users of all dialects have the advantage of signaling their community membership through their dialect. However, some dialects are shared by a larger number of speakers (e.g., GAE) than others (e.g., Pennsylvania Dutch). In that sense, knowledge of the dominant dialect enables a speaker to communicate more easily with a larger community.

Everyone who participates in the delivery of services to children with disabilities needs to be aware of dialectical variations, to honor the cultural roots from which the variations arise, and to consider these variations if questions are raised about the developmental status of a child's language skills. Later in this book, we discuss strategies for addressing questions about the language development of children from different linguistic backgrounds.

Registers

Registers are variations in the style of communication to fit the needs of a listener or of the social situation. Most adults use a variety of registers throughout the course of the day. For example, we have already discussed a register known as motherese, which results from adjustments made by speakers communicating with young children who have fewer experiences and less knowledge about language. Another kind of register is required of adults in a working situation. Think, for example, about the technical vocabulary necessary for engineers to communicate with each other about the structure and function of electronic equipment. We all are likely to use language that is more formal when communicating with acquaintances at a gathering than when communicating with a close friend over coffee. These register variations enable individuals to function effectively in different social circumstances.

The early social experiences of infants and toddlers typically are limited to routine interactions with primary caregivers at home (e.g., bathing, dressing, meal time, play, joint book-reading) and periodic activities in the community (e.g., at the grocery store, during doctor visits, in the park, at the zoo, etc.). However, as they mature, their experiences expand to include a greater variety of community outings, exposure to a larger number of conversational partners, and (in many cases) the opportunity to interact with peers and to participate in small social groups within a preschool setting. By the age

of about 3 years, children begin to use different registers for talking to adults (especially less familiar adults) and for talking to peers. This has been demonstrated in relation to a number of communicative functions.

Evidence for the use of different registers comes from studies that have explored **forms of requesting**. In English, forms of request exist on a **continuum of directness**, from very direct (e.g., "*Give me a cookie*") to indirect (e.g., "*Can you give me a cookie?*") and hinting (e.g., "*Cookies are my favorite treat*"). Requests also can vary according to whether they are accompanied by semantic aggravators or mitigators. **Semantic aggravators** include words such as *right now* and *or else* that intensify the request. **Semantic mitigators** include politeness markers (e.g., *please*) or reasons, which can soften a request.

Selecting the appropriate form of a request is influenced by the social role relationships between the person requesting and the person of whom the request is made. If the requestor is younger, or if the person of whom a request is made has a position of authority over the person requesting, then the choice of a linguistic form typically moves in the direction of an indirect request with semantic mitigators. If the request is likely to require extra effort on the part of the person being asked, then the choice of a linguistic form is likely to include reasons and expressions of appreciation.

Not surprisingly, developmental studies show that 2-year-olds tend to produce direct requests (e.g., *Gimme cookies*) and need or want statements (e.g., *need juice, want cookies*). However, between 2 and 3 years of age, children begin to use politeness markers more often if a listener is older, bigger, less familiar, dominant, or the possessor of a desired privilege (Ervin-Tripp, 1986). By the age of 3 years, modal auxiliary verbs begin to appear in the formulation of indirect requests (e.g., *Can I have a crayon?*). At 4 years, requests become even more indirect (e.g., *Don't forget to bring some popcorn*) and may be accompanied by justifications. This pattern continues at the age of 5 years, especially if the listener might deny the request (Owens, 2008). Still, preschoolers tend to use direct requests with semantic aggravators when speaking to listeners of lower status (Ervin-Tripp, 1977; Gordon & Ervin-Tripp, 1984), knowing full well that direct forms sound "bossier" while the more indirect forms sound "nicer" (Becker, 1986).

Differential use of registers has been observed during **other communicative contexts** as well. For example, Shatz and Gelman (1973) found that 4-year-olds used longer utterances with more frequent complex forms when teaching adults versus 2-year-olds how to use a toy parking garage. Similarly, Sachs and Devin (1976) observed adjustments in the language used by 4-year-olds during a free play activity across four different partners: an adult, a peer, a baby, and a baby doll. Interestingly, although preschoolers adjusted their speech when talking to younger children, their adjustments did not match the adjustments observed in motherese. Instead, the 4-year-olds tended to use a lower proportion of questions and a higher proportion of directives than typically observed in motherese.

Finally, preschoolers also have been observed to adjust their language **in consideration of a listener's perceptual abilities**. A study by Maratsos (1973) found that 3- to 5-year-olds used significantly more explicit language and fewer gestures when speaking to an adult who had her eyes closed than when speaking to an adult who was looking at the objects being discussed.

Overall, the evidence shows that the development of register variations begins early during the preschool period.

Summary of Early Pragmatic Development

In summary, the development of pragmatics in the emerging and early language skills of young children reflects remarkable growth in relation to the expression of communicative intent, the formulation of extended discourse, and knowledge of dialects and registers. These skills are a crucial part of the oral language base that supports children's participation in a wider range of social contexts during the elementary school years.

INTEGRATION OF LANGUAGE SKILLS

Our discussion of language development addressed individual components of language separately, but language develops as an integrated whole. To appreciate the interrelationships between different components of language, please consider the case of a 3-year-old boy named George, whose speech was only about 50% intelligible. Recall that 75% intelligibility normally is expected of children by the age of 3 years. Because George's speech was only 50% intelligible, his utterances frequently were misunderstood, As a result, he became a passive communicator, answering simple questions but rarely initiating new topics or extending previously established conversational topics. When George did try to communicate a more complex idea, his peers and caregivers spent more time trying to understand his messages than responding to their content. This resulted in fewer opportunities to hear good language models for topics of interest, and consequently, George's grammatical development began to lag. Soon, George's preschool peers began to avoid him because he was difficult to understand and they thought he talked like a baby. Sometimes he was excluded from participation at birthday parties or other play dates. This exclusion further reduced George's opportunities to learn about appropriate ways to communicate in different social situations. Without support, it is very likely that George's language skills would have continued to lag and he would have been at a distinct disadvantage by the time he entered elementary school. Fortunately, his lagging language growth was identified by an astute preschool teacher, and he was referred for a full speech-language evaluation. During the evaluation, he failed a hearing screening, which eventually resulted in his referral to a medical professional. The medical professional discovered a serious middle ear condition that compromised George's hearing sensitivity. Fortunately, the condition was treatable, and George's hearing quickly improved. As his hearing improved, so did his ability to benefit from exposure to appropriate language models. With clearer language models, George's auditory discrimination improved, and this affected his articulation. He began to notice the difference between his own speech and the speech of others, and this helped him to improve his own speech production. Greater intelligibility increased George's desirability as a communication partners. His peers began to seek him out, and he became a more assertive communicator. As his own communication became more assertive and intelligible, others began to expand

and extend George's conversational topics. This further supported George's grammatical growth. By the time George entered kindergarten, the quality of his speech, language, and communication was indistinguishable from that of his classmates.

CONCLUSION

In this chapter, we summarized children's interrelated accomplishments in the semantic, phonological, grammatical, and pragmatic components of language. For most children, the motivation to communicate is a major force in the integration of skills across language domains. As children's experiences increase, so does their range of potential conversational topics and conversational partners. The desire to communicate about an expanded range of topics requires an ongoing and rapid expansion of word learning. The ability to communicate successfully with a more diverse range of communicative partners requires intelligible speech and a style of language that is referentially clear. Referential clarity can be improved both by the growth in vocabulary and the acquisition of grammatical forms. As children reach the later preschool years, the content of their intended messages becomes more complex and extensive. To accommodate this, they begin to acquire narrative forms.

All along the way, caregivers support communicative growth by engaging their children in joint activity routines, following their children's focus of attention, and using patterns of motherese to scaffold, expand, and extend their children's communicative performance within the zone of proximal development. One of the most important child-caregiver activities is joint book reading. During joint book reading, children have the opportunity to learn about topics removed from the here and now and to hear a more literate language style. This style of language includes a more diverse vocabulary and it models narrative structures. Exposure to this style serves as a model for oral narrative development and as a building block for the later development of literacy skills.

The example of 3-year-old George provided in the previous section of this chapter shows how each part of language is interrelated and that, in most cases, growth is motivated by the desire to communicate successfully about an increasing range of topics with an increasing variety of communicative partners. These abilities prepare a child to participate in kindergarten with a new teacher and a new group of peers. Kindergarten is a time when many children are introduced more systematically to preliteracy skills, and the oral language skills that are acquired prior to kindergarten provide children with a solid basis for benefiting from literacy experiences.

REFLECTION QUESTIONS

1. Define the concepts in Table 4–22 and give an example of each. Whenever possible give an example that is different from one in the chapter.

2. Describe the difference between an icon, index, and a symbol. Give examples of each that are different from the examples in this chapter.

3. How are metaphor, simile, idiom, and proverb alike? How are they different?

4. What is the advantage of the ECM in comparison to the domain-specific, social-interactionist, and domain-general models? Describe four variables that are presumed by the ECM to affect the abstractness of a word's referent.

5. What is the difference between communicative and linguistic comprehension?

6. How do the first 25 words differ from the first 50 words?

7. What is the vocabulary spurt and what factors seem to contribute to it?

8. Describe some different categories of words and indicate which are learned sooner than others. What factors influence how early categories of words are learned?

9. Describe contexts of child-caregiver interaction that are especially helpful for word learning. Describe specific child-caregiver interaction patterns that support children's word learning.

10. Describe different manners of articulation and give examples of words beginning with sounds representing each manner of articulation.

TABLE 4–22. Concepts in Language Development

Concepts Related to Semantics	Concepts Related to Phonology	Concepts Related to Grammar	Concepts Related to Pragmatics
word	phone	grammar	speech act
onomatopoetic words	phoneme	morphology	communicative intent
deictic words	consonant	syntax	verbal behavior
lexical words	vowel	morpheme	discourse
function words	diphthong	MLU	dialogue
semantic categories	coarticulation	semantic relations	narrative
basic level category	phonetic inventory	telegraphic speech	macrostructure
taxonomic relationships	place of articulation	phrase	microstructure
nonliteral meanings	manner of articulation	clause	private speech
homonyms	voicing	compound sentence	metacognitive awareness
heterophones	syllable	complex sentence	executive functions
underextension	open/closed syllables	passive sentence	dialects
overextension	intelligibility	IPLP	registers
semantic network	simplification process	overregularization error	theory of mind
semantic constraints	phonological awareness		

11. Describe different places of articulation and give examples of words beginning with sounds representing each place.

12. Describe changes in children's speech intelligibility between 24 and 48 months.

13. Describe whole-word and segment-change phonological processes and provide examples of each that are different from the examples given in the book. Describe the individual variations that may apply to children's use of phonological simplification processes.

14. Explain the procedures and limitations of the traditional framework for describing the development of speech sounds.

15. How did Brown arrive at stages of MLU? What are the major characteristics of each stage?

16. What is the difference between reflexive object relations and semantic relations? Describe some common semantic relations and give examples of each that are different from the examples in this chapter.

17. Describe some syntactic forms that are not acquired in comprehension until the late preschool period and even early elementary school period.

18. Describe communicative intentions that can be expressed with and without language. Then describe communicative intentions that can only be expressed with language. Provide examples of each.

19. What is the difference between linguistic competence and communicative competence?

20. Describe patterns of adult-addressed speech that seem to support children's development of dialogue discourse.

APPLICATION EXERCISES

1. Find five children's books that illustrate true story sequences (including at least one episode) using a wordless picture sequence.

2. Spend some time with a preschooler during play activities with age-appropriate toys. Engage the child in dialogue discourse and invite the child to retell a story after reviewing a wordless picture book. Record utterances during each speaking task. Transcribe the dialogue and the narrative by typing the utterances into a text editing program. Summarize your transcripts in the following ways: Make a list of the number of different words and word categories represented in the transcript. Use Brown's (1973) rules to calculate MLU during dialogue. Count the number of child utterances that maintain the topic of the adult's previous utterance. Classify the child's utterances in dialogue according to categories of communicative intent. Describe the child's narrative by counting the number of words, the number of different words, and the number of story elements within the narrative. Compare your results to the expectations suggested by the developmental sequences described in this chapter. Compare your results to the results of other students who observed children at the same or different ages.

3. Write the orthographic transcription of the words represented by IPA symbols. Then, use the symbols C (consonant) and V (vowel) to describe the syllable structure of the words represented by English letters.

   a. /bʌbəl/

   b. /bejbɪ/

   c. /fɪlədəlfɪjə/

   d. /igəlz/

   e. /kəmpjutɚ/

f.	spoon	k.	strings
g.	chip	l.	hi
h.	fish	m.	years
i.	lady	n.	sheets
j.	crown	o.	lamb

REFERENCES

Anglin, J. M. (1977). *Word, object, and conceptual development.* New York, NY: W.W. Norton.

Anglin, J. M. (1978). From reference to meaning. *Child Development, 49,* 969–976.

Anglin, J. M. (1995). Classifying the world through language: Functional relevance, cultural significance, and category name learning. *International Journal of Intercultural Relations, 19,* 161–181.

Anselmi, D., Tomasello, M., & Acunzo, M. (1986). Young children's responses to neutral and specific contingent queries. *Journal of Child Language, 13,* 135–144.

Aslin, R. N., Saffran, J. R., & Newport, E. L. (1998). Computation of conditional probability statistics by 8-month-old infants. *Psychological Science, 9,* 321–324.

Austin, J. L. (1962). *How to do things with words.* Oxford, UK: Oxford University Press.

Avrutin, S. (1999). *Development of the syntax-discourse interchange.* Dordrecht, Netherlands: Kluwer Academic.

Baldwin, D. (1993). Infant's ability to consult the speaker for clues to word reference. *Journal of Child Language, 20,* 395–418.

Baldwin, D. (1995). Understanding the link between joint attention and language. In C. Moore & P. Dunham (Eds.), *Joint attention. Its origins and role in development* (pp. 131–158). Hillsdale, NJ: Erlbaum.

Baldwin, D., & Meyer, M. (2007). How inherently social is language? In E. Hoff & M. Shatz (Eds.), *Blackwell's handbook of language development* (pp. 87–106). Malden, MA: Blackwell.

Baldwin, D., & Tomasello, M. (1998). Word learning: A window on early pragmatic understanding, In E. V. Clark (Ed.), *Proceedings of the Stanford child language research forum* (pp. 3–23). Palo Alto, CA: Center for the Study of Language and Information.

Bankson, N. W., & Bernthal, J. E. (2004). Phonological assessment procedures. In J. E. Bernthal & N. W. Bankson (Eds.), *Articulation and phonological disorders* (5th ed., pp. 201–267). Boston, MA: Pearson, Allyn, and Bacon.

Baron-Cohen, S. (2000). Theory of mind and autism: A fifteen year review. In S. Baron-Cohen, H. Tager-Flusberg, & D. J. Cohen (Eds.), *Understanding other minds: Perspectives from developmental cognitive neuroscience* (pp. 3–20). Oxford, United Kingdom: Oxford University Press.

Baron-Cohen, S., Tager-Flusberg, H., & Cohen, D. J. (Eds.). (1993). *Understanding other minds: Perspectives from autism.* Oxford, United Kingdom: Oxford University Press.

Baron-Cohen, S., Tager-Flusberg, H., & Cohen, D. J. (2000). *Understanding other minds: Perspectives from developmental cognitive neuroscience* (2nd ed.). Oxford, UK: Oxford University Press.

Bartsch, K., & Wellman, H. (1995). *Children talk about the mind.* New York, NY: Oxford University Press.

Bates, E., Camaioni, L., & Volterra, V. (1975). The acquisition of performatives prior to speech. *Merrill-Palmer Quarterly, 21*, 205–216.

Bates, E., Dale, P., & Thal, D. (1995). Individual differences and their implications for theories of language development. In P. Fletcher & B. MacWhinney (Eds.), *The handbook of child language* (pp. 96–151). Oxford, UK: Blackwell.

Bauman-Waengler, J. (2004). *Articulatory and phonological impairments: A clinical focus* (2nd ed.). Boston, MA: Pearson Education.

Beals, D. E. (1997). Sources of support for learning words in conversation: Evidence from mealtimes. *Journal of Child Language, 24*(3), 673–694.

Becker, J. (1986). Bossy and nice requests: Children's production and interpretation. *Merrill-Palmer Quarterly, 32*, 393–413.

Behrend, D., Rosengren, K. S., & Perlmutter, M. A. (1992). Parental scaffolding and children's private speech: Differing sources of cognitive regulation. In R. M. Diaz & L. E. Berk (Eds.), *Private speech: From social interaction to self-regulation* (pp. 85–100). Hillsdale, NJ: Erlbaum.

Benedict, H. (1979). Early lexical development: Comprehension and production. *Journal of Child Language, 6*, 183–200.

Berk, L. (1992). Children's private speech: An overview of theory and the status of research. In R. M. Diaz & L. E. Berk (Eds.), *Private speech: From social interaction to self-regulation* (pp. 17–53). Hillsdale, NJ: Erlbaum.

Berk, L. (1994). Why children talk to themselves. *Scientific American, 271*(5), 78–83.

Berk, L. (2005). *Infants, children, and adolescents* (5th ed.). Boston, MA: Pearson, Allyn, & Bacon.

Berk, L. (2006). *Child development* (7th ed.). New Delhi: Prentice-Hall of India.

Berk, L., & Landau, S. (1993). Private speech of learning disabled and normally achieving children in classroom academic and laboratory contexts. *Child Development, 64*(2), 556–571.

Berk, L., & Spuhl, S. (1995). Maternal interaction, private speech, and task performance in preschool children. *Early Childhood Research Quarterly, 10*, 145–169.

Berko, J., & Brown, R. (1960). Psycholinguistic research methods. In P. H. Mussen (Ed.), *Handbook of research methods in child development* (pp. 517–557). New York, NY: Wiley.

Bernthal, J. E., & Bankson, N. W. (2004). *Articulation and phonological disorders* (5th ed.). Boston, MA: Pearson, Allyn, and Bacon.

Bivens, J. A., & Berk, L. E. (1990). A longitudinal study of the development of elementary school children's private speech. *Merrill-Palmer Quarterly, 36*, 443–463.

Bleile, K. (1995). *Manual of articulation and phonological disorders.* San Diego, CA: Singular.

Bloom, L. (1973). *One word at a time: The use of single word utterances before syntax.* The Hague, Netherlands: Mouton.

Bloom, L. (1993). *The transition from infancy to language: Acquiring the power of expression.* New York, NY: Cambridge University Press.

Bloom, L. (2000). Commentary. In G. Hollich, K. Hirsh-Pasek, & R. M. Golinkoff (Eds.), Breaking the language barrier: An emergentist coalition model for the origins of word learning. *Monographs of the Society for Research in Child Development.* Serial No. 362, *65*(3), 124–135.

Bloom, L., & Lahey, M. (1978). *Language development and language disorders.* New York, NY: Wiley.

Bloom, L., Lahey, M., Hood, L., Lifter, K., & Feiss, K. (1980). Complex sentences: Acquisition of syntactic connections and the semantic relations they encode. *Journal of Child Language, 7*, 235–261.

Bloom, L., Lightbown, P., & Hood, L. (1975). Structure and variation in child language. *Monographs of the Society for Research in Child Development, 40*, Serial Number 160.

Bloom, L., Rocissano, L., & Hood, L. (1976). Adult-child discourse: Developmental interaction between information processing and linguistic knowledge. *Cognitive Psychology, 8*, 521–551.

Bloom, P. (2000). *How children learn the meanings of words.* Cambridge, MA: MIT Press.

Bornstein, M. H., Cote, L. R., Maital, S., Painter, K., Park, S., Pascual, L., . . . Vyt, A. (2004). Crosslinguistic analysis of vocabulary in young children: Spanish, Dutch, French, Hebrew, Italian, Korean, and American English. *Child Development, 75*, 111–139.

Bornstein, M. H., Haynes, O. M., & Painter, K. M. (1998). Sources of child vocabulary competence: A multivariate model. *Journal of Child Language, 25*, 367–393.

Bowerman, M. (1978a). The acquisition of word meaning: An investigation into some current conflicts. In N. Waterson & C. Snow (Eds.), *The development of communication* (pp. 263–287). New York, NY: Wiley.

Bowerman, M. (1978b). Systematizing semantic knowledge: Changes over time in the child's organization of word meaning. *Child Development, 49*, 977–987.

Braisby, N., & Dockrell, J. (1999). Why is color naming difficult? *Journal of Child Language, 26*, 23–48.

Braunwald, S. (1995). Differences in the acquisition of early verbs: Evidence from diary data from sisters. In M. Tomasello & W. E. Merriman (Eds.), *Beyond names for things. The acquisition of verbs* (pp. 81-114). Hillsdale, NJ: Erlbaum.

Brinton, B., Fujiki, M., Loeb, D., & Winkler, E. (1986). Development of conversational repair strategies in response to requests for clarification. *Journal of Speech and Hearing Research, 29,* 75-81.

Brown, R. (1958). How shall a thing be called? *Psychological Review, 65,* 14-21.

Brown, R. (1973). *A first language: The early stages.* Cambridge, MA: Harvard University Press.

Brown, R., & Berko, J. (1960). Word association and the acquisition of grammar. *Child Development, 31,* 1-14.

Brown, R., & Frasier, C. (1963). The acquisition of syntax. In C. N. Cofer & B. Musgrave (Eds.), *Verbal behavior and learning: Problems and processes* (pp. 158-196). New York, NY: McGraw-Hill.

Brown, R., & Hanlon, C. (1970). Derivational complexity and the order of acquisition in child speech. In J. R. Hayes (Ed.), *Cognition and the development of language* (pp. 11-54). New York, NY: Wiley.

Byrne, M. C., & Hayden, E. (1980, November). *Topic maintenance and topic establishment in mother-child dialogue.* Paper presented at the meeting of the American Speech and Hearing Association, Detroit, MI.

Carey, S. (1978). The child as word learner. In M. Halle, J. Bresnan, & G. A. Miller (Eds.), *Linguistic theory and psychological reality* (pp. 264-293). Cambridge, MA: MIT Press.

Carpenter, M., Nagell, K., & Tomasello, M. (1998). Social cognition, joint attention, and communicative competence from 9 to 15 months of age. *Monographs of the Society for Research in Child Development, 63*(4), Serial No. 255.

Caselli, M. C., Bates, E., Casadio, P., Fenson, J., Fenson, L., Sander, L., & Weir, J. (1995). A crosslinguistic study of early lexical development. *Cognitive Development, 10,* 159-201.

Cerutti, D. T. (1989). Discrimination theory of rule-governed behavior. *Journal of the Experimental Analysis of Behavior, 51,* 259-276.

Champion, T. B. (1998). "Tell me somethin' good": A description of narrative structures among African American children. *Linguistics and Education, 9,* 251-286.

Chapman, K. L., Leonard, L. B., & Mervis, C. B. (1986). The effect of feedback on young children's inappropriate word useage. *Journal of Child Language, 13,* 101-117.

Chapman, R. (1981). Exploring children's communicative intents. In J. Miller (Ed.), *Assessing language production in children: Experimental procedures* (pp. 111-136). Baltimore, MD: University Park Press.

Chapman, R., & Miller, J. (1975). Word order in early two and three word utterances: Does production precede comprehension? *Journal of Speech and Hearing Research, 18,* 355-371.

Chomsky, A. N. (1965). *Aspects of the theory of syntax.* Cambridge, MA: MIT Press.

Chomsky, A. N. (1984). *Modular approaches to the study of the mind.* San Diego, CA: State University Press.

Chomsky, C. S. (1969). *The acquisition of syntax in children 5 to 10.* Cambridge, MA: MIT Press.

Clark, E. (1975). What's in a word? On the child's acquisition of semantics in his first language. In T. Moore (Ed.), *Cognitive development and the acquisition of language* (pp. 65-110). New York, NY: Academic Press.

Clark, E. (1982). The young word maker. In E. Wanner, & L. Gleitman (Eds.), *Language acquisition: The state of the art* (pp. 390-428). Cambridge, UK: Cambridge University Press.

Clark, E. (1993). *The lexicon in acquisition.* Cambridge, UK: Cambridge University Press.

Clark, E., & Sengul, C. J. (1978). Strategies in the acquisition of deixis. *Journal of Child Language, 5,* 457-475.

Cleave, P., & Kay-Raining Bird, E. (2007). Effects of familiarity on mothers' talk about nouns and verbs. *Journal of Child Language, 33,* 661-676.

Coggins, T. E., & Carpenter, R. L. (1981). The communicative intention inventory: A system for coding children's early intentional communication. *Applied Psycholinguistics, 2,* 235-252.

Cooper, J. O, Heron, T. E., & Heward, W. L. (2007). *Applied behavior analysis* (2nd ed.). Upper Saddle River, NJ: Pearson Higher Ed.

Coplan, J., & Gleason, J. (1988). Unclear speech: Recognition and significance of unintelligible speech in preschool children. *Pediatrics, 82,* 447-452.

Cowan, N. (1989). Acquisition of Pig Latin: A case study. *Journal of Child Language, 16,* 365-386.

Craig, H., Thompson, C. A., Washington, J. A., & Potter, S. L. (2003). Phonological features of child African American English. *Journal of Speech and Hearing Research, 46,* 623-635.

Cummings, S. (2003). *First words: An investigation of the nature of children's first word productions.* Master's thesis, University of Montana. Retrieved July 12, 2007, from www.umt.edu/ling/students/Grad/FirstWords.pdf

dePaola, T. (1978). *Pancakes for breakfast.* San Diego, CA: Harcourt, Brace Jovanovich.

deVilliers, J. G., Roeper, T., & Vainikka, A. (1990) The acquisition of long distance rules. In L. Frazier & J. G.

deVilliers (Eds.), *Language processing and acquisition* (pp. 257–297). Dordrecht, the Netherlands: Kluwer Academic.

deVilliers, J. G., & de Villiers, P. A. (1973). Development of the use of word order in comprehension. *Journal of Psycholinguistic Research*, *2*, 331–341.

deVilliers P., & deVilliers, J. (1974). On this that and the other: Nonegocentrism in very young children. *Journal of Experimental Child Psychology*, *18*, 438–447.

deVilliers, P. A., & deVilliers, J. G. (1979). Form and function in the development of sentence negation. *Papers and Reports on Child Language Development*, *17*, 56–64.

Diaz, R., & Berk, L. (1992). *Private speech: From social interaction to self-regulation*. Hillsdale, NJ: Lawrence Erlbaum

Dore, J. (1975). Holophrases, speech acts, and language universals. *Journal of Child Language*, *2*, 21–40.

Duncan, R. M., & Pratt, M. W. (1997). Microgenetic change in the quantity and quality of preschoolers' private speech. *International Journal of Behavior Development*, *20*, 367–383.

Eisenberg A. (1985). Learning to describe past experiences in conversation. *Discourse Processes*, *8*, 177–204.

Engel, S. (1995). *The stories children tell: Making sense of the narratives of childhood*. New York, NY: W. H. Freeman.

Ervin-Tripp, S. M. (1977). Wait for me, roller-skate. In C. Mitchell-Kernan & & S. Ervin-Tripp (Eds.), *Child discourse* (pp. 164–188). New York, NY: Academic Press.

Ervin-Tripp, S. (1979). Children's verbal turn-taking. In E. Ochs & B. Schieffelin (Eds.), *Developmental pragmatics* (pp. 391–414). New York, NY: Academic Press.

Ervin-Tripp, S., & Gordon, D. (1986). The development of requests. In R. Schiefelbusch (Ed.), *Language competence: Assessment and intervention* (pp. 73–81). San Diego, CA: College-Hill Press.

Farrar, M. J., & Maag, L. (2002). Early language development and the emergence of a theory of mind. *First Language*, *22*, 197–213.

Fenson, L., Dale, P. S., Reznick, J. S., Bates, E., Thal, D. J., & Pethick, S. J. (1994). Variability in early communicative development. *Monographs of the Society for Research in Child Development*, *59*(Serial No. 242).

Fenson, L., Dale, P. S., Reznick, J .S., Thal, D. J., Bates, E., Hartung, J. P., . . . Reilly, J. S. (1993). *Technical manual for the MacArthur Communicative Development Inventory*. San Diego, CA. Singular.

Ferguson, C. A., & Farwell, C. B. (1975). Words and sounds in early language acquisition. *Language*, *51*, 419–439.

Fernyhough, C., & Meins, E. (2009). Private speech and theory of mind: Evidence for developing interfunctional relations. In A. Winsler & C. Fernyhough (Eds.), *Private speech, executive function, and the development of verbal self-regulaiton* (pp. 95–104). New York, NY: Cambridge University Press.

Flavell, J. H. (1992). Perspectives on perspective taking. In H. Beilin & P. B. Pufall (Eds.), *Piaget's theory: Prospects and possibilities. The Jean Piaget symposium series* (pp. 107–139). Hillsdale, NJ: Erlbaum.

Flavell, J. H. (1999). Cognitive development: Children's knowledge about the mind. *Annual Review of Psychology*, *50*, 21–45.

Flavell, J. H. (2004). Theory of mind development: Retrospect and prospect. *Merrill-Palmer Quarterly*, *50*(3), 274–290.

Flavell, J. H., & Miller, P. H. (1998). Social cognition. In D. Kuhn & R. S. Siegler (Eds.), *Handbook of child psychology: Vol 2. Cognition, perception, and language* (4th ed., pp. 851–898). New York, NY: Wiley.

Forbes, J., & Poulin-Dubois, D. (1997). Representational changes in young children's understanding of familiar verb meanings. *Journal of Child Language*, *24*, 389–406.

Frost, L., & Bondy, A. (2006). A common language: Using B. F. Skinner's *Verbal Behavior* for assessment and treatment of communication disabilities in SLP-ABA. *Journal of Speech-Language Pathology and Applied Behavior Analysis*, *2–3*, pp. 103–110. http://www .behavior-analyst-today.com/SLP-ABA-VOL-1/SLP-ABA-1-2.pdf

Furrow, D., & Lewis, S. (1987). The role of the initial utterance in contingent query sequences: Its influences on responses to requests for clarification. *Journal of Child Language*, *14*, 467–479.

Gallagher, T. (1977). Revision behaviors in the speech of normal children developing language. *Journal of Speech and Hearing Research*, *20*, 303–318.

Garvey, C., & Hogan, R. (1973). Social speech and social interaction: Egocentrism revisited. *Child Development*, *44*, 562–568.

Gelman, S. A., Coley, J. D., Rosengren, K. S., Hartman, E., & Pappas, A. (1998). Beyond labeling: The role of maternal input in the acquisition of richly structured categories. *Monographs of the Society for Research in Child Development*, *62*(1 Serial No. 253).

Gentner, D. (1982). Why nouns are learned before verbs. Linguistic relativity versus natural partitioning. In S. A. Kuczaj (Ed.), *Language development: Vol. 2. Language, thought, and culture* (pp. 301–334). Hillsdale, NJ: Erlbaum.

Gerken, L. (2002). Early sensitivity to linguistic form. *Annual Review of Language Acquisition*, *2*(1), 1–36.

Ginsberg, H., & Opper, S. (1969). *Piaget's theory of intellectual development: An introduction.* Englewood Cliffs, NJ: Prentice-Hall.

Gleitman, L. (1990) The structural source of verb meaning. *Language Acquisition, 1*(1), 3-55.

Goldfield, B. (2000) Nouns before verbs in comprehension vs. production: The view from pragmatics. *Journal of Child Language, 27,* 501-520.

Goldfield, B., & Reznick, J. S. (1990). Early lexical acquisition: Rate, content, and the vocabulary spurt. *Journal of Child Language, 17,* 171-183.

Goldin-Meadow, S., Seligman, M., & Gelman, R, (1976). Language in the two-year-old. *Cognition, 5,* 189-202.

Goldstein, B., & Iglesias, A. (2004). Language and dialectal variations. In J. E. Bernthal & N. W. Bankson (Eds), *Articlulation and phonological disorders* (5th ed., pp. 348-375). Boston, MA: Pearson, Allyn, & Bacon.

Goldstein, M. H., King, A. P., & West, M. J. (2003). Social interaction shapes babbling: Testing parallels between birdsong and speech. *Proceedings of the National Academy of Sciences, 100,* 8030-8035.

Golinkoff, R. (1983). The preverbal negotiation of failed messages: Insights into the transition period. In R. M.Golinkoff (Ed.), *The transition from prelinguistic to linguistic communication* (pp. 1-25). Hillside, NJ: Erlbaum.

Golinkoff, R., Hirsh-Pasek, K., Cauley, K., & Gordon, L. (1987). The eyes have it: Lexical and syntactic comprehension in a new paradigm. *Journal of Child Language, 14,* 23-34.

Golinkoff, R., Mervis, C., & Hirsh-Pasek, K. (1994). Early object labels: The case for a developmental lexical principles framework. *Journal of Child Language, 14,* 23-46.

Goodman, J. C., McDonough, L., & Brown, N. (1998). The role of semantic content and memory in the acquisition of novel nouns. *Child Development, 69,* 1330-1344.

Gordon, D., & Ervin-Tripp, (1984). The structure of children's requests. In R. Schiefelbusch & J. Pickar (Eds.), *The acquisition of communicative competence* (Vol. 3, Language Intervention Series, pp. 295-321). Baltimore, MD: University Park Press.

Graf Estes, K. M., Evans, J., Alibali, M. W., & Saffran, J. R. (2007). Can infants map meaning to newly segmented words? Statistical segmentation and word learning. *Psychological Science, 18,* 254-260.

Greer, R. D., & Ross, D. E. (2008). *Verbal behavior analysis: Inducing and expanding new verbal capabilities in children with language delays.* New York, NY: Pearson, Allyn & Bacon

Grice, H. P. (1975). Logic and conversation. In P. Cole & J. L. Morgan (Eds.), *Syntax and semantics, Vol. 3: Speech acts.* New York, NY: Academic Press.

Hale, C. M., & Tager-Flusberg, H. (2003). The influence of language on theory of mind: A Training study. *Developmental Science, 6*(3), 346-359.

Halliday, M. A. K. (1975). *Learning how to mean: Explorations in the development of language.* New York, NY: Arnold.

Halliday, M. A. K., & Hassan, R. (1976). *Cohesion in English.* New York, NY: Longman.

Hart, B. (1991). Input frequency and children's first words. *First Language, 11*(32), 289-300.

Hart, B., & Risley, T. R. (1995). *Meaningful differences in the everyday experience of young American children.* Baltimore, MD: Paul H Brookes.

Heath, S. B. (1983). *Ways with words: Language, life, and work in communities and classrooms.* Cambridge, UK: Cambridge University Press.

Heath. S. B. (1986). Taking a cross-cultural look at narratives. *Topics in Language Disorders, 7*(1), 84-95.

Hegde, M. N. (1980). Issues in the study and explanation of language behavior. *Journal of Psycholinguistic Research, 9,* 1-22.

Hegde, M. N. (2008). Meaning in behavior analysis. *Journal of Speech-Language Pathology and Applied Behavior Analysis, 2*(4)-3(1), 1-24.

Hegde, M. N. (2010). Language and grammar: A behavioral analysis. *Journal of Speech-Language Pathology and Applied Behavior Analysis, 5*(2), 90-114.

Hirsh-Pasek, K., & Golinkoff, R. M. (1996). *The origins of grammar: Evidence from early language comprehension.* Cambridge, MA: MIT Press.

Hirsch-Pasek, K., & Golinkoff, R. M. (2000). Word learning: icon, index, or symbol? In R. M. Golinkoff, K. Hirsh-Pasek, L. Bloom, et al. (Eds.), *Becoming a word learner: A debate on lexical acquisition* (pp. 3-18). New York, NY: Oxford University Press.

Hirsh-Pasek, K., & Golinkoff, R. M. (2006). *Action meets word: How children learn verbs.* New York, NY: Oxford University Press.

Hirsh-Pasek, K., Golinkoff, R., Hennon, E., & McGuire, M. (2004). Hybrid theories at the forefront of developmental psychology: The emergentist coalition model of word learning as a case in point. In D. G. Hall & S. R. Waxman (Eds.), *Weaving a lexicon* (pp. 173-204). Cambridge. MA: MIT Press.

Hoff, E. (2003). The specificity of environmental influence: Socioeconomic status affects early vocabulary development via maternal speech. *Child Development, 74*(5), 1368-1378.

Hoff, E. (2005). *Language development.* Belmont, CA: Wadsworth

Hoff, E., & Naigles, L. (2002). How children use input to acquire a lexicon. *Child Development, 73*(2), 418-433.

Hollich, G. J., Hirsh-Pasek, K., & Golinkoff, R. M. (2000). Breaking the language barrier: An emergentist coalition model for the origins of word learning. *Monographs of the Society for Research in Child Development*, *65*(3, Serial No. 262).

Hughes, C., & Graham, A. (2002). Measuring executive functions in childhood: Problems and solutions? *Child and Adolescent Mental Health*, *7*, 131–142.

Hughes, D., McGillivray, L., & Schmidek, M. (1997). *Guide to narrative language: Procedures for assessment.* Eau Claire, WI: Thinking Publications.

Hulit, L., & Howard, M. (2006). *Born to talk: An introduction to speech and language development.* Boston, MA: Upper Saddle River.

Huttenlocher, J. (1974). The origins of language comprehension. In R. Soslo (Ed.), *Theories in cognitive psychology: The Loyola symposium* (pp. 331–368). New York, NY: Wiley.

Huttenlocher, J., Smiley, P., & Charney, R. (1983). The emergence of action categories in the child: Evidence from verb meaning. *Psychological Review*, *90*, 72–93.

Jaswal, V. K., & Markman, E. M. (2001). Learning proper and common names in inferential versus ostensive contexts. *Child Development*, *72*, 768–786.

Justice, L. J., & Ezell, H. K. (2002). *The syntax handbook: Everything you learned about syntax but forgot.* Eau Claire, WI: Thinking Publications.

Keenan, E. O., & Klein, E. (1975). Conversational competence in children. *Journal of Child Language*, *1*, 163–184.

Kemmer, S., & Barlow, M. (2000). Introduction: A usage-based conception of language. In M. Barlow & S. Kemmer (Eds.), *Usage-based models of language* (pp. 7–28). Stanford, CA: CLSI.

Kent, R. D. (1992). The biology of phonological development. In C. A. Ferguson, L. Menn, & C. Stoel-Gammon (Eds.), *Phonological development: Model, research, implications* (pp. 65–90). Timonium, MD: York Press.

Kessel, F. S. (1970). The role of syntax in children's comprehension from ages six to twelve. *Monographs of the Society for Research in Child Development*, *35*(6), 1–95.

Kuczaj, S. (1982). *Language development, Vol. 1: Syntax and semantics.* Hillsdale, NJ: Lawrence Erlbaum.

Kuhl, P. K. (2000). Colloquium Paper: A new view of language acquisition. *Proceedings of the National Academy of Sciences*, *97*(22), 11850–11857. Retrieved January 4, 2010, from http://www.ncbi.nlm.nih.gov/pmc/articles/PMC34178/#B102#B102

Kuhl, P. K. (2004). Early language acquisition: Cracking the speech code. *Nature Reviews Neuroscience*, *5*, 831–843.

Landau, B., Smith, K., & Jones, S. (1988). The importance of shape in early lexical learning. *Cognitive Development*, *3*, 199–321.

Leonard, L., Newhoff, M., & Meselam, L. (1980). Individual differences in early child phonology. *Applied Psycholinguistics*, *1*, 7–30.

Leopold, W. (1939-1949). *Speech development of a bilingual child.* Evanson, IL: Northwestern University Press.

Liles, B. (1993). Narrative discourse in children with language disorders and children with normal language: A critical review of the literature. *Journal of Speech and Hearing Research*, *36*, 868–887.

Liles, B. Z. (1993). Narrative discourse in children with language disorders and children with normal language: A critical review of the literature. *Journal of Speech and Hearing Research*, *36*, 868–882.

Maguire, M., Hirsh-Pasek, K., & Golinkoff, R. M. (2006). A unified theory of word learning: Putting verb acquisition in context. In K. Hirsh-Pasek & R. M. Golinkoff (Eds.), *Action meets word* (pp. 364–391). New York, NY: Oxford University Press.

Mallott, R. W., Whaley, D. L., & Mallott, M. E. (1997). *Elementary principles of behavior* (3rd ed.). Upper Saddle River, NJ: Prentice Hall

Maratsos, M. P. (1974). Children who get worse at understanding the passive: A replication of Bever. *Journal of Psycholinguistic Research*, *3*, 65–74.

Markman, E. (1987). How children constrain the possible meanings of words. In U. Neisser (Ed.), *Concepts and conceptual development: Ecological and intellectual factors in categorization* (pp. 255–287). Cambridge, UK: Cambridge University Press.

Markson, L., & Bloom, P. (1997). Evidence against a dedicated system for word learning in children. *Nature*, *385*, 813–815.

McCabe, A., & Bliss L. S. (2003). *Patterns of narrative discourse: A multicultural, lifespan approach.* Boston, MA: Allyn & Bacon.

McCabe, A., & Peterson, C. (1991). Getting the story: A longitudinal study of parental styles in eliciting narratives and developing narrative skill. In A. McCabe & C. Peterson (Eds.), *Developing narrative atructure* (pp. 217–254). Hillsdale, NJ: Lawrence Erlbaum.

McCabe, A., & Rollins, P. R. (1994). Assessment of preschool narrative skills: Prerequisite for literacy. *American Journal of Speech-Language Pathology*, *3*(1), 45–56.

McDonough, L. (2002). Basic-level nouns: First learned but misunderstood. *Journal of Child Language*, *29*, 357–377.

McLaughlin, S. F. (2006). *Introduction to language development* (2nd ed.). Clifton Park, NY: Thomson Delmar Learning.

McLaughlin, S. F., & Cullinan, W. L. (1981). An empirical perspective on language development and language training. In N. J. Lass (Ed.), *Speech and language: Advances in basic research ad practice* (Vol. 5, pp. 249–310). New York, NY: Academic Press.

McLeod, S., & Bleile, K. (2003, November). *Neurological and developmental foundations of speech acquisition.* Invited presentation, American Speech-Language and Hearing Association Convention. Chicago, IL. Retrieved from http://www.speech-language-therapy.com/ASHA03McLeodBleile.pdf

Menn, L., & Stoel-Gammon, C. (2005). Phonological development: Learning sounds and sound patterns. In J. Berko Gleason (Ed.), *The development of language* (6th ed., pp. 62–111). Boston, MA: Pearson, Allyn & Bacon.

Menyuk, P., Liebergott, J. W., & Schultz, M. C. (1995). *Early language development in full term and premature infants.* Hillsdale, NJ: Erlbaum.

Mervis, C. B. (1987). Child-basic object categories and early lexical development. In U. Neisser (Ed.), *Concepts and conceptual development: Ecological and intellectual factors in categorization* (pp. 201–233). Cambridge, UK: Cambridge University Press.

Mervis, C. B. (1998). Child-basic object categories and early lexical development. In U. Neisser (Ed.), *Concepts in conceptual development: Ecological and intellectual factors in categorization* (pp. 201–233). New York, NY: Cambridge University Press.

Mervis, C. B., & Bertrand, J. (1993). Acquisition of early object labels: The roles of operating principles and input. In A. Kaiser & D. B. Gray (Eds.), *Enhancing children's communication: Research foundations for intervention* (pp. 287–316). Baltimore, MD: Paul H. Brookes.

Mervis, C. B., & Mervis, C. (1982). Leopards are kitty-cats: Object labeling by mothers for their thirteen-month-olds. *Child Development, 53,* 267–273.

Mervis, C. B., & Mervis, C. (1988). Role of adult input in young children's category evolution: An observational study. *Journal of Child Language, 15,* 257–272.

Michaels, S. (1983). The role of adult assistance in children's acquisition of literate discourse strategies. *Volta Review, 85,* 72–85.

Miller, G. A. (1999). On knowing a word. *Annual Review of Psychology, 50,* 1–9.

Miller, J. F. (1981). *Assessing language production in children: Experimental procedures.* Baltimore, MD: University Park Press.

Miller, J. F., Chapman, R. S., Branston, M. B., & Reichle, J. (1980). Language comprehension in sensorimotor stages V and VI. *Journal of Speech and Hearing Research, 22,* 284–311.

Miller, L. K. (1997). *Principles of everyday behavior analysis* (3rd ed.) Boston, MA: Brooks/Cole.

Minami M., & McCabe, A. (1995). Rice balls versus bear hunts: Japanese and European North American family narrative patterns. *Journal of Child Language, 22,* 423–466.

Mintz, T. H., & Gleitman, L. R. (2002). Adjectives really do modify nouns: The incremental and restricted nature of early adjective acquisition. *Cognition, 84,* 267–293.

Moerk, E. L. (1992). *A first language taught and learned.* Baltimore, MD: Paul H. Brookes.

Moerk, E. L. (1994). Corrections in first language acquisition: Theoretical controversies and factual evidence. *International Journal of Psycholinguistic Research, 10,* 33–58.

Morgan, J., & Demuth, K. (1996). *Signal to syntax: Bootstrapping from speech to grammar in early acquisition.* Hillsdale, NJ: Erlbaum.

Mowrer, O. (1960). *Learning theory and symbolic processes.* New York, NY: Wiley.

Müller, U., Jacques, S., Brocki, K., & Zelazo, P. D. (2009). The executive functions of language in preschool children. In A. Winsler, C. Ferrybough (Eds.), *Private speech, executive functioning, and the development of verbal self-regulation* (pp. 73–100). Cambridge, UK: Cambridge University Press.

Naigles, L. (1997). Are English-speaking one-year-olds verb learners, too? In E. Clark (Ed.), *Proceedings of the 28th annual child language research forum* (pp. 199–212). Palo Alto, CA: CSLI.

Naigles, L., & Hoff, E. (2006). Verbs at the very beginning. In K. Hirsh-Pasek & R. Golinkoff (Eds.), *Action meets word: How children learn verbs* (pp. 336–363). Oxford, NY: Oxford University Press.

Naigles, L., & Hoff-Ginsberg, E. (1998). Why are some verbs learned before other verbs? Effects of input frequency and structure on children's early verb use. *Journal of Child Language, 25,* 95–120.

Nelson, K. (1973). Structure and strategy in learning to talk. *Monographs of the Society for Research in Child Development,* Serial No. 147, 1–2.

Nelson, K. (1974). Concept, word and sentence: Interrelations in acquisition and development. *Psychological Review, 81,* 267–295.

Nelson, K. (1977). The conceptual basis of naming. In J. Macnamara (Ed.), *Language learning and thought.* New York, NY: Academic Press.

Nelson, K. (1988). Constraints on word learning? *Cognitive Development, 3,* 221–246.

Newport, E. I. (1976). Motherese: The speech of mothers to young children. In J. Castellan, D. Pisoni, & G. Potts (Eds.), *Cognitive theory* (pp. 177–210). New York, NY: Wiley.

Ninio, A. (1995). Expression of communicative intents in the single-word period and the vocabulary spurt. In K. E. Nelson & Z. Reger (Eds.), *Children's language* (Vol. 8, pp. 103–124). Mahwah, NJ: Erlbaum.

Ninio, A., & Snow, C. (1999). The development of pragmatics: Learning to use language appropriately. Invited chapter, in T. K. Bhatia & W. C. Ritchie (Eds.), *Handbook of language acquisition* (pp. 347–383). New York, NY: Academic Press.

Owens, R. (2008). *Language development: An introduction* (7th ed.). Boston, MA: Pearson, Allyn & Bacon.

Pan, B. A. (2005). Semantic development. In J. B. Gleason (Ed.), *The development of meaning.* (pp. 112–147). Boston, MA: Pearson, Allyn & Bacon.

Peirce, C. S., Jartshorne, C., & Weiss, P. (Eds.). (1932). *Collected papers of Charles Sanders Peirce.* Cambridge, MA: Harvard University Press.

Peña-Brooks, A., & Hegde, G. (2000). *Assessment and treatment of articulation and phonological disorders in children.* Austin, TX: Pro-Ed.

Perner, J. (1991). *Understanding the representational mind.* Cambridge, MA: The MIT Press.

Perner, J., Leekam, S., & Wimmer, H. (1987). Three-year-olds' difficulty in understanding false belief: Cognitive limitation, lack of knowledge, or pragmatic misunderstanding? *British Journal of Developmental Psychology*, 5, 125–137.

Peterson, C. (1994). Narrative skills and social class. *Canadian Journal of Education/Revue Canadienne de l'Education*, 19(3), 251–269.

Peterson, C., & McCabe, A. (1983). *Developmental psycholinguistics: Three ways of looking at a child's narrative.* New York, NY: Plenum.

Philips, J. R. (1973). Syntax and vocabulary of mothers' speech to young children: Age and sex comparisons. *Child Development*, 44, 182–185.

Pinker, S. (1984). *Language learnablity and language development.* Cambridge, MA: Harvard University Press.

Plunkett, K. (1997). Theories of early language acquisition. *Trends in Cognitive Sciences*, 1(4), 146–153.

Preece, A. (1987). The range of narrative forms conversationally produced by young children. *Journal of Child Language*, 14, 353–373.

Quine, W. V. O. (1960). *Word and object: An inquiry into the linguistic mechanisms of objective reference.* Cambridge, UK: Cambridge University Press.

Reich, P. (1986). *Language development.* Englewood Cliffs, NJ: Prentice-Hall.

Repacholi, B., & Gopnik, A. (1997). Early reasoning about desires. Evidence from 14- and 18-month-olds. *Developmental Psychology*, 33, 12–21.

Rollins, P. R., Pan, B. A., Conti-Ramsden, G., & Snow C. E. (1994). Communicative skills in children with specific language impairments: A comparison with their language-matched siblings. *Journal of Communication Disorders*, 27, 188–201.

Rosenbaum, P. (1967). *The grammar of English predicate construction.* Cambridge, MA: MIT Press.

Sachs, J., & Devin, J. (1976). Young children's use of age-appropriate speech styles in social interaction and role-playing. *Journal of Child Language*, 3, 81–98.

Sander, E. (1972). When are speech sounds learned? *Journal of Speech and Hearing Disorders*, 37, 55–63.

Santelmann, L., Berk, S., Austin, J., & Lust, B. (2002). Continuity and development in the acquisition of inversion in yes/no questions: dissociating movement and inflection. *Journal of Child Language*, 29, 813–842.

Schmidt, C. L. (1996). Scrutinizing reference: How gesture and speech are coordinated in mother-child interaction. *Journal of Child Language*, 23, 279–305.

Schober-Peterson, D., & Johnson, C. J. (1989). Conversational topics of four-year-olds. *Journal of Speech and Hearing Research*, 32, 857–870.

Searle, J. (1969). *Speech acts: An essay in the philosophy of language.* New York, NY: Cambridge University Press.

Shatz M., & Gelman, R. (1973). The development of communication skills: Modifications in the speech of young children as a function of the listener. *Monographs of the Society for Research in Child Development*, 38(5, Serial No. 152).

Skinner, B. F. (1957). *Verbal behavior.* New York, NY: Apple-Century-Crofts.

Skinner, B. F. (1974). *About behaviorism.* New York, NY: Alfred A. Knopf.

Slobin, D. I. (1971). Introduction. In D. I. Slobin (Ed.), *The ontogenesis of grammar: A theoretical symposium* (pp. 3–14) New York, NY: Academic Press.

Slobin, D. I. (1973). Cognitive prerequisites for the development of grammar. In C. Ferguson & D. Slobin (Eds.), *Studies of child language development.* New York, NY: Holt, Reinhart, & Winston.

Smiley, P., & Huttenlocher, J. (1995). Conceptual development and the child's early words for events, objects, and persons. In M. Tomasello & W. Merriman (Eds.), *Beyond names and things: The acquisition of verbs* (pp. 21–62). Hillsdale, NJ: Erlbaum.

Smith, C., & Sachs, J. (1990). Cognition and the verb lexicon in early lexical development. *Applied Psycholinguistics*, 11, 409–424.

Smith, L. B. (1995). Self-organizing processes in learning to learn words: Development is not induction. In C. A. Nelson (Ed.), *The Minnesota Symposia on Child Psychology.* (Vol. 28, pp. 1–32). Mahwah, NJ: Erlbaum.

Snow, C. E. (1972). Mothers' speech to children learning language. *Child Development*, 43, 549–565.

Snow, C. E. (1999). Social perspectives on the development of language. In B. MacWhinney (Ed.), *The emergence of language* (pp. 257–276). Mahwah, NJ: Erlbaum.

Snow, C. E., de Blauw, A., & Van Roosmalen, G. (1979). Talking and playing with babies: The role of ideologies of child-rearing. In M. Bullowa (Ed.), *Before speech: The beginning of interpersonal communication* (pp. 268–288). Cambridge, UK: Cambridge University Press.

Snow, C. E., & Goldfield, B. A. (1983). Turn the page please: Situation-specific language acquisition. *Journal of Child language, 10,* 551–569.

Snow, C. E., Pan, B., Imbens-Bailey, A., & Herman, J. (1996). Learning how to say what one means: A longitudinal study of children's speech act use. *Social Development, 5,* 56–84.

Sodian, B., Taylor, C., Harris, P. L., & Perner, J. (1991). Early deception and the child's theory of mind: False trails and genuine markers. *Child Development, 62,* 468–483.

Soja, N. (1994). Young children's concept of color and its relation to the acquisition of color words. *Child Development, 65,* 918–937.

Stampe, D. (1969). *The acquisition of phonetic representation.* Paper presented at the Fifth Regional Meeting of the Chicago Linguistic Society, Chicago, IL.

Stein, M. L., & Glenn, C. (1979). An analysis of story comprehension in elementary school children. In R. Freedle (Ed.), *New directions in discourse processing* (pp. 53–120). Norwood, NJ: ABLEX.

Stoel-Gammon, C. (1998). The role of babbling and phonology in early linguistic development. In A. M. Wetherby, S. F. Warren, & J. Reichle (Eds), *Transitions in prelinguistic communication* (pp. 89–110). Baltimore, MD: Paul H. Brookes.

Stoel-Gammon, C. (2007). Phonological development. In E. Hoff & M. Shatz (Eds.), *Blackwell handbook of language development* (pp. 238–256). Malden, MA: Blackwell.

Stoel-Gammon, C., & Cooper, J. (1984). Patterns of early lexical and phonological development. *Journal of Child Language, 11,* 247–271.

Stoel-Gammon, C., & Dunn, C. (1985). *Normal and disordered phonology in children.* Baltimore, MD: University Park Press.

Sundberg, M., & Partington, J. (1998). *Teaching language to children with autism and other developmental disabilities.* Pleasant Hill, CA: Behavior Analysts.

Tager-Flusberg, H. (2005). Putting words together: Morphology and syntax in the preschool years. In J. Berko Gleason (Ed.), *The development of language* (pp. 148–190). Boston, MA: Pearson, Allyn & Bacon.

Tanz, C. (1980). *Studies in the acquisition of deictic terms.* Cambridge, UK: Cambridge University Press.

Templin, M. (1957). *Certain language skills in children.* Minneapolis, MN: University of Minnesota Press.

Tomasello, M. (1995). Joint attention as social cognition. In C. Moore & P. J. Dunham (Eds.), *Joint attention: Its origins and role in development* (pp. 103–130). Hillsdale, NJ: Erlbaum.

Tomasello, M. (2002). Do young children have adult syntactic competence? *Cognition, 74,* 209–253.

Tomasello, M., & Farrar, M. J. (1986). Joint attention and early language. *Child Development, 57,* 1454–1463.

Tomasello, M., Farrar, M. J., & Dines, J. (1984). Children's speech revisions for a familiar and an unfamiliar adult. *Journal of Speech and Hearing Research, 27,* 359–363.

Tomasello, M., Mannle, S., & Kruger, A. (1986). The linguistic environment of one to two year old twins. *Developmental Psychology, 22,* 169–176.

Tomasello, M., & Todd, J. (1983). Joint attention and lexical acquisition style. *First Language, 4,* 197–212.

Umiker-Sebeok, D. J. (1979). Preschool children's intra-conversational narratives. *Journal of Child Language, 6,* 91–109.

Valian, V. (1981). Linguistic knowledge and language acquisition. *Cognition, 10,* 323–329.

Vellman, A. Mangipudi, L. & Locke, J. (1989). Prelinguistic phonetic contingency. *First Language, 9,* 169–173.

Vihman, M. M. (2004). Later phonological development. In J. E. Bernthal & N. W. Bankson (Eds.), *Articulation and phonological disorders* (5th ed., pp. 105–137). Boston, MA: Pearson, Allyn & Bacon.

Vygotsky, L. (1962). *Thought and language.* Cambridge, MA: MIT Press. (Original work published in Russian in 1934).

Wales, R. (1986). Deixis. In P. Fletcher & M. Garman (Eds.), *Language acquisition* (2nd ed., pp. 401–428). New York, NY: Cambridge University Press.

Wanska, S. K., & Bedrosian, J. L. (1985). Conversational structure and topic performance in mother-child interaction. *Journal of Speech and Hearing Research, 28,* 579–584.

Waterson, N. (1971). Child phonology: A prosodic view. *Journal of Linguistics, 7,* 179–221.

Waxman, S. R., & Lidz, J. L. (2006). Early word learning. In W. Damon, R. Lerner, D. Kuhn, & R. Siegler (Eds.), *Handbook of child psychology* (6th ed., Vol. 2, pp. 229–335). Hoboken, NJ: Wiley.

Weir, R. (1962). *Language in the crib.* The Hague, The Netherlands: Mouton.

Wellman, H. M. (1991). From desires to beliefs: Acquisition of a theory of mind. In A. Whiten (Ed.), *Natural theories of the mind* (pp. 19–38). Oxford, UK: Blackwell.

Wellman, H. M., Cross, D., & Watson, J. (2001). Meta-analysis of theory-of-mind development: The truth about false belief. *Child Development, 72,* 655–684.

Werker, J., Fennell, C. T., Corcoran, K. M., & Stager, C. L. (2002). Infants' ability to learn phonetically similar words: Effects of age and vocabulary size. *Infancy, 3,* 1-30.

Westby, C. (1994a). Sociocommunicative bases of communication development. In W. O. Haynes & B. B. Shulman (Eds.), *Communication development: Foundations, processes, and clinical applications* (pp. 199-229). Englewood Cliffs, NJ: Prentice-Hall.

Westby, C. (1994b). Communication refinement in school-age and adolescence. *Communication development: Foundations, processes, and clinical applications* (pp. 230-256). Englewood Cliffs, NJ: Prentice-Hall.

Wetherby, A. M., Cain, D. H., Yonclas, D.G., & Walker, V. G. (1988). Anaysis of intentional communication in normal children from the prelinguistic to the multiword stage. *Journal of Speech and Hearing Research, 31,* 240-252.

Wetstone, H., & Friedlander, B. (1973). The effect of word-order on children's responses to simple questions and commands. *Child Development, 44,* 734-740.

Wilcox, M. J., & Webster, E. J. (1980). Early discourse behavior: An analysis of children's responses to listener feedback. *Child Development, 51,* 1120-1125.

Wode, H. (1977). Four early stages in the development of L1 negation. *Journal of Child Language, 4,* 87-102.

Woodward, A., Markman, E., & Fitzimmons, C. (1994). Rapid word learning in 13- and 18-month-olds. *Developmental Psychology, 30,* 553-566.

Wooten, J., Merkin, S., Hood, L., & Bloom, L. (1979, March). *Wh-questions: Linguistic evidence to explain the sequence of acquisition.* Paper presented at the biennial meeting of the Society for Research in Child Development, San Francisco, CA.

Youngblade, L. M., & Dunn, J. (1995). Individual differences in young children's pretend play with mothers and siblings: Links to relationships and understanding of other people's feelings and beliefs. *Child Development, 66,* 1472-1492.

Zivin, G. (1979). Removing common confusions about egocentric speech, private speech, and self-regulation. In G. Zivin (Ed.), *The development of self-regulation through private speech* (pp. 13-39). New York, NY: Wiley.

CHAPTER 5

Language Development: Later Linguistic Skills

LATER LINGUISTIC PERIOD: PARAMETERS

Language continues to develop in dramatic ways as children transition through the school years. Development is prompted by (among other things) the experience of schooling itself, the growth of reasoning skills, the extended range of social experiences in which children engage, children's expanding range of knowledge about the world, and literacy experiences. Major achievements are seen in oral language and in the development of literacy skills. Oral language is refined with respect to the vocabulary and grammatical skills needed to communicate about an expanding range of topics at increasing levels of complexity with a more diverse range of communicative partners. Pragmatic skills expand to include extended and increasingly decontextualized discourse patterns in various dialogue, narrative, and expository genres. A developing awareness about the structure and functions of language itself increases at the phonological level and across all components of language. Literacy skills emerge on the basis of a solid foundation of entry-level oral language skills and emergent literacy development. For the first three school years, reading and writing are the focus of deliberate teaching and learning. However, by third to fourth grades, these skills become tools for learning about a universe of other topics and con- necting with a wide network of people. In a world rich with electronic communication options, the impact of literacy skills has expanded in ways never before experienced. Within this framework, the acquisition of language skills throughout the school years is no less awesome than the emergence of language itself.

LATER LINGUISTIC PERIOD: PURPOSES

In this chapter we summarize: (a) key developments in oral language during the elementary, middle, and high school years and (b) the emergence and development of literacy skills. As in previous chapters, the development of oral language skills is discussed in relation to the lexical system, phonology, grammar, and pragmatics. A recurrent theme in this discussion is that oral language and literacy are intimately intertwined and that each exerts an influence on the other throughout the school years.

PRIMARY ACCOMPLISHMENTS: LEXICON AND SEMANTICS

Our discussion of lexical development focuses on quantitative features of vocabulary development and qualitative changes in the growth of word meanings. Special consideration is given to the growth of double meanings, the literate lexicon, figurative meanings, word definitions, and linguistic humor. The section concludes with a consideration of experiences known to support lexical growth.

Vocabulary Growth

The importance of vocabulary development cannot be overstated. Not only is word knowledge key for self expression, interpersonal communication, and learning, it also is a crucial building block for the initial development of literacy skills. In fact, vocabulary knowledge in kindergarten and first grade is a significant predictor of reading comprehension in the middle and secondary grades (Cunningham & Stanovich, 1997; Scarborough, 1998).

Despite its importance, the measurement of vocabulary skills is more challenging than it may seem. During the initial stages of language acquisition, reliable estimates of children's lexical knowledge can be obtained by interviewing their caregivers (e.g., Fenson et al., 2007). However, by the time children reach school age, it is no longer possible for caregivers to keep track of every word their children learn. Instead, the average rate of vocabulary development is estimated by researchers who test children's knowledge of representative samples of words. These estimates vary widely depending on how the word samples are derived, the tasks that are used to observe children's performance, and the criteria for crediting word knowledge. For example, when word knowledge is estimated by word definitions it is possible to underestimate the knowledge of younger children who may know a word's meaning but not know how to define it. An extensive review of these and related issues is provided by Anglin, Miller, and Wakefield (1993).

Extending the work of previous researchers, Anglin et al. (1993) studied the vocabulary development of first, third, and fifth graders using a methodology that reduced the sources of variance in previous studies. Their word sample was selected systematically from *Webster's Third New International Dictionary of the English Language* (1981), an unabridged dictionary offering the most comprehensive, readily available inventory of the total number of words in the language. Furthermore, each word selected for the sample represented one of six word types: (1) **root words**—words consisting of a single free morpheme (e.g., *flop, pep, loft*); (2) **inflected words**—root words with suffixes that do not change the lexical meaning of the word (e.g., words with verb tense markers such as *soaking*, and plurals such as *reports*); (3) **derived words**—root words with an affix (prefix or suffix) that changes the word's meaning even though it may remain semantically related to the original word (e.g., *incomparable*); (5) **literal compounds**—words formed by two independent root words whose meanings can be deduced from the meanings of the individual roots (e.g., *outgrow*); and (6) **idioms**—words whose meanings cannot be deduced by analyzing the root words (e.g., *carrying on* means misbehaving).

Children were interviewed individually and asked to demonstrate their knowledge of individual words by: (a) providing a definition, (b) using a word in a sentence, and (c) selecting the correct definition from four carefully constructed choices. Credit for knowing a word was given if a child responded correctly on at least one of the three task levels. The raw scores of all children within a grade level were used to compute an average raw score for that grade level. Each average raw score was then multiplied by a factor to arrive at an estimated mean number of total words. Results showed that the number of known words increased from about 10,000 in first grade to about 40,000 by fifth grade, suggesting that children acquire an average of approximately 10,000 words a year. Studies by other researchers estimate that older children and youth acquire from 3,000 to 5,000 new words each year, resulting in at least 80,000 different words by the time they graduate from high school (Miller & Gildea, 1987; Nagy & Herman, 1987). However, the results of Anglin et al.'s (1993) study suggest that this may be an underestimate.

Another important discovery made by Anglin et al. (1993) pertains to the differential growth of word types. Specifically, the estimated growth rate for derived words is markedly higher than that of the three other word categories, particularly in fifth grade. Fifth graders recognize the morphological structure of words and use this information to figure out word meanings. However, the estimated growth rate for idioms remains below all other word types even at fifth grade.

Qualitative Changes in Word Meanings

The growth of lexical skills during school age involves more than just an accumulation of words. We also see two types of changes in the growth of meaning. One type, **horizontal development**, involves an expansion of knowledge about the meanings of individual words (McNeill, 1970). For example, during the early language development period, a child may have learned the word *dog* for referring to his or her own pet and to other dogs in the neighborhood. With increasing experience, that same child is likely to learn that a dog is a mammal; there are different kinds of dogs; and dogs serve different functions (e.g., as pets, as guides for people with visual impairments, etc.). Word meanings also expand as children learn that an individual word can have more than one kind of referent. For example, *fly* can refer to an insect, to the action of a bird, to the zipper on trousers, and so forth.

We also see changes in **vertical development** as represented by the growth of knowledge about the relationships between words (McNeill, 1970). For example, students learn to recognize relationships between words based on taxonomic categories (e.g., *dog, animal, canine, mammal*, etc.). They become aware of words that represents points on a continuum (e.g., *small, medium, large*); words that function as synonyms (e.g., *little, small*); words that are associated by context (e.g., *school, teacher, desks, books, computers*, etc.); by metalinguistic features (e.g., nouns, verbs, adjectives, etc.) and by other potential traits. Changes in horizontal development contribute to changes in vertical development. For example, as students learn about the morphological structure of individual words (e.g., *unhappy = un + happy*) they begin to recognize morphological relationships between different words (e.g., <u>un</u>*common*, <u>un</u>*usual*, <u>un</u>*becoming*, <u>un</u>*believable*, etc.).

Vertical development has been conceptualized within the framework of **semantic networks** (also known as **semantic webs**) (Pan, 2005). Theoretically, semantic networks consist of nodes and links between the nodes. Nodes typically consist of nouns and links usually consist of verbs. As children acquire more semantic information, the number of nodes increases as does the number of connections between nodes. Theoretically, the connection between nodes is bidirectional to support both divergent and convergent processing. **Divergent processing** is the ability to access many related concepts when exposed to an individual word. For example, hearing the word *snow* may trigger numerous associated concepts such as *cold, gloves, earmuffs, snowman*, and others. **Convergent processing** is the ability to make inferences about a topic based on hearing a number of related words. For example, hearing words such as *sun, beach, palm tree, coconut, island*, and *volcano* might lead you to think about Hawaii. The organization of semantic networks is a lifelong dynamic process as new words are continually entering the lexicon.

Learning Words with Double Meanings

The comprehension and use of words with **double meanings** (also known as **polysemous forms**) deserves special attention for several reasons. First, such words are pervasive in the English language (Nippold, 1995), and the ability to understand them is essential to every day communication. Second, the ability to appreciate double meanings plays an especially important role in the comprehension of academic instruction, the understanding of figurative language (discussed in a separate section, below), and the appreciation of humor (also discussed separately, below). Finally, students with language impairments may have special difficulty in comprehending double meanings, so this is an area of importance for both teachers and speech-language pathologists alike.

The recognition of double meanings requires the cognitive flexibility to ignore one meaning of a word and the linguistic resources to search for another. An appreciation of double meanings normally begins in preschool when children learn that some words have more than one kind of referent. For example, they might know that *bark* refers to the sound that a dog makes and to the outer covering of a tree trunk. As in the example of *bark*, the double meanings understood by preschoolers typically involve concrete referents. However, by the age of about 8 years, children begin to appreciate that double meanings can include psychological referents as well (e.g., *sharp, bright, warm, sweet, bitter*). By the age of 9 to 10 years, the ability to describe these meanings begins to emerge, and by 13 to 14 years these descriptions sound adultlike (e.g., "He's hard like a rock 'cause you can't move him or change him") (Wiig, 1989). Moreover, 13- and 14-year-olds can verbalize the relationship between the two meanings of these words (e.g., *Warm temperature and warm people are alike because they are comfortable*).

A number of words in the academic lexicon have different meanings than when used in casual contexts. For example, Table 5–1 lists 32 polysemous words associated with math. Additionally, Nippold (1995) noted three polysemous terms (*up, above, lower*) whose meanings may be challenging to students in mathematics and music classes. The primary meanings of these words refer to spatial relationships (e.g., going *up* the stairs; reaching *above* the second shelf; sitting on the *lower* level). However, in mathematics, their meanings refer to quantitative concepts (e.g., counting *up* to 10; finding a number *above* 50; getting a *lower* score) and in music their meanings refer to acoustic indexes (e.g., going *up* an octave; singing *above* the noise; having a *lower* voice). When working with students who have language impairments, it is important to be aware of polysemous terms and to verify the children's understanding of the secondary meanings.

Literacy and Lexicon

At school age, there is a shift from learning to talk to talking to learn (Westby, 1985). Throughout their academic journey, students are expected to understand the language of instruction, verbalize the content of their knowledge, describe their reasoning processes, and reflect on language itself. These emerging skills require a new set of lexical tools. Several sets of such lexical items were identified by Nippold (1998), including: (a) **adverbs of likelihood** (e.g., *possibly, probably, definitely*) and **adverbs of magnitude** (e.g., *somewhat, rather, extremely*), (b) **metalinguistic and metacognitive verbs** (e.g., *concede, infer, conclude*), and (c) **factive verbs** (e.g., *know, notice*) and **nonfactive verbs** (e.g., *think, believe*). Acquisition of these words occurs over a protracted period between first grade and high school. Examples of research conducted to assess these forms are summarized below, based on Nippold (1998).

Adverbs of Likelihood

Hoffner, Cantor, and Badzinski (in Nippold, 1998) provided 5- to 8-, and 10-year-olds with short vignettes followed by comprehension questions. Each question required the students to discriminate between the meanings of two adverbs. One vignette included the words *probably* and *definitely* to describe how likely each different character would be to perform an action (e.g., *Lori will probably go skating. Robin will definitely go skating*). The comprehension questions then referred back to the probability of an action (e.g., Which girl do you think went skating?). Results showed that performance increased with age. The 5-, 7-, 8-, and 10-year-olds performed with 53%, 65%, 79%, and 93% accuracy, respectively. Additionally, it was easier for students to discriminate between *definitely* and *possibly* and between *definitely* and *probably* than between *possibly* and *probably*.

Adverbs of Magnitude

Adverbs of magnitude are also acquired over a protracted time period. Bashaw and Anderson (in Nippold, 1998) examined the development of nine such adverbs (*slightly, somewhat, rather, pretty, quite, decidedly, unusually, very, extremely*). The participants were children from grades 1 through 6, 8, 10, and 12. College students were also tested.

TABLE 5–1. Math Words With Double Meanings

average	mass	power	row
cancel	match	prime	scale
correspondence	mean	product	score
cycle	multiply	quarters	share
double	odd	represent	table
even	order	relationship	take-away
factor	pattern	root	times
foot	place	round	volume

Results showed that first and second graders discriminated among some of the word pairs (e.g., *slightly* vs. *extremely large*). Older students made increasingly more discriminations (e.g., *somewhat* vs. *rather large*). However, some discriminations were missed even by college students (e.g., *quite* vs. *decidedly large*).

Metaverbs

Metalinguistic verbs (e.g., *assert, predict, interpret*) and **metacognitive verbs** (e.g., *remember, doubt, assume*) are used to talk about thought and verbal processes, respectively. A study by Arlington and Olson (in Nippold, 1998) examined the comprehension of these verbs (known collectively as **literate verbs**) by students in sixth, eighth, tenth, and twelfth grades and college. Each student was provided with a short vignette about the behavior of individuals that illustrated a type of thinking or language use. Each vignette was then followed by a choice of four statements containing literate verbs, and students were asked to choose the statement that applied to the individual(s) in the vignette. Once again, comprehension improved gradually with age. The mean accuracy scores for sixth, eighth, tenth, twelfth graders and college students were 45%, 42%, 59%, 71%, and 92%, respectively.

Knowledge Verbs

Factive (e.g., *know, forget*) and **nonfactive** (*think, believe*) verbs differ in the extent to which the object of knowledge is known to be true (factive) or not entirely certain (nonfactive). Scoville and Gordon (in Nippold, 1998) studied the comprehension of five factive verbs (*know, forget, be sorry, be happy, be surprised*) and five nonfactive verbs (*think, be sure, figure, say, believe*) in students at the ages of 5, 8, 11, 14, and 20 years. The 5- and 8-year-olds demonstrated little understanding of the difference between factive and nonfactive verbs. However, accuracy improved with age. This protracted rate of development suggests that even high school students may be confused at times by the use of these verbs (e.g., *Physicists believe that Pluto is not a true planet* vs. *Physicists know that Pluto is not a true planet*).

Figurative Meanings

Figurative meanings (also known as **nonliteral meanings**) are expressed by **metaphors** (e.g., *You're an angel*), **similes** (e.g., *The street is like a sheet of ice*), **idioms** (e.g., *a frog in my throat*), and **proverbs** (e.g., *Haste makes waste*). As with polysemous forms, the ability to interpret figurative language requires a listener to ignore one referent and search for an alternative. Additionally, a listener must recognize the equivalence of key features that apply across two seemingly different contexts. Consider the expression, "*The beltway is a parking lot.*" This statement evokes features of meaning associated with the concepts of two seemingly different referents: a *beltway* and a *parking lot*. To understand the metaphor, a person must attend selectively to only those features that could overlap between the two (i.e., many cars close together, standing still) and to ignore a host of other features that do not apply.

In elementary and high school, students are exposed to figurative language with increasing frequency during classroom instruction (e.g., Lazar, War-Leeper, Nicholson, & Johnson, 1989) and while reading textbooks (e.g., Nippold, 1998; Nippold, Moran, & Schwarz, 2001) For example, Lazar et al. studied the frequency and types of multiple meaning expressions addressed to children in kindergarten through eighth grade. They found that that an average of 37% of utterances produced by teachers in kindergarten through eighth grade include utterances with multiple meaning expressions. For metaphors, similes, and idioms, this includes an average of 13% of the teachers' utterances. Of the three figurative forms, idioms are the most prevalent across the grade range.

Developmentally, the comprehension and production of **figurative language emerges gradually**. As indicated in the previous chapter, preschoolers sometimes express themselves in ways that appear nonliteral, as in *My leg is soda watering* (i.e., to indicate the feeling of pins and needles when her leg fell asleep) or *I did a bum burp* (after passing gas). More likely, however, such expressions reflect children's creativity in communicating meanings for which they lack conventional words. The referents of these expressions tend to be concrete and the frequency of their use decreases as vocabulary increases (Owens, 2008).

The comprehension and production of true nonliteral semantic forms actually emerges during the later school years. Some of the forms that are used most frequently in a child's speech community are likely to be acquired first, and some of these forms may be understood, initially, as unanalyzed units (Owens, 2008). Sensory metaphors (e.g., *She's cold as ice*) tend to be acquired earlier than more abstract forms (e.g., *She's floating*). Similarly, idioms with more **transparent meanings** (e.g., *skating on thin ice*) typically are acquired sooner than those with more **opaque meanings** (e.g., *to beat around the bush*) (Nippold & Rudzinski, 1993). Owens (2008) noted that **world knowledge** can help to support the interpretation of nonliteral language. For example, *fishing for compliments* and *smooth sailing* may mean more to someone who has fished or sailed than to someone unfamiliar with these activities. To the extent that world knowledge is gained through reading and the media, children's increasing access to literature and movies also supports the acquisition of nonliteral meanings.

Nippold, Moran, and Schwarz (2001) examined the relationship between **idiom comprehension**, reading comprehension, and listening comprehension in a group of 12-year-olds. Reading comprehension and listening comprehension were assessed by standardized tests. The idiom comprehension test was designed by the examiners to include a representative sample of idioms at all levels of familiarity. For each item, comprehension was assessed by providing a short narrative in which the idiom was embedded, followed by a forced choice multiple-choice question about the idiom's meaning. Students also were asked to rate their familiarity with each idiom. Results showed that good performance on the idiom comprehension task was correlated with idiom familiarity and with good performance on the reading and listening comprehension scores.

Of all nonliteral forms, **proverbs** (also known as maxims or adages) are the last to be mastered. When asked to explain their meanings, children as old as 8 to 10 years still interpret proverbs literally. For example, if asked to explain the meaning of *One swallow does not make a summer*, an 8-year-old may say that swallowing won't turn the season into summer. One potential obstacle to proverb comprehension is that some proverbs involve unusual syntactic forms (e.g., *There is none so blind as he who will not see*). However, most proverbs are expressed in more common syntactic forms, and the basic challenge for proverb comprehension is at the semantic/conceptual level.

In one of the earliest developmental studies of proverbs, Nippold, Martin, and Erskine (1988) examined the relationship between proverb comprehension and analogical reasoning across four grade levels (fourth, sixth, eighth, tenth). Each question on the comprehension task included a statement with an embedded proverb (e.g., *Mother said, "Don't count your chickens before they hatch"*) and required the student to select one of four contexts in which the statement would have made sense (e.g., [1] Jimmy has told his mother that he would like to buy her a new dress; [2] Jimmy has told his mother that he would rather play baseball than go to school; [3] Jimmy has told his mother that when he grows up, he's going to be rich and famous, and [4] Jimmy has told his mother that he's the smartest boy in his class). Analogical reasoning was assessed through a standardized test involving pictures rather than words. Each analogy followed the form A is to B as C is to ?. For example (using pictures), car is to street as boat is to _____ (sky, railroad tracks, river, or airport). Results showed that children at all grade levels responded correctly to at least half of the proverb questions, and that the number of correct responses improved across grades. They also showed that there is a systematic positive correlation between improvements in proverb comprehension and analogical reasoning performance across all four grades.

In a later study, Nippold and Haq (1996) showed that familiarity and the degree of abstraction influence the comprehension of proverbs by students in fifth, eighth, and eleventh grades. Using a forced choice response format, they included concrete-familiar proverbs (e.g., *a rolling stone gathers no moss*), concrete-unfamiliar proverbs (e.g., *a caged bird longs for the clouds*), abstract-familiar proverbs (*Two wrongs don't make a right*), and abstract-unfamiliar proverbs (e.g., *Of idleness comes no goodness*). Results showed that the performance of students increased with grade level. Additionally, proverbs that were familiar or concrete were easier to understand than those on the other end of the continuum. The authors interpreted these findings as support for the **metasemantic hypothesis**, which holds that the comprehension of proverbs develops, in part, through active analysis of the words contained therein. Furthermore, the finding of better performance on more familiar proverbs was interpreted as support for the language **experience hypothesis**, which holds that comprehension develops, in part, through meaningful exposure to proverbs.

Comprehension development of all figurative forms involves a dynamic interplay between top-down pragmatic and bottom-up semantic processing (Nippold, Moran, & Schwartz, 2001). A listener attends to the language and to the nonverbal context in which a form is used to arrive at cues regarding a communicator's intent. Semantically, the listener considers the expression for possible cues. When pragmatic cues are limited, the listener must scrutinize the expression more carefully. When forms are extremely opaque (e.g., *raining cats and dogs*) the listener must scrutinize the context more carefully. If both contextual and linguistic information are limited, then a listener may compare the current use of the expression with memories of its previous use.

Word Definitions

The ability to formulate word definitions is of interest for both academic and practical reasons. For example, the formulation of accurate, clear, and concise word definitions is correlated with academic achievement, literacy skill development, and performance on IQ tests (Chall, 1987; Snow, Cancini, & Gonzalez, & Shriberg, 1989). On a more practical level, word definitions are often the first step in orienting a listener to a discussion about a particular topic. To that extent, they serve an important organizing role in extended discourse.

Various types of definitions are produced by people in formal and less formal situations (Makau, 1990). On the less formal end of the continuum, there are **definitions by negation** (e.g., "That test was a *bear*, and I don't mean the animal"), **definitions by comparison** (e.g., "A bat is like a mouse with wings"), **definitions by example** (e.g., "For example, *Bienenstich* is a favorite German pastry"), and **operational definitions** (e.g., "*turn* means to

rotate 360 degrees"). On the most formal end of the continuum is the **Aristotelian definition**, which requires a speaker to classify the referent according to its superordinate category and then to note the features that distinguish the referent within that category. So, *dog* might be defined as "an animal that has fur, four legs, a tail, and barks." Definitions often occur within the context of other meaningful discourse. However, in school, students may be asked to give definitions as an academic exercise outside of a communicative context.

The formulation of word definition tasks includes both linguistic and metalinguistic components (see Nippold, 1995). The speaker must have knowledge of labels for referring to general categories and specific features. Additionally, he or she must understand the structure of a definition and organize the verbal information accordingly.

High quality definitions should be able to serve both as a semantic and syntactic substitute for the word being defined (Bierwisch & Kiefer, 1970). For example, a definition for *pretty* might be "beautiful," and the word *beautiful* could serve as a substitute for the word *pretty* in a sentence like, "She is *pretty*." To formulate a definition that meets these criteria, a child must be able to analyze and coordinate both semantic content and syntactic structure. For example, depending on the context, the word *towering*, could be defined as "rising to great height," "very high," "extremely tall," or "imposing" (Johnson & Anglin, 1995).

Word definitions are considered semantically precise when they follow the Aristotelian format described above. Syntactic precision is achieved when the formulation of the definition matches the part of speech of the word being defined. For example, the noun *table* could be defined by a noun phrase as "a piece of furniture consisting of a smooth flat surface fixed on legs." Verb and adjective definitions are more variable. Some will include reference to a superordinate term (e.g., when the verb *table* is defined as "removing something from consideration"), and others will be defined by synonyms (e.g., when *large* is defined as "big").

Most early developmental studies focused on children's definition of nouns (see Markowitz & Franz [1988] and Nippold [1995] for a review). Those that explored the development of semantic content reported that children's earliest definitions often consist of personal, contextualized illustrations of a word's meaning (e.g., to define *bicycle* a child might say *I ride my bicycle*). As children mature, their definitions begin to include perceptual or functional features of the referent but fail to include the defining attributes (e.g., for *bicycle* a child might say, *you can sit on the saddle*). At the next stage, children learn to provide enough features to capture the word's meaning (e.g., *a bicycle is a vehicle with two wheels, a pedal, and a handle bar*). Studies that have explored the forms of children's definitions note that early definitions rarely include a superordinate term. When superordinate terms begin to be used, they tend to be general (e.g., *bread is something that you use to make a sandwich*) and become more precise later in development (e.g., *socks are clothing for your feet*). The semantic and formal aspects of definitions both develop gradually but not necessarily in synchrony. Coordination of both is the final step, as children learn to create true Aristotelian object-definitions.

In a later investigation, Johnson and Anglin (1995) examined the definitions produced by first, third, and fifth graders for a range of word types (nouns, verbs, adjectives) and for words varying in morphological compositions (root words, compounds, inflections, derivations, and idioms). The words were selected systematically from the bold-faced words in *Webster's Third New International Dictionary* (1981) and arranged in order of increasing difficulty based on the comprehension performance of children at each grade level. Only the words that children understood were then included on the sample for which they were asked to give definitions. The definitions were obtained during individual interviews, and each word was addressed through a hierarchy of questions (i.e., [1] "What does the word _____ mean?" [2] "Can you tell me anything more about what the word _____ means?," [3] "Can you use the word _____ in a sentence?," [4] "What does the word _____ mean in the sentence?," and [5] a multiple choice probe). Only responses to question 1 or 4 were included in the analysis. Finally, each definition was coded for quality on a four-point scale reflecting the coordination of semantic accuracy (generality, precision) and grammatical form (i.e., noun phrases used to define nouns,

verb phrases used to define verbs, etc.). Table 5–2 provides a description of the coding system and examples of children's definitions at all levels of quality for three different word types (noun, verb, adjective).

The results of Johnson and Anglin's (1995) study indicated that children at all grade levels produce some definitions with high semantic quality, and that the proportion of these definitions increases from 30% to 42% to 51% at first, third, and fifth grades, respectively. In absolute terms, the authors estimated that the number of high quality definitions in the repertoire of school age children increases from about 259 words in first grade to about 5,689 words by fifth grade. When word definitions were analyzed in relation to a word's grammatical category (noun, verb, adjective), a larger proportion of high quality definitions was observed for nouns than for adjectives or verbs. When considered in relation to word type (root, compound, derived, inflected), a larger proportion of high quality definitions was observed for compound and root words than for inflected or derived words. These results were interpreted to support the theory that the semantic and grammatical aspects of expressed word definitions develop separately before they are coordinated in high quality definitions. The relatively greater proportion of high quality definitions related to nouns (root words and compounds) was interpreted to reflect both cognitive and experiential factors. In other words, it may be easier to recall superordinate categories for nouns than to place other word types (adjectives, verbs) in a more general context. Second, the proportion of nouns in the English language is considerably higher than the proportion of other word types, so children naturally have more experience with nouns. Third, teachers are more likely to target noun definitions than definitions of other word types. Finally, dictionaries often do not include derived forms as bold entries. Instead, they are noted as options in relation to root words, hence the explicit definitions of derived forms must be inferred.

In a different study, Storck and Looft (1973) investigated the definitions produced by children, adolescents, and adults within nine different age groups between 6 and 66+ years. Participants were asked to define 45 words from the *Stanford-Binet Intelligence Scale*. These words represented a range of difficulty levels and included various parts of

TABLE 5–2. Examples of Noun, Verb, and Adjective Definitions Across the Range of Quality Categories

Code	Definition of Code	Examples		
		Closet (Noun)	*Improve* (Verb)	*Mucky* (Adjective)
1	Contextualized expressed knowledge	"Mom always tells me to put my coat and boots in the closet, but it's hard to find room in there. We have so much junk."	"If someone's report card had no marks and then the second term came up and he had really good marks that means he improved. Improved on my writing."	"It's some things that are better. Some pigs are mucky from the mud."
2	Generalized expressed knowledge without precise content and conventional form	"You put your clothes in. And you put all the rest of the stuff in there. And you put all your jimmies and stuff in."	"Well, you have to get better at something in order to get a certain mark. You have to improve at something. Improve at something to get a better mark. I have to improve my math mark in order to pass."	"Some people go in and the cows go in muck. It's sand with lots of water in it. Mucky. Sometimes children get mucky."
3a	Generalized expressed knowledge with precise content but not conventional form	"You hang clothes in it. And you wear clothes. Closets have doors. You keep bowling balls and stuff in it."	"Improve means if you have something that you're getting better on. Something like if you're reading and you're getting better on it and better each day."	"It means you're all dirty. You have like mud or something covered on you. it's something dirty."
3b	Generalized expressed knowledge with conventional form but not precise content	"It's a place where you store your clothes and your games. And sometimes it's a place that you're not really supposed to see from the outside so that they can be quite messy."	"Oh, they mean do better [on my work habits]."	"Yucky. Gooshy."
4	Generalized expressed knowledge with both precise content and conventional form	"A closet is a storage room where you hang clothes. Or you can put stuff and play hide and seek and everything."	"Do something better. You have to improve in your school work."	"Dirty. Muddy. Like it's full of dirt and you don't really want to get it in your clothes and it's like a wet dirt."

Source: Adapted from C. J. Jonson and J. M. Anglin (1995). Qualitative developments in the content and form of children's definitions. *Journal of Speech and Hearing Research, 38*, Appendix B, p. 629.

speech (nouns, verbs, adjectives). As expected, the proportion of accurate definitions, including the proportion of definitions that mentioned a general category term, increased up to the age of 25 and remained stable until 55 years. After the age of 55 it gradually declined.

Finally, and not surprisingly, there is evidence that words with concrete referents (e.g., *dog*) are easier to define than words with abstract referents (e.g., *justice*), regardless of age. For example, McGhee-Biclack (in Nippold, 1998) asked 10-, 14-, and 18-year-olds to define eight nouns with concrete referents (e.g., *flower, book, car*) and eight nouns with abstract referents (e.g., *freedom, courage, wisdom*). Results showed that, across all age groups, nouns with concrete referents were defined correctly more often than words with abstract referents. Furthermore, nouns with concrete referents were defined mainly in reference to general categories and specific characteristics (e.g., "a *flower* is a plant with colorful petals") whereas nouns with abstract referents were defined mainly in reference to their specific characteristics (e.g., "*freedom* means you can do what you want to do"). However, 18-year-olds (but not 14- or 10-year-olds) produce some definitions with general category terms for words with abstract referents.

Verbal Humor

The ability to share and appreciate humor with one's peers is an important aspect of social development, and like the comprehension of double meanings, requires a person to ignore an expected meaning and search for an alternative one. The humor typically turns on the surprise of discovering an unexpected alternative meaning. Table 5–3 summarizes six different types of linguistic ambiguity and provides examples of each. Included are phonological ambiguity (based on similar sounding words), semantic ambiguity (based on double word meanings), syntactic ambiguity (based on double meanings represented by alternate phrase structures), metalinguistic ambi-

guity (based on a shift in focus from meaning to form), and pragmatic ambiguity (based on a shift in expectation from one discourse genre to another).

The understanding of these forms of ambiguity emerges gradually (e.g., Bernstein, 1986; Fowles & Glanz, 1977; Lund & Duchan, 1983; Schultz & Horibe, 1974; Westby, 1994) and extends throughout the school years depending on the complexity of the semantic or syntactic features involved. Prior to the age of 6 years, children's humor centers on nonverbal slap-stick, pie-in-the-face events. Verbal humor based on phonological ambiguity emerges at about 6 to 8 years. Lexical ambiguity is recognized between about 8 to 10 years, and the appreciation of humor based on syntactic ambiguity is understood by 10 to 12 years.

As would be expected, humor based on comprehension of idioms is the last to be mastered. Spector (1996) studied the ability of third, fourth, and fifth graders to detect and explain humor based on idioms. Thirty students from each grade were presented with 12 very short humor vignettes to analyze, and children were asked to underline the idiom and then write an explanation of its meaning. Results showed that students at all three grade levels identified and explained idioms appropriately, but the percent correct increased for both variables across grade levels. Identification was accurate for an average of 54%, 64%, and 86% of vignettes analyzed by third, fourth, and fifth-graders, respectively, and correct explanations were provided for an average of 34%, 45%, and 59% of idioms at each grade level, respectively. One limitation of this study is that the variables of familiarity and abstractness were not systematically represented.

TABLE 5–3. Linguistic Ambiguity in Verbal Humor

Phonological ambiguity—Ambiguity based on similar sounding words

    e.g., Q: How do turtles talk to each other?

        A: By using shell phones

    e.g., Q: What can make an octopus laugh?

        A: Ten tickles

    e.g., Q: What did the Jedi say to the English teacher?

        A: Metaphors be with you!

    e.g., A rubber band pistol was confiscated from algebra class because it was being used as a weapon of math disruption.

TABLE 5–3. *continued*

Lexical ambiguity—ambiguity based on multiple word meanings

e.g., The magician got so mad he pulled his hare out.

e.g., Q: What building has the most stories?
A: A library

Syntactic ambiguity—ambiguity based on an alternate phrase structures

e.g., Tell me how long cows should be milked.
They should be milked the same as short ones, of course.

e.g., She was engaged to a man with a wooden leg but broke it off.

e.g., Time flies like an arrow, but fruit flies like a banana.

Metalinguistic ambiguity—ambiguity based on alternating attention to the form vs. meaning

e.g., Q: What do you call a fish without an eye?
A: Fsh

e.g., Q: What's the end of everything?
A: G

e.g., Q: What 11-letter English word does everyone pronounce incorrectly?
A: "Incorrectly"

e.g., Q: What kind of cheese is made backward?
A: Edam

e.g., Q: What occurs once in a minute, twice in a moment, and never in a thousand years?
A: The letter "m"

e.g., Q: What seven letters did Mother Hubbard say when she opened her cupboard?
A: O I C U R M T

e.g., Dictionary update: *Sarchasm*—The gulf between the author of sarcastic wit and the person who doesn't get it.

Figurative ambiguity—ambiguity based on literal vs. conventional interpretations of figurative language

e.g., Q: Why did Snoopy quit the comic strips?
A: Because he was tired of working for Peanuts.

e.g., There was a fight in a candy store. Two suckers got licked.

Pragmatic ambiguity—ambiguity based on alternative discourse genres (e.g., joke telling vs. information sharing)

e.g., Q: Why did the chicken cross the road?
A: Because he wanted to get to the other side.

e.g., Q: What did the grape say to the elephant?
A: Nothing. Grapes can't talk.

Sources: Adapted from C. Westby (1994). Communication refinement in school age and adolescence. In W. O. Haynes & B. B. Shulman (Eds.), *Communication Development: Foundations, Processes, and Clinical Applications* (pp. 341–383). Englewood Cliffs, NJ: Prentice-Hall. D. Bernstein (1986). The development of humor: Implications for assessment and intervention. *Topics in Language Disorders, 6*, 65–71.

Factors That Encourage Lexical Development

Reading

Throughout the early elementary years, spoken language, including language spoken in the context of joint book-reading, is the most powerful influence on children's vocabulary growth. However, by approximately nine years (and often sooner), the ability to read becomes a powerful additional factor. Research shows that children who read often and read with comprehension acquire significantly larger vocabularies than children who are less motivated to read and do so less skillfully (e.g., Miller & Gildea, 1987; Nagy, Herman, & Anderson, 1985; Perera, 1986). Print, unlike casual conversation, tends to include consistently well-formed sentences, clear linguistic cohesion, and a larger variety of unique words. As children read to learn the many components of their academic curriculum, they encounter words for increasingly abstract concepts. For all of these reasons, print becomes a richer source of semantic information than oral conversation.

Writing

Unlike most contexts of verbal communication, written language generally offers the advantage of time to make thoughtful, reflective, and deliberate choices in the selection of words. There is a tendency to avoid redundancy, so a writer may consult a thesaurus to look for different ways of referring to the same meaning. Much can be learned about semantic options in this process, and children have many opportunities to do this as part of their education.

Schooling

By design, schooling exerts a powerful influence on children's language growth, even more so than language experiences in the home. Huttenlocher, Levine, and Vevea (1998) measured the growth of children's language (vocabulary and syntax) at four points between the beginning of kindergarten and the end of first grade. Results showed that the children made more gains in language during each school year (between October and April) than during the intervals between April and October. As

word learning is a major part of the educational process in any content area, this is not surprising. Many words are learned through **direct instruction** as teachers name concepts, provide definitions, give examples, and engage children in activities that invite the use of new information. Furthermore, by second grade, children learn to use the **dictionary** (and the computer) to find word meanings. As indicated above, children also learn to define words on their own (e.g., Kurland & Snow, 1997; Miller & Gildea, 1987). These are all effects of schooling.

Contextual Cues

Imagine that you have walked into a room where a speaker is sharing the following personal experience with her friends:

Hungarians enjoy eating dios bukta at the end of a festive meal. When I was a child, I still remember the delicious smell wafting from the oven when my grandmother prepared this treat. My mother still makes it sometimes too, but she fasts for a whole day to justify the calories.

Even if you have never heard of *dios bukta* before, a reasonable conclusion would be that it refers to some kind of rich, Hungarian pastry. This inference is reasonable because the words that surround *dios bukta* refer to it as a baked treat, with lots of calories, that is eaten by Hungarians at the end of a festive meal. To confirm your hypothesis, you would want to hear *dios bukta* used in another context but in the present context, your conclusion would be justified. This process of using contextual cues to arrive at a guess about the meaning of a novel word has been characterized as **contextual abstraction** (Nippold, 1998) or **incidental word learning** (Carlisle, 2005; Rice, 1990). Contextual abstraction differs from **fast mapping** (a word-learning process used by preschoolers) because the word's meaning must be inferred from the linguistic context rather than nonlinguistic contextual cues.

According to Carlisle (2005), 90% of the words students learn each year are acquired through incidental encounters in oral and written discourse contexts. Since printed text tends to include a greater number of unique words than conversational language, children are more likely to encounter unique words while reading than during conversation. Teachers support students in contextual analysis by making them aware of the strategies they can use to make inferences about word meanings (e.g., Sinatra & Dowd, 1991) and by providing them with application practice (e.g., Nippold, 1998).

Rice (1990) uses the phrase **quick incidental learning** (**QUIL**) to refer to contextual vocabulary learning and has conducted several studies on this topic (e.g., Oetting, Rice, & Swank, 1995; Rice & Woodsmall, 1988). School-aged children were introduced to novel words in the context of story narratives, and follow-up assessments confirmed that the children had learned accurate features of meaning associated with the target words. However, other researchers have noted that the overall comprehension abilities and the proximity of a novel word to a helpful defining context can affect the accuracy of incidental learning. Cain and Oakhill (2003) found that 7- and 8-year-olds with good comprehension skills are better than same-age peers with poor comprehension skills at integrating information from different parts of a text to arrive at an appropriate meaning for a novel word, even though both groups of students were equally skilled at decoding. The task in Cain et al.'s study involved reading a narrative rather than hearing it, but it is likely that a similar pattern would result if the story narrative had been presented orally.

Morphological Analysis

Recall that morphology refers to the system of rules that determine changes in the structure of words depending on their grammatical and semantic functions. A **morpheme** is the smallest unit of meaning in our language. **Free morphemes** are root words that may occur independently (e.g., *base, ball, cup, cake*), or in combination as compound words (e.g., *baseball, cupcake*). **Bound morphemes** are affixes (prefixes, suffixes) that may be attached to a root word as an inflection to modulate the meaning of a root word (e.g., *walking, walked, walks*) or as derivational form to change its meaning (e.g., *gardener, noncompliant*). Also recall that **grammatical morphemes** (e.g., plural markers, tense markers, markers of possession, etc.) are acquired over a protracted period of time beginning at about 24 months

and extending over the preschool period. Additionally, children demonstrate their understanding of **compounding** and some **derivational forms** when they coin words (e.g., "plantman" for *gardener*; "nailer" for *hammer*; "jellying" for *spreading jelly*).

During the school years, we see additional growth in the variety of derivational forms that children learn and in the extent to which children use their knowledge of morphology to analyze meanings of novel words (Anglin, Miller, & Wakefield, 1993; Nagy, Herman, & Anderson, 1985). For example, we know from the results of Anglin et al.'s study (discussed earlier in this chapter) that the ability to make use of morphological cues increases dramatically between third and fifth grade. We also know that the use of morphological analysis to make inferences about word meanings is addressed through direct instruction in elementary school (Nippold, 1998; White, Power, & White, 1989). When children hear a sentence like, *John is a skilled rutcher*, they can use their knowledge of morphology to recognize the parts of this word (*rutch + er*) and to deduce that "rutch" probably refers to a kind of action and that John is a person who performs this action skillfully. They will then need to refer to other contextual cues to identify the nature of the action. Consider the following two stanzas from *Jabberwocky* by Lewis Carroll (1871/1987):

> Twas brillig, and the slithy toves
> Did gyre and gimble in the wabe:
> mimsy were the borogoves,
> And the mome raths outgrabe.
> Beware the Jabberwock, my son!
> The jaws that bite, the claws that catch!
> Beware the Jubjub bird, and shun
> The frumious Bandersnatch!
>
> (Carroll, 1871/1987, pp. 1–2)

What can you infer about the setting and characters in this poem despite the high proportion of unconventional words? What information can you glean from the grammatical morphemes? Based on this information, how would you describe the toves? The popularity of this poem among children speaks to their growing metalinguistic awareness of the morphological structure or **metamorphological awareness**.

PRIMARY ACCOMPLISHMENTS: PHONOLOGY

Two kinds of changes occur in the phonological systems of elementary school students. Both have a crucial impact on the development of reading. One kind of change pertains to the production of words and the other pertains to the continuing development of metaphonological awareness. Each is summarized below.

Developmental Changes in Word Production

By the time they enter first grade, most children have mastered the rules of the phonological system to the extent that their conversational speech is both 100% intelligible and almost 100% free of speech production errors. Even adults sometimes mispronounce words, so we would not expect a school-aged child to produce flawless speech. However, some children continue to have relatively consistent residual problems with the more difficult, later-to-be-acquired sounds, including liquids (/r/, /l/), fricatives (/s, z, θ, ð, ∫, ʒ/), and affricates (/t∫, dʒ/), especially when some of these sounds occur in clusters of consonants within words (e.g., Vihman, 1988). Depending on the frequency and consistency of these errors, some students benefit by support services from a speech-language pathologist (SLP). Schools generally offer screenings to identify the children who demonstrate the need for this support.

Some children whose speech is otherwise free of errors may have difficulty in pronouncing phonologically complex words, including words with both multiple syllables and consonant clusters (e.g., *aluminum, spaghetti, stethoscope,* etc.). Typical children and adults sometimes mispronounce multisyllabic words during complex speaking tasks. However, school age children who have consistent and persistent difficulties in the production of such words in all speaking tasks should be referred for a speech-language evaluation. The persistence of consistent speech production errors on complex phonological forms throughout the early elementary school years is a sign of risk for learning disabilities (Paul, 2007), and support services can help.

In addition to resolving residual phonological errors, school age children improve in their ability to understand speech in noisy environments. This improvement reflects their growing knowledge about the phonological system itself (see phonological awareness, below) as well as continued growth of vocabulary, grammar, and the ability to infer a speaker's communicative intent (e.g., Vihman, 1988). Improvements of this type continue to at least the age of 15 years.

Growth of Phonological and Phonemic Awareness

Phonological awareness is a type of **metalinguistic awareness** involving the ability to look beyond word meanings to reflect on the phonological structure of words. It is a broad term referring to the awareness of syllable structure as well as the awareness of phoneme structure. Awareness of syllable structure is indicated by a child who can clap for the number of syllables in a word. Awareness of phoneme structure is indicated by a child who can count the number of sounds within a word. In contrast to phonological awareness, **phonemic awareness** refers more narrowly to the awareness of specific sounds within words. For example, phonemic awareness is indicated by a child who can specify the first sound in a word (e.g., *ball* starts with /b/).

The growth of phonological and phonemic awareness is a crucial milestone during the early school years as it suggests that children have developed solid phonological representations of words. The accurate performance of various phonological awareness tasks is strongly correlated with later reading achievement in cultures that use an alphabetic reading system. A sampling of these tasks is provided in Table 5–4.

Awareness of syllabic units (e.g., rhyming, counting syllables) emerges and is mastered sooner than awareness of phonemic units. Lieberman, Schankweiler, Fischer, and Carter (1974) studied the emergence of these skills in 4-, 5-, and 6-year-olds. They found that phonological awareness emerges at 4 years and is mastered by 6 years. However, phonemic awareness was not evident until the

TABLE 5–4. Phonological Awareness Tasks

Rhyme awareness—A child is provided with two spoken words (e.g., *ring, sing*) and asked to say "yes" or "no" to indicate if the words rhyme.

Rhyme production—A child is provided with a model word (e.g., *sock*) and asked to identify a similar sounding word (e.g., *lock*).

Syllable awareness—A child is provided with a word (e.g., *suitcase*) and asked to clap once for each syllable.

Syllable deletion—A child is asked to say a word (e.g., *sunflower*) and then to say it again without its first syllable

Instructor: Say the word *sunflower*

Student: sunflower

Instructor: Say it again without the *sun*

Student: flower

Syllable segmentation—A child is provided with a word (e.g., *cat*) and asked to segment the word's initial consonant (/k/) from its rime (i.e., vowel + final consonant, /æt/) (e.g., Treiman, 1985)

Sound awareness—The child is provided with a word (e.g., *knit*) and asked to count the number of sounds within the word.

Initial phoneme identification—A child is provided with a model word (*soap*) and asked to produce its first sound (e.g., /s/).

Final phoneme identification—A child is provided with a word (*cup*) and asked to produce the final phoneme (e.g., /p/).

Phoneme deletion—A child is asked to say a word and then to say it again without the first sound. (This follows the same format as syllable deletion, above)

Initial phoneme substitution—A child is asked to say a word (e.g., *top*) and then to substitute the beginning sound (/t/) with another sound (e.g., /m/).

age of 5 years and had not been fully mastered by age 6. In our discussion about the development of reading skills (below) we look more closely at the importance of phonological awareness as a foundation for the acquisition of decoding skills in cultures that use an alphabetic cipher.

PRIMARY ACCOMPLISHMENTS: MORPHOLOGY AND SYNTAX

Children arrive in first grade with a basic syntactic system already acquired. A list of entry-level skills follows:

- Ability to produce all **basic sentence types** (declarative, interrogative, negative, imperative).

- Ability to **embed phrases** into sentences, including **prepositional phrases** (e.g., *Look at the car to your right*), **infinitive phrases** (e.g., *Help me to find my shoes*), **participial phrases** (e.g., *Pedaling hard, Suzanne won the race*), and **gerund phrases** (e.g., *Skiing with friends is my favorite pastime*).

- Ability to produce **complex sentences** by **embedding clauses** within sentence constituents (e.g., *I know where the cat is hiding*) and by **conjoining clauses** with subordinating conjunctions (e.g., *After we finish lunch, we can play a game*).

- Ability to create **compound sentences** by conjoining two independent clauses with a coordinating conjunction (e.g., *I am going to draw and my sister is going to paint*).

- Ability to create **complex-compound sentences** by conjoining two independent clauses and at least one dependent clause (e.g., *I have a game this afternoon, but I'll call you when it's over*).

These skills are the foundation for many refinements yet to develop. Throughout the school years, students are challenged to engage in critical thinking by examining, describing, comparing, contrasting, inducing, deducing, predicting, imagining, concluding, and summarizing information and ideas. These higher level cognitive tasks require higher-level verbal skills for their expression. The refinements in grammar that are seen during the elementary school period contribute to this skill set. Development is supported by children's exposure to the more literate language style used by teachers during classroom instruction, by direct grammar instruction, by engagement in reading for learning and pleasure, and by practice in formulating written discourse, which can be done with more reflection and planning than spontaneous conversation.

We cover the issues associated with later language development at three levels. First, we summarize quantitative changes that involve the grammatical system as a whole. Next, we present an overview of key grammatical forms that contribute to the quantitative changes. Then, we look more closely at the developmental challenges associated with a small subset of these forms. Readers who are interested in a more comprehensive and detailed description of later grammatical development are encouraged to consult the following excellent sources: Justice and Ezell (2002); Nippold (2007); Scott, (1988), Scott and Stokes (1995).

Quantitative Changes

Sentence Length

Sentence length has been measured by collecting a language sample, counting the number of words and utterances, and then calculating the average number of words per utterance. Methods of this type have been used to examine language samples produced by large numbers of children with the consistent finding of a slow, steady increase in the average length of utterances throughout the school years (Hunt, 1965, 1970; Klecan-Aker & Hedrick, 1985; Loban, 1976; O'Donnell et al., 1967; Richardson, Calnan, Essen, & Lambert, 1976). As a rule, the average length of spoken utterances matches chronologic age until about 9 years (Scott & Stokes, 1995). In other words, the average length of a spoken utterance produced by a typical 8-year-old is about eight words per utterance. However, by the age of about 9 years, the rate of increase begins to slow down. During adolescence, the average length of spoken utterances is about 10 to 12 words. The average length of written sentences mirrors this developmental pattern, ranging from 7 to 14 words between third and twelfth grades, respectively.

One limitation of this information is that utterance length is affected by the specific speaking and writing tasks during which a language sample is collected. For example, children tend to produce a larger number of words per sentence when they are producing narratives or giving explanations than when they are engaged in dialogue discourse (Leadholm & Miller, 1992; Nippold, Hekseth, Duthie, & Mansfield, 2005). Similarly, the average number of words per sentence varies in written language depending on genre. For example, students tend to produce longer sentences when they are writing persuasive texts than when they are writing narratives or descriptive texts (Crowhurst & Piche, 1979). In fact, when compared with narrative and descriptive genres, persuasive discourse is the most sensitive to developmental changes in average sentence length (Crowhurst, 1980). Ultimately, sentence length must always be evaluated in consideration of the speaking or writing task and not be interpreted as an isolated value.

Clause Density

Another quantitative measure of syntactic growth is **clause density**, which refers to the average number of clauses (main and subordinate) per sentence. Recall that a **main clause** is a group of words with a subject and a predicate. It can stand alone as a sentence (*Erin completed the marathon*) or be introduced by a coordinating conjunction (e.g., *I'm making the cake and Kathy is making the frosting.*) A **subordinate clause** is introduced by a subordinating conjunction (e.g., *while, because,* etc.) or a relative pronoun (e.g., *who, which,* etc.) and must be connected to a main clause (e.g., *while he waited for the train, Jose completed the crossword puzzle*).

Similar to sentence length, measures of clause density are based on language sample analysis. In this case, the sample is analyzed by counting the total number of T-units per sentence (or the total number of C-units per utterance) and then dividing by the total number of sentences (or utterances). Developmentally, the mean clause density for children in grades 3, 5, 6, and 11 is 1.22, 1.29, 1.39, and 1.52, respectively (Scott, 1988), and in the written language of twelfth graders it is 1.68 (Scott & Stokes, 1995).

Increases in clause density are based on children's more frequent use of two grammatical processes that emerged during the preschool period: clausal embedding and clausal conjoining. The new development during the school years is the frequency of embedding as well as the variety of subordinating conjunctions and relative pronouns used to connect subordinating clauses to a main clause. Table 5–5 summarizes the five types of subordinate clauses including the subordinating conjunctions and relative pronouns that are used to connect these clauses to an independent clause.

Overview of Later Grammatical Development

Scott and Stokes (1995) and Nippold (2007) described numerous grammatical patterns that can serve as qualitative **indices** of later language development. Table 5–6 summarizes these patterns and provides examples. The patterns involve elaborations at all levels of grammatical structure, including phrases, clauses, complex sentences, and intersentential cohesion (see example below).

Phrase structure elaborations include the use of grammatical devices for expanding noun phrases (NPs) and verb phrases (VPs). For example, as children mature, they expand NPs more often by using multiple modifiers before a noun (e.g., *the bright yellow flashing light*). VP expansion occurs more

often through the addition of modal auxiliaries (e.g., *could, would, should, might, must*) to the verb structure (e.g., *I could work on my art project if you must use the computer*). Additionally, older children more frequently elaborate adverb phrases (e.g., *The high school orchestra performed incredibly well and won the regional competition*).

Changes in clause structure are observed in the language of school age children with an increase in the number of prepositional phrases that serve an adverbial function. Consider this sentence: *We searched under every rock for several hours on Tuesday in the heat with no success.* This sentence includes a subject (*we*), a verb (*searched*), and no less than five prepositional phrases, all of which function as adverbials to specify the place, time, and manner in which the action took place.

A number of patterns are used increasingly to expand complex sentences. Some of these patterns involve subjects and others involve predicates. For example, nominal clauses are used with increasing frequency as the sentence subject. Such clauses may begin with a subordinating conjunction (e.g., *Why he pulled the trigger is a mystery to me*) or with an infinitive verb (*To enter the race at this late date could be risky*). Appositives (explanations following a noun) are used more often as well (e.g., *Paul, an expert diver, would be qualified to join the recovery effort*). Similarly, there is an increasing and more varied use of relative clauses (e.g., the light *that is produced during a fireworks show*). Relative clauses are used occasionally by preschoolers to modify the object of a sentence, although with frequent errors in the choice of the relative pronoun (e.g., *I like the crayon what you have*). By school age, children produce relative clauses accurately, use them more often, and use them to modify both the subject and the object of a sentence (e.g., *Gianina, who is an accomplished artist, completed several paintings that are on display in a gallery*). The use of a relative clause following a subject noun is known as **center-embedding**. It is worth noting here that center-embedded clauses are more difficult for younger students to understand because they require a listener to remember the subject while thinking about the modifiers before hearing the predicate.

Predicate structures within complex sentences also expand in the language of school age children.

TABLE 5–5. Five Types of Subordinate Clauses and Common Subordinating Conjunctions

Types	Grammatical Function	Examples
Nominal clause (Noun clause)	Serves as a noun. Introduced by a subordinating conjunction[1,2]	*What I think is not important.* *Why he did it is still a mystery.*
Relative clause (Adjectival clause)	Modifies a preceding noun or pronoun. Introduced by a relative pronoun[2]	*I like roller coasters that make me dizzy.* *Here's the book [that] I read.*
Adverbial clause	Specifies the time, manner, place, condition, or reason for an action. Introduced by a subordinating conjunction[1]	*When I wake up, I drink a cup of coffee.* *He ate as if it were his last meal.* *Wherever you go, remember to give me a call.* *If you want me to call, give me your number.* *She fell down because she was running too fast.*
Comparative Clause	Compares information in the dependent clause with information in the main clause. Introduced by a subordinating conjunction[1]	*Elvis is a bigger star than John is.* *I invited as many people as I could find.*
Infinitive Clause	Includes the infinitive form of the verb (*to + V*). It does not require a subordinating conjunction. An infinitive clause may be bare (lacking an overt subject), and the infinitive itself may be bare (lacking an overt *to*). Infinitive clauses may function as nominals, adjectivals, or adverbials.	e.g., Nominal infinitive clause *To visit Dubai is one of my fondest dreams.* e.g., Adjectival infinitive clause *That is a dessert to die for.* e.g., Adverbial infinitive clause *Renee moved over to make room.*

[1]**Common subordinating conjunctions**			[2]**Common relative pronouns**	
after	*since*	*where*	*who*	*what*
although	*that*	*whereas*	*whoever*	*whatever*
as	*though*	*wherever*	*whom*	*which*
as well as	*unless*	*whether*	*whomever*	*whichever*
because	*until*	*while*	*whose*	*that*
if	*when*	*why*		

Source: Adapted from [1]L. M. Justice & H. K. Ezell (2002).*The Syntax Handbook.* Eau Claire, WI: Thinking Publications, pp. 32, 217–221; [2]F. Parker & K. Riley (1994).*Linguistics for Non-Linguists.* Boston, MA: Allyn & Bacon, p. 203.

For example, there is an increased use of adverbial clauses (e.g., *The rescue crew found the climbers after several hours of intensive search.*) Moreover, the specific subordinating conjunctions used to introduce these clauses include increasingly more advanced forms (e.g., *unless, even though, whereas*).

TABLE 5–6. Features of Syntactic Growth in School-Age Children and Adolescents

Levels	Grammatical Features	Description	Examples
Phrase Structure	Complex noun phrase (NP) premodification	Two or more modifiers occur between the beginning of the noun phrase and the noun itself	e.g., _the first, multicolored_ blaze of light e.g., _every large, four-legged_ insect
	NP postmodification.	A noun is followed by a prepositional phrase or relative clause to specify or elaborate the referent	e.g., the cat _with the long white whiskers_ e.g., the woman _who drove the red car_
	Complex verb phrase (VP) structure	Use of modal auxiliaries Perfect _have + en_	e.g., We _should_ have stopped e.g., We _have_ already eat_en._
	Adjective phrase (AdjP) expansion	A qualifier plus an adjective	e.g., The serving size was _extremely large_ e.g., The view was _unbelievably beautiful_
	Adverb phrase (AdvP) expansion,	A qualifier plus an adverb	e.g., He breathed _very heavily_ e.g., She spoke _barely audibly_
Clause Structure	Increasing numbers of adverbial elements	Prepositional phrases that serve an adverbial function	e.g., Most insects hide _from the heat under the rocks in the desert during the day_
Complex Sentence (Subordination)	Left-branching (preposed) adverbial clauses	Clauses that precede the main clause of the sentence	e.g., _Under the conditions of increased snowfall and low visibility,_ the meeting is likely to be canceled.
	Center-embedded relative clauses	Relative clauses that refer to the subject of the sentence.	e.g., The light _that reflected on the water_ was enough to illuminate the space.
	Nominal clauses as subjects	The use of dependent clauses in the role of sentence subject	e.g., _Why she couldn't come to the meeting_ was not made known to us.
	Later developing adverbial subordinate conjunctions	Conjunctions that qualify the time, condition, or circumstances of an action	e.g., _unless, even though, whereas,_ etc. e.g., _As long as_ you are willing to help, we can finish this project today.
	Appositives	Explanations that follow a noun to clarify its meaning	e.g., My cousin, _the English teacher,_ enjoys reviewing manuscripts.
	Combinations of clause types in one sentence	Any combination of independent and subordinate clauses in a single sentence	e.g., Before we met for our last family reunion in Germany, I didn't know that my cousin, an anesthesiologist by profession, was also an accomplished artist, who produces extremely interesting paintings and sculptures.

continues

TABLE 5–6. *continued*

Levels	Grammatical Features	Description	Examples
Discourse Structure	Adverbial conjuncts and disjuncts	Cohesion devices used to link sentences based on some logical relationship.	e.g., *My dog destroyed the neighbor's garden. Consequently, he is no longer allowed to leave our property.*
	Ellipsis patterns	Deleting information that was stated previously	e.g., *Speaker 1: What did you order?* *Speaker 2: [I ordered] Lentil soup*
	Word-order variations for theme and focus	Selecting a sentence form to match a point of emphasis	e.g., Basic sentence: *She left because of him.* Sentence clefting for emphasis: *It was he who caused her to leave*

Source: Adapted from In C. M. Scott and S. L. Stokes (1995). Measures of syntax in school-age children and adolescents. *Language, Speech, and Hearing Services in Schools, 26,* Table 1, p. 312.

At the level of extended discourse (e.g., telling personal narratives, giving descriptions, giving directions, etc.) children increasingly use grammatical markers to establish **intersentential cohesion** (i.e., logical relationships between the information contained in consecutive sentences). For example, they increasingly use conjunctive adverbs such as *accordingly, consequently, moreover* (e.g., *Petra was late for class. Consequently she missed the test.*). Children are also using word-order variations more often to emphasize a particular point within discourse. For example, consider the difference between the following sentences:

1. Helen reorganized the books on the library shelves.

2. It was Helen who reorganized the books on the library shelves.

3. It was the books on the library shelves that Helen reorganized.

By clefting parts of sentence 1, it is possible to emphasize the subject (as in sentence 2) or the object (as in sentence 3) for emphasis consistent with the logic of the discourse.

These indexes of growth during later language development are by no means exhaustive of all the changes that take place. However, they provide a good overview of the types of changes observed. As students progress through high school, they are more apt to use a combination of these strategies within a single sentence, thereby increasing the clausal density and sentence length even further.

All grammatical refinements that we have discussed progress simultaneously and over a protracted period of time. To illustrate some of the issues that affect the learning curve, we provide a more detailed picture of the developmental trajectory for a few selected grammatical forms.

Selected Developmental Examples

As indicated above, the ability to connect increasingly complex clauses within and across sentences is one of the hallmarks of later language development. An additional important achievement is the growth of grammatical flexibility—that is, the ability to cast the same message within different syntactic structures so that selected features of content can be emphasized as intended within discourse. We now consider refinements in the use of cohesion devices, subordinate clauses, and passive voice as an aspect of this development.

Refinements in the Use of Grammatical Cohesion Devices

Cohesion refers to the joining together of linguistic segments. Among the grammatical tools available for this purpose are conjunctions and conjunctive adverbs. **Conjunctions** are words that function to join linguistic segments within a sentence whereas **conjunctive adverbs** are words that function to establish logical relationships between sentences. Table 5-7 lists the words associated with each function. We summarize the refinement of conjunctions first and conjunctive adverbs in the next section.

Technically, conjunctions can be used at various levels (e.g., to join words to words, phrases to phrases and clauses to clauses). For the purposes of this discussion, we limit our focus to the use of conjunctions for joining clauses with sentences. Not only do conjunctions serve as a kind of grammatical glue for connecting these segments, they can also make explicit the nature of the semantic relationship between those segments.

As indicated in Table 5-7, conjunctions are typically classified as coordinating, subordinating, or correlative (Justice & Ezell, 2002). **Coordinating conjunctions** are used to join clauses of equal importance (e.g., *Christina is swimming **and** Daniel is playing tennis*). **Subordinating conjunctions** are used to connect a subordinate clause with relatively less weight to a main clause of greater importance (e.g., *Please give me a call **when** you have a minute*). **Correlative conjunctions** are pairs of words that must be used together within a sentence. One example is the *either-or* contrast (e.g., *Your job is **either** to dry the dishes **or** to clean the table.*).

Knowledge of conjunctions is important for the development of literacy skills, and educators should be aware of children's performance levels (Nippold, 1998). Several studies indicate that there is a protracted period of mastery of these forms during elementary, middle, and even high school. For example, Roberts (in Nippold, 1998) studied the understanding of coordinating (*and, but, for*) and subordinating (*although, because, if, when*) conjunctions by fourth, fifth, and sixth graders.

TABLE 5–7. Conjunctions and Conjunctive Adverbs

Coordinating Conjunctions		Subordinating Conjunctions			Correlative Conjunctions
for	*but*	*after*	*since*	*where*	*both . . . and*
and	*or*	*although*	*that*	*whereas*	*either . . . or*
and then	*yet*	*as*	*though*	*wherever*	*neither . . . nor*
nor	*so*	*as well as*	*unless*	*whether*	*whether . . . or*
		because	*until*	*while*	*as . . . as*
		if	*when*	*why*	*if . . . then*
		even if			

		Conjunctive Adverbs		
accordingly	*even so*	*in contrast*	*notwithstanding*	*that is*
additionally	*for example*	*in fact*	*on the contrary*	*then*
also	*further*	*in deed*	*otherwise*	*therefore*
alternatively	*furthermore*	*in other words*	*rather*	*thus*
as such	*hence*	*likewise*	*similarly*	
besides	*however*	*moreover*	*so that*	
consequently	*in addition*	*nevertheless*	*still*	

Source: L. Justice and H. K. Ezell (2002). *The syntax handbook.* Eau Claire, WI: Thinking Publications, pp. 104, 130–132.

Each student completed the Connective Reading Test, which included items based on sentences taken from the children's textbooks. For each item, students were presented with the beginning of a sentence (e.g., "*He saw the car, but _____*") and asked to choose one of four options for completing the sentence. The students' responses showed that an understanding of these conjunctions is acquired gradually. The proportion of fourth, fifth, and sixth graders who performed correctly on this task ranged from 57%, 66%, and 75%, respectively.

As indicated previously, **adverbial conjuncts** are used to establish logical connections between sentences. Examples include *moreover, consequently,* and *furthermore.* These words occur frequently in textbooks and in the oral language style of teachers. Between the ages of 6 and 12 years, students use a small number of the more common adverbial conjunct forms (e.g., *so, then, though*) (Scott, 1984). However, an increase in the variety of these forms is observed with increasing age. Nippold, Schwarz, and Undlin (1992) studied the use and understanding of 10 adverbial conjuncts (*therefore, however, consequently, rather, nevertheless, furthermore, moreover, conversely, contrastively, similarly*) by adolescents and young adults. Production of the forms was assessed in a writing task which required each participant to complete a sentence (e.g., *Last night, David borrowed his father's car without permission, Consequently, _____*). Comprehension was assessed by asking each participant to select one of four adverbial conjunct choices to complete a sentence as in the following example (Nippold et al., p. 35):

Wood products are one of the chief exports in Sweden. Swedish furniture is sold to many people in Europe and the United States. Much of this furniture is made in the city of Stockholm. _____, the furniture makers in Stockholm depend heavily on forest resources.

A. *Moreover*   C. *Furthermore*
B. *Consequently*   D. *However*

The participants' performance of both tasks improved with increasing age. The mean ages of the groups were 12, 15, 19, and 23 years. The accuracy of their performance on the writing task was 45%, 50%, 50%, and 64%, respectively, and the accuracy of their performance on the reading task was 79%, 85%, 85%, and 94%, respectively. These results show not only increasing accuracy with age but also that comprehension emerges sooner than production.

Refinements in the Use of Dependent Clauses

During the preschool period, children learned to use the coordinating conjunction *and* to express additive, temporal, causal, and adversative relations (see the previous chapter for examples of this). During early school age, they continue to use *and* in this way when telling stories or sharing events. In fact, from 50% to 80% of children's sentences in narrative speaking tasks begin with *and*. However, as they approach the age of 11 to 14 years, this percentage drops to about 20% in oral language and 5% in written expression (Scott, in Owens, 2008).

With a decrease in the use of *and* there is an increase in the use of subordinate clauses to express relational meanings. Subordinate clauses can serve four grammatical functions: nominal (to function as a noun), adjectival (to function as an adjective), adverbial (to function as an adverb), or comparative (to establish a comparison with the premise of the main clause). Table 5–8 presents examples of each. However, there is a learning curve associated with the use of these forms, and children with language impairments often have special difficulties in processing them (Kuder, 2008). Next, we provide developmental descriptions of three types of clauses: temporal clauses, causal construction, and infinitive clauses.

Temporal clauses are introduced by subordinating temporal conjunctions (e.g., *before, after, during*). They can be used to introduce a sentence or they can be embedded within the sentence frame. Three examples follow:

1. *<u>Before you watch the game,</u> please finish your calculus homework.*

2. *Please do your art project <u>after writing your spelling words.</u>*

3. *<u>When you have completed your reading assignment,</u> it will be time for lunch.*

Notice that in each of these sentences, the conjunction that introduces the clause specifies the sequenc-

TABLE 5–8. Grammatical Functions Served by Subordinating Clauses

Function	Example
Nominal	*That Mike is an incorrigible punster was known to us all.*
Adjectival	*Christine, who is one of the nicest people I know, is also the smartest.*
Adverbial	*Before the big jump, Olga checked the function of her parachute.*
Comparative	*Although a convertible would be more fun, an SUV seems more practical.*

ing of actions named in the sentence. For example, in sentence 1, the clause *before you go outside* specifies the order in which the listener should *finish* his or her math work and go outside.

During the early elementary school years, some students use **nonsyntactic comprehension strategies** to interpret sentences of this type. One such strategy is to ignore the meaning of the subordinating conjunction and to perform the named actions in the **order of mention**. This strategy leads to an incorrect interpretation of sentences 1 and 2, and a correct interpretation of sentence 3. For example, two actions are mentioned in sentence 1: going outside and doing math work. The subordinating conjunction (*before*) indicates the intended order in which the actions are to be completed, and it is opposite to the order of mention. However, in sentence 3 the order of mention is the same as the intended order, so a student using the order of mention strategy would interpret the sentence accurately. A second strategy used by some children is to focus on the named actions and **do what is usually done** within the routine of the day. For example, a student who is told, "*Before you line up for recess please put on your coat*" is likely to respond correctly even though the order of mention does not match the order of expected performance. Eventually, children begin to pay attention to the subordinating conjunctions and to regulate their actions according to these linguistic cues. However, teachers of young elementary school students should be aware of the potential for misunderstanding.

Subordinate clauses expressing causal relationships also serve an adverbial function. In these

sentences, an outcome is typically described in the main clause. This is followed by a description of the explanation in the dependent clause, introduced by the subordinating conjunction *because*. Developmentally, children first provide reasons within discourse:

Parent: Why is the vase broken?

Child: Cause it fell down.

To use *because* as a subordinating conjunction in a complete sentence requires an understanding of the actual sequence in which cause-effect relationships occur and knowledge about the linguistic conventions for representing the order, which is often the reverse of the actual sequence. For example, imagine an actual cause-effect sequence in which you kick a ball, causing it to roll. Although it is possible to say, "*Because I kicked the ball, it rolled*," it is more conventional in casual conversation to explain the event by saying, "*The ball rolled because I kicked it.*"

During the preschool period, children use *and* to conjoin clauses that represent cause-effect sequences (Bloom, Lahey, Hood, Lifter, & Feiss, 1980). For example, they may say, "*I went outside in the rain and I got wet.*" The conjunction *because* eventually enters the lexicon, but, until the age of about 7 years, it is treated by children as functionally equivalent to *and* (Corrigan, 1975). Hence, during the early elementary school years students may produce sentences such as, *I scraped my knee cause it's bleeding.* Data regarding children's mastery of causal sentences vary depending on how the skill was observed. Emerson (1979) reported that children do not fully understand sentences with casual clauses until the age of about 10 or 11. Peterson and McCabe (1985) reported that children can make accurate judgments about the form of a causal sentence by the age of 8 years and even sooner if the task is clear and if contextual information is provided to support their judgments. In an abundance of caution, comprehension and production of causal sentences should not be taken for granted during the early elementary school years.

Another type of subordinate clause used with increasing frequency as children mature is the **infinitive clause**, which contains the infinitive form of a verb (e.g., *to run, to help, to know, to ask, to promise*, etc.). The infinitive form of a verb is considered a type of **nonfinite verb** because it does not require tense markers. Infinitive clauses are a bit quirky for several reasons. First, unlike the other subordinating clauses in Table 5–5, infinitive clauses are not introduced by a subordinating conjunction. Second, sometimes infinitive clauses contain a **bare infinitive** because *to* is missing (e.g., *Help me find my shoe*). Third, unlike the other subordinate clauses, infinitive clauses can serve three different grammatical functions: (a) nominal (e.g., *To err is human*), (b) adjectival (e.g., *This is a dessert to die for*), and (c) adverbial (e.g., *Drive past the first stop sign to find the fork in the road*). However, regardless of grammatical function, infinitive clauses can be embedded into sentence frames to help condense information and eliminate redundancy. Consider the following sentences:

1. *Carolyn came over.*

2. *Carolyn told us about the concert.*

3. *Carolyn came over to tell us about the concert.*

Notice that sentence 3 combines sentences 1 and 2 by embedding the infinitive clause as an adverbial within a primary sentence frame. In this sense, the use of infinitive clauses contributes to the growth of clause density during school age.

By first grade, children typically understand and produce true infinitive clauses with some degree of success. However, challenges remain in some semantic contexts, and they are related to one last quirky feature of infinitive clauses. Unlike any other clause, infinitive clauses sometimes lack an overt subject. Consider these examples:

1. *Bruce asked Helga to play the piano.*

2. *Bruce wants to play golf.*

In example 1, the subject of the infinitive phrase is *Helga*. However, in example 2, there is no overt subject within the infinitive clause. This is known as a **bare clause**. A strategy for determining the subject of a bare clause is known as the **minimal distance principle** (**MDP**). According to this principle, the subject of an infinitive is the closest preceding noun. This principle generally holds true, whether we have a bare infinitive clause or an infinitive clause with a named subject (e.g., *Mom wants John to clean his room*). However, the MDP does not apply in some semantic contexts. In fact, the MDP never applies when the infinitive clause follows the verb *promise,* and it applies following the verb *ask* only when *ask* means *tell.* Consider these examples:

1. *John told Nancy to park the bike.* (MDP applies)

2. *John asked Nancy to park the bike.* (MDP applies)

3. *John asked Nancy where to park the bike.* (MDP does not apply)

4. *John promised Nancy to park the bike.* (MDP does not apply)

For this reason, comprehension of infinitive clauses is not mastered until school age. The results of a study by C. Chomsky (1969) indicate that sentences with *tell* (which always follow the MDP) and with *ask* (where *ask* functions as a polite form of *tell*) are first understood at about 5 years. Sentences with *promise* (which never follow the MDP) are understood at about 7 years, and sentences with *ask* (where *ask* functions to introduce a wh-question) are understood at about 9 years. Other studies have reported a similar pattern (e.g., Kessel, 1970).

Refinements in the Use of Passive Voice

Until this point, we have been discussing grammatical forms that contribute to the overall increase in clausal density. We now turn to the grammatical feature of passive voice. We highlight this feature for three reasons. First, the ability to use passive voice increases a speaker's grammatical flexibility. For example, passive voice allows a speaker to de-emphasize the agent of an action. To illustrate, consider these two sentences:

1. *I ate the last piece of that delicious pecan pie.* (active voice)

2. *The last piece of that delicious pecan pie was eaten.* (passive voice)

Notice how passive voice allows the speaker to tell the truth but also to avoid being exposed as the culprit who ate that very least delicious piece of pecan pie. Another reason for choosing this feature is that passive voice is often used in written texts and in the more literate language style used by teachers during classroom instruction. Moreover, passive sentence structure contains features that are challenging for some children, and teachers should be aware of this.

To appreciate the development of passive voice at school age, it is helpful to review aspects of this form that influence children's comprehension and production. Consider the following examples:

1. *The receptionist answers the phone.* (Basic active sentence)

2. *The phone is answered by a receptionist.* (Full nonreversible passive sentence)

3. *The phone is answered.* (Truncated passive sentence)

4. *The cat was chased by the dog.* (Reversible passive sentence)

5. *The boy was tripped by <u>a branch</u>.* (Passive with an inanimate agent)

6. *The ball was kicked by <u>the girl</u>.* (Passive with an animate agent)

7. *The game was <u>lost</u> by the Bears.* (Passive with a state verb)

8. *The ball was <u>hit</u> by the batter.* (Passive with an action verb)

9. *The cake was bak<u>ed</u>.* (Passive with a verb taking *-ed* in the participial form)

10. *The candy was eat<u>en</u>.* (Truncated passive with a verb taking *-en* in the participial form)

11. *The boy was <u>hit</u>.* (Truncated passive with a verb taking no ending in the participial form)

12. *The picture was painted <u>with a brush</u>.* (Truncated passive with embedded adverbial phrase)

13. *The key <u>might</u> have been lost by the guest.* (Passive with modal auxiliary verb)

Example 1 is a simple active declarative sentence, included for purposes of comparison. Sentence 2 is a passive sentence with exactly the same meaning as sentence 1. Notice that the passive sentence includes a noun phrase (*the phone*), a verb phrase (*is answered*), and a prepositional phrase (*by a receptionist*). When all three of these components are present in a passive sentence, we characterize it as a **full passive** sentence. However, when the sentence only includes the noun phrase and the verb phrase (examples 3, 9-12) it is classified as a **truncated passive** sentence.

Second, notice that the grammatical subject, verb, and object of the active sentence (example 1) correspond to the semantic agent, action, and object, respectively. However, this is not the case in the full passive sentence (example 2). Here, the grammatical subject (*telephone*) is actually the semantic object, and the grammatical object of the preposition *by* (*the receptionist*) represents the semantic agent. It is no wonder that this is a source of confusion for children during the early stages of passive sentence comprehension (see below).

Third, passive sentences are sometimes classified as either reversible or nonreversible depending on the semantic features of the subject and object nouns. Example 4 illustrates a **reversible passive** because the meaning of the sentence would remain plausible if the subject (*cat*) and the object (*dog*) were reversed. However, example 2 illustrates a **nonreversible passive** sentence because it would not make sense if the subject and object were reversed. In other words, one can easily imagine that the phone was answered by the receptionist but not that the receptionist was answered by the phone.

Fourth, from a semantic perspective, passive sentences can be formulated with **inanimate agents** (e.g., *a branch* in example 5) or **animate agents** (e.g., *a girl* in example 6). The predicate may be a **state verb** (e.g., *lost* in example 7) or an **action**

verb (e.g., *hit* in example 8). Finally, there are aspects of verb structure that can further complicate the comprehension and production of passive sentences. For example, the verb phrase can be expanded by adding an adverbial clause, as in example 13.

Developmentally, mastery of passive voice occurs over a protracted period of time. In the previous chapter we noted that children's initial attempts to interpret passive sentences involve the use of **nonsyntactic comprehension strategies** which do not always lead to the correct interpretation. For example, to understand a reversible passive (*The dog chased the cat*), preschoolers are inclined to use the **order-of-mention strategy**, assuming that the grammatical SVO sequence correlates with the semantic agent, action, object sequence, respectively. Unfortunately, this leads them to incorrect interpretations. A more helpful approach is the **plausible-event strategy**, which typically is used by preschoolers to interpret **nonreversible passives** (e.g., *The castle was built by the children*). However, this strategy is based on cognitive knowledge and not on linguistic processing. By school age, typical children begin to use true **syntactic comprehension strategies** to interpret passive sentences.

We also noted in the previous chapter that children begin to express passive voice within conversational contexts by using **truncated passive** forms that omit the agent of action (e.g., *The vase got broken*). **Full passives** (*The vase got broken by me*) also emerge during the preschool years but are not mastered until early school age. The noun or pronoun subject of these early forms almost always refers to an inanimate object, and state verbs (*lost, left*) tend to predominate (Owens, 2008). Gradually, action verbs are included as well (e.g., *It got smashed*). Eventually, children learn to produce passive sentences with animate subjects and a larger variety of verb types. However, children may continue to have problems sorting out when a verb requires an *-en* ending (e.g., *The food was eat<u>en</u> by the dog*) and when it requires an *-ed* ending (e.g., *John was help<u>ed</u> by his mother*) (Redmond, 2003). In the case of irregular verbs, no ending is required at all (e.g., *The bread was <u>cut</u> by the baker*), and this must also be sorted out. According to Owens (2008), commission errors (e.g., *He was <u>cutted</u> by the axe*) sometimes persist into early adolescence.

The types of passive sentences and the frequency with which they are used depend on the extent to which children are inclined to (or required to) use a more literate language style (see pragmatics, below) and it is undoubtedly influenced by their exposure to this style in classroom instruction and in print.

Final Note

Our review of grammatical development shows that although children arrive in first grade with a set of basic grammatical skills, there is continued growth and refinement in their expressive and receptive grammatical repertoires throughout the school years. Quantitatively, this is reflected by gradual increases in average sentence length and clause density. The specific refinements that contribute to these quantitative changes occur at all levels of grammatical processing: phrases, clauses, sentences, and intersentential cohesion. As a result of these refinements, children possess the grammatical tools needed to talk about increasingly complex ideas and relationships between ideas with a reasonable degree of grammatical flexibility.

Many of the same factors that influence the development of semantic skills also influence the refinement of grammatical forms. Included are exposure to the literate language style of teachers, direct English instruction, and engagement in literacy experiences. The last item is crucial for several reasons. First, reading offers more frequent opportunities to process low-frequency grammatical structures than oral discourse. Second, the opportunity to see a static visual representation of grammatical structures allows a reader to reflect and re-read if needed. Similarly, writing offers the opportunity to think about the selection of grammatical forms and experiment with different ways of formulating messages. This is especially convenient with the use of electronic text editing software. All of these experiences are increasingly frequent for school age children, and they are bound to have an enormous impact on spoken language.

The development of grammatical fluency (and fluency in all aspects of language) is always a work in progress. Not even adult utterances are 100% error free. Moreover, all speakers produce false starts, hesitations, and revisions in their spoken language at one time or another. This combination of patterns is sometimes characterized as a **verbal maze** (Loban, 1976; MacLachlan & Chapman, 1988; Nippold, 1998). Here is an example:

I was like . . . my friend had a . . . last night . . . yesterday we . . . there was this party last week and there were . . . there was, um, . . . there was this guy who played guitar.

However, when errors of this type occur frequently enough to create a consistent interference with communication, teachers should refer a student for a speech-language evaluation. Although the linguistic fluency of verbal utterances can be affected by many things (e.g., complexity of ideas, aggravating circumstances, emotional content, etc.), there is evidence that students with lower overall language proficiency present with more instances of mazing than students with language skills in the average to above-average range of proficiency (Loban, 1976).

Finally, sentences are the building blocks of longer pieces of discourse. At school age, students are engaged in telling stories reporting experiences, describing, summarizing, analyzing, and reflecting on larger chunks of information. This involves the ability to formulate, sequence, and tie sentences together in ways that serve the needs of a particular discourse task. We turn now to a discussion of these and other issues at the discourse level associated with later pragmatic development.

PRIMARY ACCOMPLISHMENTS: PRAGMATICS

As children and youth mature, their pragmatic repertoires grow to accommodate more sophisticated communicative demands. For example, they become more proficient conversational partners by learning to maintain topics for longer stretches, to change topics in a more graceful manner, to adjust their language more effectively relative to the needs of a conversational partner, and to integrate well-formed narratives into conversational contexts. They also learn the discourse rules associated with an academic environment, the literate language style that is used with increasing frequency as part of academic instruction, and the formulation of extended discourse segments. Additionally, changes occur in the use of language for reflecting on language itself (metalinguistic function) and for reflecting on thought (metacognitive function). In this section, we highlight selected developmental refinements in the pragmatic repertoire during the elementary and high school years.

Improvement in Conversational Skills

Conversation is a kind of discourse, and all **discourse** involves an exchange of information with one or more conversational partners for some purpose. Different discourse styles or **genres** are used depending on the content of the interaction (**referential dimension**) and on the nature or roles of the conversational partner(s) (**rhetorical dimension**) (Westby, 1994). For example, we adjust the style of our language in one way when conversing with a close friend and another way when taking one's turn in a classroom discussion.

Referential Dimension

Good conversational skills play an important role in children's access to interactions with peers (Ninio & Snow, 1999). Recall that the foundation for conversational discourse is acquired during the preschool period. Later development involves, among other things, refinements in the use of topic management skills and conversational repair strategies.

Topic management includes such skills as topic introduction, maintenance, extension, change, reintroduction, and others. Several investigators have described developmental changes across school-aged children and youth in topic management patterns (Brinton & Fujiki, 1984; Schober-Peterson & Johnson, 1983). Collectively, these investigators found that, with increasing maturity, children and youth tend to initiate fewer topics over the same length of conversational time. They tend to discuss individual topics over a larger number of conversational turns, and they tend to produce a larger number of novel utterances about the same topic. Table 5–9 illustrates this trend based on data from Brinton and Fujiki (1984). These researchers compared patterns of topic manipulation during dyadic

TABLE 5–9. Topic Manipulation Patterns of School-Age Children

Topic Manipulation Pattern	5 years	9 years	22–26 yrs
Mean number of topics introduced	23.50 [1](SD = 5.99)	23.33 (SD = 7.28)	13.17 (SD = 5.67)
Mean number of topics reintroduced	22.83 (SD = 9.22)	20.50 (SD = 3.21)	6.00 (SD = 3.74)
Mean percentage of topics maintained	79%	84%	96%
Mean number of utterances per maintained topic	5.08 (SD = .82)	6.34 (SD = 1.42)	10.69 (SD = 2.75)
Mean number of novel utterances per maintained topic	4.13 (SD = 0.54)	6.07 (SD = 1.33)	10.62 (SD = 2.71)
Mean number of topic shadings	4.83 (SD = 1.86)	6.00 (SD = –2.19)	10.50 (SD = 3.27i)

SD = Standard deviation.

Source: Based on B. Brinton and M. Fujiki (1984). Development of topic manipulation skills in discourse. *Journal of Speech and Hearing Research, 27,* pp. 354–356.

conversations between individuals within three age groups: 5-year-olds, 9-year-olds, and young adults. It should be noted, however, that there are considerable variations in the performance of different individuals within an age group. There also are variations in the performance of the same individual in different contexts. For example, the same person may introduce more or fewer topics and discuss individual topics over a longer or shorter number of volleys depending on the topic that is being discussed (referential context) and on an individual's relationship to the conversational partner (rhetorical context). For these reasons, there is no prototype to serve as a developmental end point for the acquisition of conversational skills (Hoff, 2009).

Dorval and Eckerman (1984) examined developmental changes in the quality of topically related utterances generated by children, youth, and adults within the context of small social peer groups. Each group consisted of 6 participants (3 male, 3 female), and three groups represented each of five grades and age ranges: second grade (7–8 years), fifth grade (10–11 years), ninth grade (14–15 years), twelfth grade (17–18 years), and college level (early 20s). Each group met twice weekly for 12 sessions with a nondirective adult leader who invited the partici-

pants to use the time as they wished for the purpose of getting to know each other. All meetings were tape-recorded, and utterances produced during the eighth meeting were used as the data for the study. Utterances were transcribed and segmented into speaking turns. Turns were then coded for subcategories of topic relatedness and for focus.

Several patterns were found in the data. First, as expected, there was a decrease with age in the proportion of turn relations that fail to sustain topics. These included unrelated turns and tangential turns. An **unrelated turn** is one in which a speaking turn bears no relation to the previous or recent turns in the conversation. This is illustrated by Turn 3 below:

Turn 1 (Speaker 1): *I wonder where John is?*

Turn 2 (Speaker 2): *Here he comes.*

Turn 3 (Speaker 1): *Did you see my bike?*

A **tangential turn** is one in which the speaker's utterance refers to a different topic but one that is related to an aspect of the original topic as in Turn 2, below:

Turn 1 (Speaker 1): *My dad and I went fishing yesterday*.

Turn 2 (Speaker 2): *My dad bought a new car*.

Note that tangential turns are sometimes used deliberately to change topics. Therefore, this pattern is also known as **topic shading** (Brinton & Fujiki, 1984) and would never be expected to disappear completely.

Dorval and Eckerman's (1984) second finding was an increase across groups in the proportion of topic relations of increasing sophistication. These included factually related turns and perspective-related turns. A **factually related turn** is a turn that extends a topic by adding substantive information, as in Turn 2 of the following example:

Turn 1 (Speaker 1): *Mrs. Jones is our substitute teacher*.

Turn 2 (Speaker 2): *This is her second day with our class*.

A **perspective related turn** is one in which the topic of conversation is a person and the speaker refers to the person's point of view. An example is illustrated in Turn 2, as follows:

Turn 1 (Speaker 1): *Mrs. Jones is the substitute teacher*.

Turn 2 (Speaker 2): *By the end of today she may wish she had stayed at home*.

Perspective related turns were first observed in the conversation of twelfth graders and occurred with increasing proportion in the conversations of the young adults.

The third finding reported by Dorval and Eckerman (1984) was an increase in the proportion of **focused turns** across groups. A focused turn is one that expresses agreement, disagreement, question, answer, and/or direction. The proportion of all types of focused turns in the conversations of groups gradually increased as follows: 34% by second graders; 45% by fifth graders; 38% by ninth graders; 51% by twelfth graders; and 52% by young adults. However, when focused turns were further analyzed with respect to subtypes, results showed that some subtypes increased with development while

others decreased. Specifically, there was a gradual increase in the proportion of focused turns expressing agreements, questions, and answers, and a gradual decrease in the proportion of focused turns expressing disagreements and directives.

Nippold (2007) and Reed (2005) summarized developmental changes in conversational performance during adolescence. Based on a study by Larson and McKinley (1998) they reported that interruptions increase significantly with age level. However, the kinds of interruptions that are produced typically have a constructive effect on the discussion in that some interruptions are positive (e.g., *Yeah, I know what you mean*) and some are negative (e.g., *I don't understand*) (Nippold, 2007, p. 291).

Conversational Repair

Another aspect of conversational skill is the ability to **repair misunderstandings**. Recall that children begin responding to requests for clarification at 20 months and continue to do so with increasing skill throughout the preschool period by using a small number of repair strategies that may or may not be helpful to the conversational partner (Brinton, Fujiki, Loeb, & Winkler, 1986; Gallagher, 1977; Garvey, 1977; Langford, 1981). For example, if they make a statement and their conversational partner says, *What?*, preschoolers may repeat the same utterance more loudly or articulate the same utterance more precisely. They may add or delete a word, or use a different word with a similar meaning (Gallagher, 1977). However, in comparison to school-age children, younger children have more difficulty inferring the reason for a misunderstanding and may still fail to provide the specific information needed to achieve successful repair.

Brinton, Fujiki, Loeb, and Winkler (1986) studied developmental changes in conversational repair by observing 10 children across four age groups: 2:7 (years: months) to 3:10; 4:10 to 5:10; 6:10 to 7:10; and 8:10 to 9:10. Each child was asked to describe a pictured scene to an adult who could not see the picture. Periodically, the adult responded to a child's descriptive statement by initiating a **stacked repair sequence**. The sequence consisted of three consecutive nonspecific requests for clarification, beginning with *Huh?* After a child responded to the first request, the adult posed the second (*What?*); and after the second response, the adult posed the third (*I don't understand*). Here is an example of the dialogue in a three-part stacked repair sequence.

Child's original statement: *Some guy is holding a package*

Adult's first clarification request: *Huh?*

Child's first clarification: *A guy is holding a package*

Adult's second clarification request: *What?*

Child's second clarification: *A young man is holding a package in his hand.*

Adult's third clarification request: *I don't understand*

Child's third clarification: *There's a man. He has a package. It might be a present.*

In the above example, the child's first clarification is a **repetition** of the initial statement. Given the nature of the clarification request, which was neutral and nonspecific, repetition is a reasonable repair strategy. The second clarification includes a **revision** of the first (i.e., *man* instead of *guy*) and an **addition** (i.e., *holding in his hand* instead of just *holding*). Revision is a reasonable alternative if simple repetition did not yield success. In the third clarification, a **cue** is provided regarding one of the referents in the original statement (i.e., *It might be a present* referring to the package).

Each participant in Brinton et al.'s (1986) study had an equal number of opportunities to respond to three-part stacked repair sequences. However, they performed differently depending on age. All of the participants used repetition as a clarification strategy, especially in response to the initial request in each sequence. However, 9-year-olds were the most persistent in responding to all three stacked clarification requests. They used the largest variety of clarification strategies, used the cue strategy significantly more often than any of the other age groups, and produced the smallest number of inappropriate responses. The youngest children gave a high proportion of inappropriate responses to the second and third requests in the stacked repair sequences, and the 5-year-olds gave a high proportion of inappropriate responses to the third request

in the sequence. These patterns suggested that while children under the age of 9 years may recognize that clarification is needed, they have more difficulty than 9-year-olds in understanding why their first or second repairs were unsuccessful. By the age of 9 years, children are better able to interpret the second and third request in a stacked repair sequence as an indication that the conversational partner needs a different kind of information, and their repertoire of response strategies includes a greater variety of options to meet this need.

Rhetorical Dimension

We noted several times that aspects of conversational style will change depending on the referential and rhetorical dimensions of a communicative event. Here, we address some changes in style related to the rhetorical dimension under the umbrella of conversational discourse. Nippold (2007) and Reed (2005) described variations in the communicative style of adolescents across different types of communication partners. Based on a study by Raffaelli and Duckett (1989), Nippold (2007) noted that youth between the ages of 10 to 15 years spend increasing amounts of time socializing with friends in person and on the phone, and their conversational topics differ depending on the communicative partner. For example, as they mature, adolescents are increasingly more likely to discuss personal issues and peer concerns with friends rather than with family. Based on a study by Larson and McKinley (1998) it was further noted that when adolescents talk to each other, they use a larger range of question types, rely on figurative language more often, introduce a wider variety of unique topics, and use more abrupt topic shifts than when they are engaged in conversations with adults.

Reed, McLeod, and McAllister (1999) asked a sample of 100 students (41 male, 59 female) between the ages of 14:4 and 16:4 to rank 14 different communication skills in importance in two situations: (1) when communicating with a peer and (2) when communicating with a teacher. The participants were normally achieving Australian teenagers enrolled in an intermediate tenth grade English class. The 14 skills and mean rank orders are provided below, based on Reed et al., p. 387.

Importance for Communicating with a Peer	Importance for Communicating with a Teacher
Nonverbal Comprehension	Turn-Taking
Perspective Taking	Perspective Taking
Vocal Tone Interpretation	Logical Communication
Vocal Tone Expression	Clarification
Topic Selection	Vocal Tone Expression
Tact	Tact
Logical Communication	Vocal Tone Interpretation
Turn-Taking	Narrative
Clarification	Eye Contact
Eye Contact	Topic Selection
Narrative	Nonverbal Comprehension
Humor Comprehension	Topic Maintenance
Topic Maintenance	Humor Comprehension
Slang Usage	Slang Usage

Several interesting patterns emerged from these data. The adolescents considered nonverbal comprehension, humor comprehension, and topic selection to be significantly more important in their own communication when talking with peers than when talking with teachers. On the other hand, they considered clarification and turn-taking to be significantly more important when talking to their teachers than when talking to their peers. Interestingly, perspective taking ranked high as a valued skill for communicating with both types of communication partners.

Some related patterns were reported in a longitudinal study mentioned earlier by Larson and McKinley (1998). The purpose of this study was to explore patterns of conversational behavior related to the age of the participants and to the gender of their communication partners. The participants in this study included eight typically developing adolescents (4 boys, 4 girls) from middle class backgrounds. Observations began when the adolescents were in seventh grade (12–13 years of age) and continued until they reached the twelfth grade (17–18 years of age). Each student was observed periodically during two 10-minute conversations, one with a friend (usually a peer of the same sex) and one with an unfamiliar adult of the opposite sex. One finding showed that the participants used more communicative functions designed to entertain and to persuade someone to feel, believe, or do something when conversing with their peers than when conversing with an adult. However, no changes were found in the proportion of entertainment or persuasion functions expressed by the adolescents as they matured.

To summarize, changes in social conversation occur as children mature through elementary school and high school. These changes are reflected in topic manipulation patterns, responses to requests for clarification, and the ability to make adjustments in communicative style relative to the needs of the conversational partner. Another important adjustment concerns the style of language used in the classroom. We address this in a separate section to highlight the important role of language in supporting academic and social success.

Development of Classroom Discourse

As students move through elementary and high school, they are expected to understand and honor the rules of discourse within academic settings. Some of these rules are typically learned without direct instruction. In that sense, they are considered part of the "hidden curriculum" of the academic culture (e.g., Bieber, 1994; Hemmings, 2000; Myles, Trautman, & Schelvan, 2004). Other rules of discourse, such as those resulting in a more literary language style, are learned through direct instruction as well as exposure (e.g., van Kleeck, 2004; Westby, 1994). Key features of the hidden curriculum and of literate language style are summarized in this section on discourse development.

Mastering the Hidden Curriculum

The term *curriculum* typically refers to the content and deliberate study of particular subject matter. The first grade math curriculum refers to instructional content on the topic of math, and it is the object of direct instruction at first grade. In contrast, the phrase "**hidden curriculum**" refers to social/cultural skills (including situation-specific patterns of communication) that are normally acquired through spontaneous observational learning without much direct instruction.

Classroom discourse structure is one of the situation-specific social skills acquired by school-age children (Paul, 2007). For example, children learn that the teacher chooses the topic of discussion and students must comment on it when called on to do so. They learn that the teacher will decide who will be called on, what they will talk about, and how long they will have the floor. Moreover, students learn to read the teacher's nonverbal cues to determine when they can volunteer to offer a response and when their turn has ended. They also become aware of behavior that is not valued by the teacher, such as talking out of turn, changing the topic, or failing to respond when called on. Most children learn these rules despite the fact that only a fraction of them is ever verbalized by the teacher (Hoover & Patton, 1997).

One particular discourse routine included in the hidden curriculum is known as the **structured school lesson** (Duchan, 2004). This short, three-part discourse pattern is initiated by a teacher's question directed to the class or to a particular student. The question is then followed by a student's response, which is then evaluated for quality and accuracy by the teacher. This sequence of initiation, response, and evaluation (IRE) occurs frequently throughout the school years across the entire curriculum. Through repeated exposure and participation, students quickly develop a generalized understanding (schema) of the IRE structure. This understanding, in turn, guides their expectation and participation during many different types of lessons (Mehan, 1979; Ripich & Panagos, 1985).

In the absence of explicit teaching, many aspects of the hidden curriculum are normally acquired through **spontaneous observational learning**. That is, students observe the teacher's response when their peers perform appropriately or outside of the expected discourse structure. If the teacher praises a student for raising his hand before talking, his or her classmates will learn that hand-raising is a desirable way to initiate participation in class discussions. Similarly, if a teacher reprimands a student for talking to a classmate during instruction, students who observe this interaction will learn that the teacher wants students to pay attention and not to talk to each other during a lesson. We tend to take the hidden curriculum for granted and only

think about it explicitly when there is a problem. Myles, Trautman, and Schelvan (2004) note that the rules of the hidden curriculum have probably been broken when someone begins a sentence with a phrase like, *I shouldn't have to tell you this* . . . or *Everyone knows that* . . . or *Common sense tells us that* . . . and other similar expressions (p. 5).

Students from mainstream-culture homes are typically primed to learn classroom discourse rules through the kinds of interactions that are valued and encouraged by their caregivers (e.g., van Kleeck, 2004). For example, during shared book-reading, these children are often engaged in a "**display of knowledge**" sequence in response to "**test questions**" (van Kleeck, 2004, p. 183). In other words, caregivers ask their children questions for which the caregivers believe their children know the answers. For example, after reading the title *Goldilocks and the Three Bears*, a caregiver may ask, *Who is the story about?* This pattern of experience prepares children for the most common participation structure they will later experience in a classroom (Reid, 2000; Watson, 2001). However, test questions and displays of knowledge are not a part of every child's preschool experience, as in the case of some children in nondominant culture homes (Harris, 1998; Heath, 1983; Valdez, 1996).

Failure to learn the hidden curriculum places individuals at risk for social problems, and is unfortunately characteristic of students with autism spectrum disorders (ASD) as well as other related developmental disabilities. Some of these students learn aspects of the traditional curriculum as well as or better than their typical peers. However, the hidden curriculum is extremely challenging for them because they have difficulty identifying appropriate social behavior through spontaneous observational learning. For them, the hidden curriculum must be made explicit. An important note for educators and clinicians is to be aware that mastery of the hidden curriculum is not always a guaranteed skill, and that the poor social skills of some students may reflect challenges in spontaneous observational learning rather than deliberate acts of defiance.

Literate Language Style

Another aspect of classroom discourse is literate language style. In an academic setting, children are increasingly expected to understand and formulate discourse with the characteristics of literate language style. By approximately third grade, they are exposed to this style in both oral language and print. In oral form, literate language is used with increasing frequency by teachers during class instruction. Students are expected to use this style for participating in academic discussions and for making oral presentations. In written form, literate language style appears in textbooks with increasing frequency across all content areas except English. By seventh grade, textbooks use this style exclusively. Literate language style also is used in newspapers, major reference works (e.g., encyclopedia), and on the internet (e.g., Wikipedia), and it is the style of language that students are expected to use when completing writing assignments across the curriculum (again, with the exception of English).

To appreciate the characteristics of literary language style, it is useful to compare it with **social conversation**, the dominant style of discourse in children's repertoires at the beginning of elementary school. Recall that social conversation is used to accomplish interactive goals such as commenting on conversational topics, making requests, and regulating interactive goals. It is highly **contextualized** in that the meanings of utterances are supported by extralinguistic cues such as a speaker's tone, nonverbal gestures, orientation to present objects or events, and other cues. For example, a speaker may use pronouns (e.g., *Look at him*) with gestures (e.g., pointing to a clown) to establish joint reference to a topic in the environment without ever naming the referent. This pattern of pronoun use is known as deictic **extraphoric reference**. Topics of social conversation arise spontaneously, and one leads to another through chained associations. Conversational turn-taking is generally balanced across conversational partners. Although one or the other partner may formulate short personal narratives or retell a short story, speaking turns remain balanced overall. Individual utterances may or may not consist of complete grammatical sentences, and unclear references are occasionally made. However, each conversational partner has the opportunity to request and offer clarification as needed.

Literate language style differs from social conversational style in at least five important ways. First, literate language typically is used for informational purposes rather than for social purposes, and it is structured to guide a listener's or reader's thinking about ideas that extend to **levels of abstraction**. Moffett (1968) described a continuum of discourse abstraction, including: (1) drama —recording what is happening; (2) narrative—description of what happened; (3) exposition—generalizing what happens in a situation; and (4) logical argumentation—theorizing what might happen in a situation. In comparison to conversational discourse which relies on the first two levels (drama, narrative), literate language relies more heavily on **exposition** and **argumentation**.

Second, unlike conversational topics that arise spontaneously and change frequently, the topics of literate discourse are typically planned and sustained throughout the discourse. Third, although conversational discourse occurs within a **dialogic structure** with occasional embedded narratives, literate language style makes greater use of **extended discourse** within a **monologic structure**. When literate language is used in an oral presentation, comments and questions from an audience may follow. Similarly, written texts may be debated and discussed in the literature. However, such exchanges are more delayed, more planned, and more formal than conversational dialogue.

The **macrostructure** (also known as **text structure**) of literate language differs from the macrostructure of narratives that are embedded within social conversations. Unlike narratives, which follow a similar structure regardless of subgenre, literate language may be organized by one or several different forms of **expository text structure** or **argumentative text**. Common expository structures include **descriptive**, **enumerative**, and **comparison-contrast** texts, **cause-effect** explanations, and **problem-solution** descriptions. Table 5–10 summarizes key features of each. The organization and coherence of an individual text structure is supported by **key words** (see Table 5–10) and by other **signaling devices** such as titles, headings, introductions, overviews, summaries. Recognizing text structure supports children's reading comprehension by helping them to predict the type of content a structure may hold (e.g., Moss, 2004; Slater & Graves, 1989; Westby, 1994). In that sense, it is similar to using the shape of a container (e.g., a lunch box, a soda can, a heart-shaped candy box, a violin case, etc.)

TABLE 5–10. Expository Text Structures, Functions, Graphic Organizers, and Cue Words

Text Structure	Text Function	Graphic Organizers	Examples of Cue Words
Description, Collection, Enumeration	The text provides a statement of the topic and a list of characteristics, attributes, or examples	Topic → Attribute/Example, Attribute/Example, Attribute/Example → details, details, details	Characteristics For example For instance To illustrate Including
Sequence	The text describes a sequence of events or steps for how to do something	Topic → Action 1, Action 2, Action n → details, details, details	First, second, etc. Before, after Next, last Now, later And then When, then Initially, eventually
Comparison Contrast	The text describes how two things are alike and different	Topic → Alike, Different → details details, details details	Same Alike Similar Likewise In Contrast On the other hand However
Cause-Effect Explanation	The text summarizes reasons why something happened	Topic → Antecedent, Consequence; Antecedent → Antecedent → details, details, details	Reason why As a result Consequently Because Since So that Due to Hence Reasons
Problem-Solution	The text states a problem and offers solutions	Topic → Problem (Who, what, where, when, how) → Solutions → Option 1, Option 2, Option n → details, details, details	Problem Solution Options Results Solved

Source: Adapted from C. Westby (1994). Communication refinement in school age and adolescence. In W. O. Haynes & B. B. Shulman (Eds.), *Communication development: Foundations, processes, and clinical applications* (pp. 341–383). Englewood Cliffs, NJ: Prentice-Hall, p. 362. And from B. Moss (2004). Teaching expository text structures through information trade book retellings. *Reading Teacher, 57*(8), pp. 710–718.

to predict its contents. Awareness of text structure also serves as an organizational blueprint for written discourse.

In addition to the devices that signal text coherence, literate discourse also includes **linguistic cohesion devices** such as conjunctions (e.g., *and, but, so*). These forms occur in conversation as well, however, literate language uses a greater variety of them, particularly those that signal logical relationships (e.g., *therefore, however, moreover*, etc.). They serve to establish logical relationships between sentences (**intersentential cohesion**) or segments of text rather than only connections within sentences (**intrasentential cohesion**). Other cohesion devices are summarized in Table 5–11. Recall also the examples given in our earlier description of the literate lexicon under lexical development.

A fourth and major difference between literate language style and social conversation is that the former is characterized by **decontextualization**. As such, meaning must be derived exclusively from the language without the benefit of physical contextual cues. This is particularly evident when we consider the use of pronouns, because pronouns only have meaning in literate language if they can be linked with a noun phrase in the text. This type of linkage is known as **endophoric reference**, and includes two patterns: **anaphoric reference** (referring back to a previously stated noun phrase) and **cataphoric reference** (referring forward to a noun phrase or a nominal clause yet to be stated). These patterns contrast with the deictic **exophoric reference** in conversational speech which guides a listener's attention to items in the physical environment. Examples of all three patterns are provided below for ease of comparison:

■ Exophoric Reference (used more often in conversation)

■ Deictic pattern: *There <u>it</u> is* [said as the speaker points to his key]

■ Endophoric Reference (used more often in literate texts)

■ Anaphoric pattern: *The 2008 <u>Perseid meteor shower</u> peaked during the dark hours before dawn on Tuesday, August 12th. Observers described <u>it</u> as a great show.*

■ Cataphoric pattern: *<u>It</u> was done: <u>The Supreme Court's decision had resulted in the selection of the President.</u>*

Notice that the same pronoun (*it*) is used in all three examples. However, in the exophoric deictic pattern, *it* refers to the unnamed dog in the physical environment to which the speaker is pointing. In the anaphoric reference example *it* refers to the subject noun phrase of the previous sentence (*the 2008 Perseid meteor shower*), and in the cataphoric reference example *it* refers to the entire following clause (*The Supreme Court's decision had resulted in the selection of the President*).

Decontextualization requires a speaker or writer to specify as much detail verbally as needed to communicate his or her ideas clearly and unambiguously. For this reason, and because the topics of literate language tend to be more abstract than those of conversational speech, the semantic characteristics of literate language differs from those of conversational speech. For example, literate language includes greater **lexical diversity**, as seen by the proportion of different words in a text (e.g., Malvern, Richards, Chipere, & Duran, 2004). It also has greater **lexical density**, as measured by the proportion of content words relative to the total words in a text (e.g., Strömqvist et al., 2002), and **lexical complexity**, reflected by the increased polysyllabic structure of words in a text (Berman & Nir-Sagiv, 2007). Consistent with this, Berman (2007) noted that literate language style relies more heavily on words of Latinate origin (e.g., *considerable, industrial, military*) than on everyday Germanic word stock (e.g., *dirty, sunny, sandy*).

Complex syntactic forms also support decontextualization (Berman, 2007; Westby, 1994). This may involve **verb phrase** expansion through the use of **adverbs** to express time (e.g., *simultaneously)*, manner (e.g., *mistakenly*), and degree (e.g., *excruciatingly*). It may involve the embedding of **adverbial phrases and clauses**, also to specify the time (e.g., *<u>After years of research</u>, scientists still aren't sure why low-hanging moons look unusually large to the human eye*), manner (e.g., *It is important to complete each step <u>with careful attention to detail</u>*) and degree (e.g., *To compete in the Olympics one must submit to a rigorous regimen of practice <u>with unwavering commitment</u>*.).

TABLE 5–11. A Sampling of Linguistic Cohesion Devices

Type	Definition	Examples
Reference	A semantic relation whereby the information needed for interpretation is found somewhere in the text. Cohesion lies in the continuity of reference, as the same thing is referred to more than once in the discourse.	**Pronominal** *Joe is a writer. He published a book.* **Definite article** *I bought shoes and a purse. The shoes are black.* **Demonstrative** *Philip is in the pool. You can find him there.* **Comparative** *Tim used his cell phone. The other phone was busy.*
Lexical	A relation which is achieved through vocabulary selection. Cohesion is formed by using the same word, a synonym, a superordinate word, and a general item or an associated word.	**Same word** *We vacation at the shore. The shore is fun.* **Synonym** *The girl figured it out. The child is brilliant.* **Superordinate word** *Have some cherries. Fruit is good for you.* **General word** *I gave George the tickets. The idiot lost them.* **Associated word** *She was a jogger. She wanted to win the race.*
Conjunction	A logical relation expressed between clauses that signals how what is to follow is related to what has gone before. Cohesion is achieved by using various connectors that show relationships between statements.	**Additive** *She clapped. And everyone cheered along with her.* **Adversative** *His friends were there. Yet something was missing.* **Causal** *I didn't know. Otherwise, I would have helped.* **Temporal** *She made a wish. Then she blew out the candles.* **Continuative** *You can take a break. After all, you've done the work.*
Conjunctive adverbials	Additional relations can be established by conjunctive ties involving a variety of specific transitional words.	**Consequence** *therefore, then, thus, hence, accordingly* **Likeness** *likewise, similarly* **Contrast** *but, however, nevertheless, on the other hand* **Amplification** *and again, in addition, further, moreover, also, too* **Example** *for instance, for example* **Sequence** *first, second, finally (temporal)* **Restatement** *that is, in other words, to put it differently, in sum*

TABLE 5–11. *continued*

Type	Definition	Examples
Substitution	The cohesive bond is established by the use of one word for another but repetition of the first term is avoided. The substituted word has the same structural function as that for which it substitutes.	Nominal *You should use a larger nail. I'll bring you <u>one</u>.* Clausal *Was he in an accident? Regretfully <u>so</u>.*
Ellipsis	Cohesion is established by the deletion of a phrase or a word or a clause	Verbal *Who's wearing a red shirt? John is . . .* Nominal *What kind of ice cream do you want? Strawberry . . .* Clausal *Have she finished her homework? Yes she has . . .*

Source: Adapted from G. Wallach (1988); N Gregg (1986); M. Mentis & C. A. Prutting (1987); and M. A. K. Halliday & R. Hasan (1976).

Noun phrase expansion may be used to specify a referent or to provide needed detail. This can be accomplished by the use of one or more **adjectives** (e.g., *circular, deranged, magnificent*, etc.) or by embedding clauses and phrases within the matrix sentence. **Center-embedded relative clauses** are used more often by mature speakers and writers (e.g., *A compound statement <u>that is true for every truth value of every statement included in the compound statement</u> is known as a tautology*). **Passive sentences** are also used more frequently in literate language style. Recall that these sentence forms follow an object-action-agent sequence which violates the more typical agent-action-object sequence of conversational speech style. They may be used when the speaker or writer wishes to emphasize a procedure rather than the agents of the procedure (e.g., *Water is directed into the container by a carefully engineered funneling system*).

When literate language style is used in oral discourse, listeners do have access to a speaker's tone of voice. However, as topics tend to extend beyond the here and now, oral literate style must include semantic and syntactic features with the same precision, level of complexity, and attention to decontextualization as required in print. If misunderstandings occur, the opportunity for requesting clarification will be less immediate, less spontaneous, more lim-

ited, and more formal than during conversational discourse.

A final difference between literate language style and social conversation pertains to the type of inferencing that is required for the comprehension of each genre (Westby, 1994). Social conversation and narrative language typically are associated with **pragmatic inferencing**, which involves the use of world experience to think beyond the specific referents named in an utterance. For example, if we are told, *The nurse took care of my grandfather in the ICU*, common experience suggests that the action took place in a hospital. Literate language style typically also requires the use of **logical inferencing**, which is based entirely on information contained within a text. For example, given the premise that rare birds are at risk for extinction and that there are only three known Po'ouli birds in existence, we can conclude that Po'ouli birds are at risk for extinction, even though we have never had direct contact with them.

In sum, literate language style is characterized by macrostructures and microstructure elements that are distinct from conversational discourse. Unlike social conversation, which is typically context bound, literate language is highly **decontextualized** and functions to guide thinking beyond the here and now. The aim of literate language is to be informative or persuasive rather than to support social interactions. In contrast to the more balanced turn-taking and the spontaneous generation of multiple topics included in social conversations, literate language is a more deliberate, topic-centered style expressed in monologues with macrostructures that vary depending on the specific type of information being shared. The microstructure must include linguistic elements that support topic coherence, text cohesion, and decontextualization, thereby allowing a reader or listener to derive meaning and inferences from the words alone without the benefit of contextual cues. Clearly, literate language style differs considerably from speech addressed to preschoolers and from the language that they generate. In the next section, we consider the relationship between joint book-reading and the development of literate language style.

Joint Book Reading: A Bridge to Literate Language Style

Multiple strands of influence intertwine to support the development of literate discourse in both oral and written modalities. One important strand is the preliteracy experience of **joint book-reading**. We noted in previous chapters that joint book-reading is a frequent source of entertainment for many young children and their caregivers throughout the preschool period. This also reflects the value that mainstream-culture families place on literacy and on children's acquisition of literacy skills (van Kleeck, 2004). In this section we summarize features of joint book-reading that serve as a bridge between conversational and literary language style by considering the structure of stories as well as the patterns of interactions between children and their caregivers during joint book-reading sessions. Although joint book-reading occurs primarily between children and caregivers during the preschool period, we include it here as background to the development of literate language style.

The particular books used for joint book-reading vary. Some are theme-based sequences (e.g., alphabet books) and others fictional narratives (e.g., storybooks). Our focus here is primarily on storybooks. Stories typically describe concrete events that address familiar themes and fantasies of high interest to children. Although the stories are fictional, their themes are often used to communicate abstract ideas (e.g., *The Tortoise and the Hare*). The communication of abstract ideas also is a characteristic that story narratives share with literate language style.

As indicated in the previous chapter, the elements of a story are organized according to a predictable macrostructure known as **story grammar**, which includes a setting and an episode structure (i.e., initiating event, reaction, internal response, plan, attempt, outcome, conclusion). This is true, regardless of the specific details of the settings in which different stories take place or of the specifics of the episode structure. A predictable macrostructure provides the listener or the reader with a set of expectations about the type of information to follow, and this predictability aids comprehension. Recall from our discussion of literate language style that similar advantages are associated with the structures of expository texts.

In addition to a macrostructure, each story has a **microstructure**, which consists of the linguistic elements (lexical words, sentences, and cohesion devices) used to create the elements of macrostructure. Similar to literate language style, the microstructure of stories is constructed of more specific and diverse vocabulary, more complete and complex syntax, and a larger range of linguistic cohesion markers for making explicit ties between the information in consecutive sentences.

Unlike the texts of literary discourse, children's storybooks often provide picture illustrations to serve as a rich source of nonlinguistic contextual information. However, text comprehension is the key to a true understanding of the story events, especially the characters' inner motivations, internal reactions, plans, and responses. When preschoolers have difficulty processing the text, clarification can be provided immediately and spontaneously by their caregivers. In these ways, joint book-reading offers a few of the contextual and interactive features of conversational discourse to help children process the structural and decontextualized features of literate language style.

The **child-caregiver interactions accompanying joint book-reading** are just as important as visual and auditory exposure to the story text (van Kleeck, 2004) because children learn to comprehend the stories and to recognize the structure of narrative style through these interactions. We describe typical patterns of interaction based on research involving children from mainstream-culture families and their caregivers. van Kleeck noted that these patterns represent neither the only model nor necessarily a better model than approaches to literacy and child-caregiver interaction observed in nondominant cultures. However, these patterns are known to support the acquisition of literate language style, and they are isomorphic with the experiences children encounter in early elementary school.

Based on previous research, van Kleeck (2004) identified five general teaching strategies and six language-specific teaching strategies demonstrated by mainstream-family caregivers when interacting with their children during joint book-reading. First, among the **general teaching strategies** is the **use of routines**, such as re-reading the same book. An analysis of this practice suggests that repeated opportunities to read the same book can serve as an organizational prosthetic which limits the information processing load and thereby enables a child to focus on details within the routine. Second, caregivers **gradually shift responsibility for the routine to the child**. Initially, the adult scaffolds the entire routine. As the child learns more about the routine, the adult cedes more and more of the event sequence to the child's initiative until the child performs independently. Third, caregivers **operate in the child's zone of proximal development** (ZPD). In other words, they tune their expectations of the child to within a range of skills between those that the child can perform independently and those that he or she can perform with guidance. So, if the child indicates that he or she does not understand some aspect of a story, an adult might simplify the text (e.g., reword, summarize or restate, omit information), explain inferences, or provide additional explanations of concepts, words, or story events. The fourth general strategy is to **request verbal display** by asking children to name or talk about story elements that are already within the child's repertoire. This pattern is tuned to the high end of the ZPD and provides children with opportunities for success. The fifth general strategy is to **adjust the proportion of input containing mastered versus challenging information**. Data reflecting the optimal balance are limited. However, preliminary observations suggest a balance of 70% for mastered information and 30% for challenging information is appropriate for young children. With increasing linguistic maturity, the percentages may come closer to half and half.

Of the six **language-specific interactional strategies** reviewed by van Kleeck (2004), four pertain to the content of extratextual talk and two pertain to strategies of interaction. **Extratextual talk** refers to conversation about the story as opposed to story text per se. The first extratextual strategy is to **use increasingly abstract language**. When talking about elements of a story, the questions and comments of caregivers range from concrete (e.g., asking the child to name a character or an object described in the book) to abstract (e.g., asking a child to think beyond the information given and predict what will happen next or supply an explanation for what has happened). Research indicates that, as children mature, a larger percentage of extratextual talk by caregivers becomes abstract or decontextualized (e.g., Goodsitt, Raitan, & Perlmutter, 1988; Heath, 1982, 1983; Ninio & Bruner, 1978; Snow & Ninio, 1986; van Kleeck, Alexander, Vigil, & Templeton, 1996; van Kleeck & Beckley-McCall, 2002; van Kleeck, Gillam, & Breshears, 1998; van Kleeck, Vigil, & Beer, 1998; Wheeler, 1983). Moreover, engaging children in more abstract discussions about book content was shown to be related to gains in children's development of abstract (decontextualized) language and to their later academic success (Heath, 1982, 1983; van Kleeck, Gillam, Hamilton, & McGrath, 1997; Wells, 1985). These findings are particularly germane to our discussion of the relationship between joint book-reading and literate language style.

The second extratextual strategy is for caregivers to **focus on meaning and enjoyment of print first, and then on print form in simpler form-meaning contexts**. In the context of our present discussion, this pattern highlights the initial importance that caregivers place on text comprehension over the decoding process which is also a part of literacy. Furthermore, although older preschoolers are increasingly introduced to the sound-symbol relationships, particularly when reading alphabet books (e.g., "*A is for apple.*"), this does not occur during joint book-reading around storybooks.

Third, caregivers **increasingly frame books as a unique context** by using words to describe the medium (e.g., *book, page, story, read, write, draw*) (Jones, 1996). They also talk about the "rules" for interacting with books (Snow & Ninio, 1986). For example, books control the topic. Pictures in books represent some of the topics and can be named. Book sharing is an activity that has a beginning, middle, and end. Some parents point out to their children that books have publication dates and ISBN numbers. The children in some of van Kleeck's studies responded by asking whether these were like the book's birthday and telephone number, respectively (van Kleeck, 2004). This strategy is part of the literacy socialization process (see Emerging Literacy later in this chapter).

The last extratextual pattern used by caregivers is to **adjust to the child's interests and experience**. This strategy makes the child both an apprentice and an architect in his or her own acquisition of literacy skills (Jones, 1996). In the studies reviewed by van Kleeck, parents adjusted to their child in several ways during joint book-reading. Many invited children to select the books that were read. Some added characters (e.g., a dog) to stories that did not include them because their child particularly liked those characters. However, the most important strategy within this framework was for caregivers to relate story events to their children's experience. When parents do this, children increase their own initiations and their responses to their caregivers.

In addition to the extratextual strategies used by caregivers, van Kleeck (2004) described two **interactional strategies** that caregivers use for motivating their children's meaningful participation in the joint book-reading dialogue. The first strategy is to **be semantically contingent with the child's contributions**. As in the case of social conversations, caregivers follow their children's lead during joint book-reading by imitating, syntactically expanding, or semantically extending what the children say. If a child produces an utterance that is ambiguous or not understood, his or her caregiver asks for clarification. If the child asks a question about the story, the caregiver addresses the question. The second interactional strategy is to **prompt the child's verbal participation**. This is done by asking questions and following up to make sure the child provides an answer if he or she knows it. If the child does not know an answer, caregivers follow up by

scaffolding the child's discovery of the answer. Caregivers also motivate their children's participation by providing them with positive feedback about their contributions. Overall, these patterns of contingent responding and prompting encourage high rates of participation in dialogues and make joint book-reading fun for children. More frequent participation offers a higher rate of learning opportunities, and research has demonstrated that children with higher response levels during joint book-reading develop higher prereading skills than those who participate less actively (Flood, 1977). Furthermore, evidence suggests that children whose early encounters with literacy are enjoyable tend to read more frequently and more broadly when they are older (Baker, Scher, & Mackler, 1997).

Joint book-reading continues in kindergarten and in the early elementary school years in some but not all classrooms. For more detail about the influence of joint book-reading on children's development of literacy skills please refer to a number of excellent resources on this topic (e.g., van Kleeck, 2004, 2006, 2008; Van Kleeck, Stahl, & Bauer, 2003).

Although joint book-reading has an important influence on children's development of literate language, so does the ability to formulate narrative language. We turn now to a consideration of growth in this area.

Development of Narrative Discourse

In the previous chapter we discussed the emergence of narrative language in the form of five narrative subgenres, including **recounts** (prompted descriptions of specific events experienced by the child and the conversational partner), **accounts** (spontaneous descriptions of specific events experienced by the child), **event casts** (descriptions of ongoing activity), **verbal scripts** (accounts of what typically happens in a situation), and **story narratives** (descriptions of fictional event sequences) (Engel, 1995; Heath, 1986; Hughes, McGillivray, & Schmidek, 1997; Peterson & McCabe, 1983). All of these forms involve the description of event sequences, and they are established to some degree of proficiency in the repertoires of children from mainstream families by approximately 5 to 6 years. However, a refinement of these forms continues through early elementary school and sometimes into later grades.

To formulate mature narratives, a speaker must be proficient in four areas: (1) the organization of macrostructure (e.g., story grammar); (2) access to script knowledge (for narrative content); (3) use of coherence and cohesion devices, and (4) the ability to adjust language to a listener's perspective (Johnston, 1982, 2008). Additionally, children must have the processing capabilities to employ these skills simultaneously (Johnston, 2008). Therefore, a thorough description of narrative development should address each of these dimensions in relation to the whole. It should be based on observations of children across the entire range of ages from preschool to high school (e.g., Botvin & Sutton-Smith, 1977), and it should include a consideration of cultural variations (e.g., Berman & Slobin, 1994; Bliss & McCabe, 2008).

Many studies have examined later narrative development, but the specification of norms is complicated by the tremendous individual variations that exist depending on modality, subgenres, and task structure. For example, the same child may perform at different levels of proficiency depending on whether he or she is formulating a narrative in oral or written form. Similarly, it may be easier for the same child to tell a joke or to describe a previous experience than to summarize a mystery or a science fiction story (1993; Nelson, 1993). Task structure will also affect performance. Proficiency in any aspect of storytelling may vary depending on whether a child is asked to generate a story independently, to tell a story based on one or more pictures, to retell a story after watching a movie, or to finish a story after hearing a story stem (e.g., *Once on a time, a family drove into the desert . . .*) (e.g., Eisenberg et al., 2008; Hughes, McGillivray, & Schmidek, 1997).

Given these layers of complexity and sources of variation, current findings should be regarded as works in progress. Still, a number of developmental patterns are suggested by the available evidence. In the remainder of this section, we trace the development of narratives in relation to macrostructure, script knowledge, linguistic cohesion devices, and language adjustments. We also consider the integration of narrative language within dialogue discourse,

and the links between narratives to expository text. Emphasis is placed on the development of story grammar, but other forms of narrative development also are mentioned.

Macrostructure Development

Recall that story grammar has two major parts: (1) the setting and (2) the episode structure (Stein & Glen, 1979). The setting involves an introduction of the main characters, the protagonist, the location of the story events, and the frame. The episode structure consists of one or more episodes. An episode includes an initiating event, the protagonist's internal response, a plan, an attempt, a consequence, and a reaction. Children's development of macrostructure has been studied by tracking changes in the inclusion of individual elements as well as changes reflecting levels of organization.

In a review of multiple studies conducted prior to 1982, Johnston (1982) identified seven areas of growth in story grammar elements demonstrated by children during late preschool and early school age. Specifically, children learn to include more explicit reference to the time and location of story events, increasing amounts of relevant detail, decreasing amounts of extraneous information, and fewer unresolved problems or unprepared resolutions. By the age of 8 years, children include information about the characters' emotions and thoughts, and clearer descriptions of episode structure.

As noted above, narrative discourse development not only involves the growth of individual narrative elements (e.g., description of character motivations, event sequences, cohesion devices, listener perspective, etc.), it also requires the ability to process these elements simultaneously. Before simultaneous processing abilities are fully mature, children may appear to lack skills that are actually within their repertoires but are masked by limited processing skills (Johnston, 2008). This point is illustrated in the results of a study by Shapiro and Hudson (1991), who observed the narratives of 4- and 6-year-olds under two conditions. In one condition, the story was prompted by a picture sequence clearly illustrating the key elements of macrostructure (e.g., goal, obstacle and solution). In the second condition, children also were provided with a picture sequence but with fewer cues regarding the macrostructure. Results showed that the children's use of linguistic cohesion devices was better in the narratives produced during the first task than during the second task. In other words, when more effort was needed to concentrate on a narrative's macrostructure, then aspects of linguistic form (e.g., cohesion devices) were expressed more poorly, even though the children could use these same forms when the narrative task was less demanding. Similar patterns have been reported in the performance of children with language impairments (e.g., Johnston, 2008; MacLachlan & Chapman, 1988).

Looking beyond individual elements, Botvin and Sutton-Smith (1977) conducted a structural analysis of the spontaneous stories produced by 220 children in eight age groups between 3 to 12 years. Each child's story was classified according to one of seven story grammar levels. Definitions of each level and corresponding examples are provided in Table 5–12. As expected, the frequency of narratives with greater complexity increased across the age groups. Most 3-year-olds produced narratives at level 1 (verbalization of associated events without structural coherence). By approximately 6 years, most narratives were consistent with level 3 (conjunction of two or more problem-resolution sequences without coordination of content and with little detail), and by age 8 years, most narratives reflected level 5 (conjunction and coordination of problem-resolution sequences with internal expansion of detail). Production of complex narratives with one or more embedded subplots (levels 6 and 7) emerged at the ages of about 11 to 12 years, respectively. However, there were considerable variations of performance within age groups.

Some researchers viewed children's narrative skills directly in relation to the development of **literary schemas**, the blueprints of macrostructure (Berman, 2007; Duchan, 2004; Karmiloff-Smith, 1986). These researchers propose that children develop narrative schemas gradually through repeated participation in joint book-reading and through systematic scaffolding of personal narratives. They assume that repetition will enable children to recognize the patterns underlying particular content and to use these patterns as templates to formulate their own narratives independently and with appropriate levels of detail. Karmiloff-Smith (in Westby 1988) described three phases of narrative development

TABLE 5–12. Botvin and Sutton-Smith's (1977) Seven Levels of Story Structure

Level	Characteristics	Example
1	Associated events without structural coherence	*The little duck went swimming. Then the crab came. A lobster came. And a popsicle was playing by itself.*
2	One problem-resolution sequence with or without other associated events	*An astronaut went into space. He was attacked by a monster. The astronaut got in his spaceship and flew away.*
3	Internal expansion of problem-resolution sequence through intermediate elements	*Once there was a little girl. She went walking into the woods and soon it was dark. It was so dark that she couldn't find her way back home. She cried and cried. An owl heard her and asked if she was lost. She said yes. The owl said that he would help her find her way home. He flew up in the air and looked around. After finding out which way to go, he said, "Okay, follow me." Then he led the girl out of the woods and showed her the way home. When she got back home, she was so happy. She gave the friendly owl a kiss and thanked him and told her parents she would never go walking in the woods again by herself. The end.*

TABLE 5–12. *continued*

Level	Characteristics	Example
4	Conjunction of 2 or more problem-resolution sequences without coordination of content and without expansion.	*There was this friendly lion in Asia, but he was captured and brought to a zoo. Then the lion escaped. Has walking down the road and a truck tried to run him over, but he managed to get out of the way. He began to get hungry, so he ate a rabbit.*
5	Conjunction and coordination of problem-resolution sequences with internal expansion	*Once Batman and Robin were in a haunted house. Robin fell through a trap door in the floor and landed in an underground river. Robin pressed his magic watch to signal Batman for help. Batman heard the signal and looked all over the house for Robin. Then he saw the trap door. He lowered a rope from his Bat belt and pulled Robin out of the water. Then they heard a scream. The thought it was a girl but it was Spiderman. They looked around and the screams seemed to come from the attic. Batman and Robin ran up to the attic to save the girl, but Spiderman was hiding behind the door waiting for them. When they came in Spiderman threw an extra strong Spider net over them. They tried to get out but they couldn't. "I've got you now," he said. "I'm going to kill you, and Wonder Woman and I are going to take your Batmobile and live in your Bat Cave." And when Spiderman came over to get the key, Batman hit him right in the face and knocked him down. Then Batman and Robin got out of the net and beat up Spiderman and put him in jail so he wouldn't bother them anymore. The end.*
6	Single embedding of one problem-resolution sequence within another, (i.e., the beginning of subplots).	*A man named Mr. Dirt lived in the country all by himself and owns a farm. One calf got away and went into the woods and headed for the mountains. So, Mr. Dirt went up the mountains after the calf. On the way, a bear came after Mr. Dirt. He ran up a tree and the bear climbed up the tree after him. Mr. Dirt threw his ax at the bear and hit the bear in the head. Blood poured out of his head and the bear fell down and died. A few minutes later, the calf ran over to Mr. Dirt and they went back to the farm.*
7	Similar to level 6, but includes multiple embeddings of problem-resolution sequences.	*Once upon a time there was a little fish named Josh and he was going to a fish fair and there were fishers over the fish fair and the fishermen caught everyone including Josh. Then they put all the fish in the fisher's hole and there were sharks and stingrays and a stingray was going after Josh and then a shark chased the stingray because he wanted to eat the stingray. So, the sting ray stopped chasing Josh and ran away from the shark. So the shark and the stingray got into a big fight. But then another shark gobbled up his mother and father and sister. And then the boat was sailing and sailing and sailing. There was a big storm that night. And it hit against the rocks and made a big hole in the fishers' hole and Josh escaped and went back to his house and he stayed there until he was big.*

Source: Adapted from G. Botvin and B. Sutton-Smith (1977). The development of structural complexity in children's fantasy narratives. *Developmental Psychology, 13*(4), 377–378.

that reflect this perspective. Her illustration of each phase is supported by observations of children between 4 to 9 years of age who were invited to tell a story based on the events depicted in wordless picture books. Table 5–13 describes each phase and provides a corresponding narrative production sample. Overall, these phases represent a gradual shift in text processing from data-driven (bottom-up), to conceptually-based (top-down), to bidirectional (top-down and bottom-up) patterns. Phase 1 is characterized as **procedural**. Children produce syntactically correct sentences to describe pictures in detail, but the utterances, as a group, lack organizational struc-

ture. Phase 2 is characterized as **metaprocedural**. At this phase, children use their knowledge of narrative schema to interpret the pictures and formulate a coherent text. The gist of the story is of primary importance, even at the expense of detail. Phase 3 reflects a **bidirectional processing** including both bottom-up and top-down influences. Children provide a larger number of details than in phase 2, but the details are coordinated with the top-down organization of the story elements. Based on a review of cross-linguistic studies, Berman (2007) reported that maturation of schema-based storytelling occurs at about 9 to 10 years.

TABLE 5–13. Three Phases of Narrative Development Based on Karmiloff-Smith (1986)

Phase	Characteristics	Examples from Westby (1988)
I. Procedural	Output is data drive. If the story is generated based on a wordless picture book, the child describes the content of each picture. However, although sentences may be well formed, there is no intersentential cohesion or sense of a unified text. If pronouns are used, they are used for contextual reference.	*There's a boy and a dog. He has a net and a bucket. The boy is running down the hill. He trips over the tree. And he falls in the water.*
II. Metaprocedural	The child recognizes that the story events are interrelated. He or she is now interpreting pictures rather than just describing them. Utterances are organized primarily by a top-down organization of story elements. The child's focus is on representing the gist of the story, even at the expense of detail. Pronouns are used selectively to establish linguistic reference back to the names of the main characters. Minor characters are typically named by noun phrases.	*The boy and the dog are going fishing. The boy sees a frog. He picks up his bucket and tries to catch the frog. He misses and the frog gets away.*
III. Bidirectional Processing	After considerable practice in representing the gist of stories, children are now capable of including more details about elements in the story structure. They now provide the amount of detail (or more) than they did at phase I, but the details are coordinated with the structural blue print used to organize the story.	*Once there was a boy who wanted to go fishing with his dog. He took his fishing net and his bucket. When he got to the pond, he saw a frog, so he ran down the hill, but he tripped over the tree and fell in the water. The frog was disgusted with all this. The boy tried to grab the frog, but the frog jumped away and sat on a log watching the boy.*

Sources: Based on A. Karmiloff-Smith (1986). Some fundamental aspects of language development after age 5. In P. Fletcher & M. Garman (Eds.), *Language acquisition* (2nd ed., 455–474). New York, NY: Cambridge University Press. Also based on C. Westby (1988) *Oral language and reading: Connections.* A clinical workshop presented in Denver, Colorado, October 8–9.

Changes in the appreciation and elaboration of narrative schemes are paralleled by growth in the style of narration itself. With increasing maturity, children begin to add information and perspective to transform event descriptions into artful, interesting, and personalized forms. This is known as **expressive elaboration** (Kernan, 1977), and it has been described within the framework of **high point analysis** (Labove, 1972; Labove & Waletzky, 1967; Ukrainetz et al., 2005). Here, the complicating event and resolution are viewed as the core of the narrative with a high point that emerges through the unfolding of events between the two. Expressive elaboration may be observed in the formulation of **appendages** on either side of the core, such as: (1) an **opening** to announce a narrative (e.g., *Hey, guess what!*), (2) an **abstract** to preview the content (e.g., *I nearly won the lottery*), (3) an **orientation** that includes not only the setting but also insights into the characters' relationships, personality features, and motivating circumstances, and (4) a **coda** to end the narrative (e.g., *that's all*). Expressive elaboration can also be observed in **evaluations** reflecting the narrator's thoughts, insights, and perspectives about the events. Evaluations may be offered anywhere throughout the narrative, but they are often stated after the initiating event to stop the action and to build a listener's interest and suspense toward the high point within the narrative's core.

Urkrainetz et al. (2005) studied the development of expressive elaboration in the oral narratives produced by 293 children between 5 and 12 years of age. Each child was asked to tell a story based on a short picture sequence. Expressive elaboration was found to be common in the narratives across all age groups. However, total expressive elaboration increased significantly both in presence and in frequency across the ages. To illustrate the differences in the children's performance, the researchers provided four narrative examples to match the mean performance for each age cluster of the children in their study. An example given to illustrate performance between 5 and 6 years is as follows:

Once there was a little boy. He was sleeping in his bed. And he went to go eat his breakfast and accidentally took the string out of his shoe and accidentally broke. And then he tried to go to school with the bus. But the bus leaved already. And he had to walk to school. And then the teacher said he was late. (p. 1375)

In contrast, the example given to illustrate performance at the 10- to 12-year level is as follows:

One morning a kid woke up. And his name was Todd. He got up and he looked at his clock and it turned out he was almost late for school. And so he got out of bed. And got dressed hurriedly. And he went into the kitchen. This is where he poured his favorite cereal was out. So he had to do his least favorite which is crunch-munchys. And while he was looking at the clock worrying about time he poured milk all over his cereal. After he got dressed he started to tie his shoe. And the shoelace snapped. After a long time of trying to repair the shoelace, he decided to give up. He put on his backpack ran outside and discovered his school bus had raced ahead of him. After a long and treacherous time of walking to school the teacher said he was late. And he had to spend the recess inside. (p. 1375)

Peterson and McCabe (1983) used the term **story sparkle** to characterize narratives with a rich vocabulary, complex episodes, a dramatic high point, and literate language style. According to Berman (2007), the full development of these skills can be seen at adolescence. She noted that rich, expressive elaboration is characteristic of adolescent storytellers through their use of interpretive and evaluative comments about a story's content and form.

So far, our description of macrostructure development has relied exclusively on observations of children from families of mainstream, European North American culture. The personal narratives of these children can be characterized as **topic-centered** owing to the succinct, chronologic ordering of information around a central event sequence, usually with a high point (Peterson & McCabe, 1983). However, not all cultures encourage children to develop this style of personal narrative. First, some African American children produce personal narratives that are characterized as having a **topic-associating style** (Heath, 1983). Rather than focusing on a single core event, topic-associating narratives tend to include several key events related to a single theme. These narratives tend to be longer than topic-centered narratives. Second, some speakers with Central or South American backgrounds use a **conversational style** of narrative (Bliss & McCabe,

2008). This style is derived partly from a history of mother-child interactions that are conversationally-focused rather than past-event focused (e.g., Melzi, 2000; Silva & McCabe, 1996). It places emphasis on family members and habitual events rather than the sharing of past events. As a result, personal narratives tend to be about sharing information pertaining to the narrator's family through a monologic recounting of dialogue. As with the topic-associating style, the conversational style of narration tends to be relatively long. Finally, some Asian American children use a **haiku-like narrative** style. These are short, concise, multiple-event narratives with minimal information. Pronouns are omitted when the agent of an action is clear from the rest of the text. This style derives from a history of mother-child interactions that encourage brevity through frequent interruptions during narrative speaking tasks (Minami & McCabe, 1995). For an excellent discussion and illustrations of cultural variations in narrative style, see Bliss and McCabe (2008).

Script Knowledge

We have already referred to a kind of script knowledge in our discussion of literary schemas above. However, other types of script knowledge encompass content knowledge. Johnston (1982) defined **script knowledge** as generalized knowledge about particular kinds of events based on repeated experiences in similar situations. For example, a child might have a generalized fast food restaurant script that includes recurring parts of the routine (e.g., ordering food, paying for it, sitting in a booth to eat it, conversing with family or friends during the meal, waiting for everyone to finish, placing empty containers into the trash at the end of the meal, and departing). Others characterize such scripts as generalized event representations (GERs) (Nelson, 1986; Nelson & Gruendel, 1981). Scripts are stored in long-term memory and activated in appropriate situations. With the accumulation of life experience, individuals form an increasing number of scripts that become more complex. Expectations developed on the basis of script knowledge influence an individual's perceptions, choice of what to communicate, and ability to maintain a conversational flow. Content scripts are an important complement to story grammar, which, as indicated above, is itself

an organizational frame without specific content. A literature review by Johnson (1995) includes studies documenting growth over time in the range of content themes included in children's narratives.

Overlapping with script knowledge is the development of **content schemas**, a somewhat broader category of generalized knowledge structures (Duchan, 2004; Westby, 1994). According to Westby, a **content schema** is an organization of knowledge about a given topic or domain. It includes script knowledge but also information about semantic relationships and concepts of space, time, and causality. Content schemas may represent scenes, events, or concepts and ideas. For example, the content schema for a **scene**, such as a grocery store, might include a large room consisting of aisles stocked with food, a bakery section, a section for fresh produce, shoppers, check-out lanes, and checkers. The content schema for an **event** is equivalent to the generalized event sequences (GERs) discussed above. For a **concept or idea**, such as justice, the content schema might include laws of conduct, types of crimes, the responsibility of the police, prosecutors and defense attorneys, the role of courts, and punishment. As they mature, the content schemas of children and youth become increasingly organized, complex, and hierarchical through a combination of real-world experience, observational learning, direct instruction, and reading.

As content schemas develop, they become topics for the production and comprehension of verbal and written communication, including narratives. One area of growth that is particularly germane to the development of narratives is children's increased appreciation of **cause-effect relations** throughout the school years (Johnson, 1995). Concepts of **psychological causality** also expand. During early elementary school, children understand **primary emotions** such as happiness, anger, sadness, fear, and surprise (e.g., Flavell, 2004; Westby, 1988). They recognize the types of events that would lead to these emotions, as well as the kinds of reactions that typically follow. During later elementary school, children become aware of more complex states that could be classified as **secondary** or **cognitive emotions** such as jealousy, guilt, shame, and embarrassment, and they recognize the antecedents and consequences associated with these as well. The development of this awareness supports the elaboration of elements in the narrative episode structure such as a character's reaction to an interference with his or her goals, and the development of plans to resolve the interference. The understanding of psychological causality is also linked with growth in children's theory of mind (ToM), discussed later in this chapter (Flavell, 2004).

Text Cohesion and Coherence

Storytelling requires more than the formulation of complete sentences. In addition to these, it requires the use of linguistic devices to establish meaningful relationships between sentences (**text cohesion**) and other markers to support the overall theme and macrostructure (**text coherence**) Shapiro and Hudson (1991, 1997). Key words, phrases, and content information are used to support text coherence (e.g., *Once upon a time . . .* ; *All of a sudden . . .* ; *The end*). Specific syntactic devices are used to achieve intersentential cohesion (Halliday & Hassan, 1973). Examples of syntactic cohesion devices include conjunctions (e.g., *and, but, or, because*), **conjunctive adverbials** (e.g., *nevertheless, on the other hand, at the same time*), **anaphoric pronouns**, (e.g., *his, her, this, that*), and the **definite article** (*the*). Table 5–11 provides a list of six major categories of cohesion devices, definitions of each, and examples of subtypes. The organization and cohesion resulting from the use of these markers and devices help to facilitate story comprehension (Cain, 2003).

As expected, there is an increase with age in the accurate use of cohesion devices. According to Bliss and McCabe (2008), **conjunctive cohesion** should be mastered by children between the ages of 4 and 6 years during the production of personal narratives. As noted in Table 5–11, conjunctive cohesion refers to the use of words or phrases that link utterances and events (e.g., *and, then, because, but, and so*). Furthermore, conjunctive cohesion may have either a semantic function or a pragmatic function (Peterson and McCabe, 1991). The **semantic function** is consistent with the literal meaning of the conjunctions (e.g., additive, adversative, causal, or temporal). The **pragmatic function** is in play when conjunctions are used to: (1) initiate a passage (e.g., *I bet you saw the sun coming up. But I saw these animals in the zoo*), (2) close a passage

(e.g., *So, they lived happily ever after*), (3) signal a chronologic change in ordering (e.g., *We went to Florida but first we went to Texas*), or (4) change the focus of discourse (e.g., *And then I fell down, but you know what?*) (Bliss & McCabe, 2008, p. 164). Children between 4 and 6 years of age should be able to use both types of conjunctive cohesion.

Although the use of conjunctive cohesion may emerge between 4 and 6 years, there is evidence of a more protracted period of refinement, at least in some narrative tasks. Liles (1987) studied the use of conjunctives by 40 students with and without language impairments between the ages of 7;6 (years; months) and 10;6. Each student viewed a movie and then told the story to each of two adults—one who had seen the movie and another who had not. Four types of conjunctives were targeted, including those that would be classified on semantic grounds as additive (e.g., *and*), temporal (e.g., *before, after, during*, etc.), causal (e.g., *because, so, therefore*, etc.), and adversative (e.g., *but, however*, etc.). However, the use of conjunctives was tracked with respect to both intersentential cohesion as well as cohesion between larger narrative segments. One result of this complex study was that the students at all ages (with and without language impairments) used conjunctives more skillfully to establish intersentential cohesion than to establishing cohesion between episodes (Liles, 1987).

Roth, Spekman, and Fye (1995) investigated the use of **reference cohesion**. They observed students ranging in age from 8 to 14 years. Reference cohesion involves the use of a linguistic form to signal to a listener or reader that the referent for that form is found in another sentence. The four types of reference cohesion studied by Roth et al. are based on Halliday and Hasan (1976) and summarized on Table 5–11. The participants in the study included 93 students with and without language impairment. Each student told one spontaneously generated story and one story in response to a theme-based picture. Each story was then analyzed for types of reference cohesion, accuracy, and other variables. The major age-related finding was an increase in overall correct use of reference cohesion as a function of increased age. Additionally, all students established a higher proportion of correct reference cohesion when producing the spontaneous story than when producing the theme-based story.

Communicative Adjustments

The ability of speakers to adjust their language according to listener needs was discussed in the previous chapter in relation to the sociolinguistic skill known as **register variations**. For example, we noted that toddlers and preschoolers use more frequent politeness markers if a listener is older, bigger, less familiar, dominant, or the possessor of a desired privilege (Ervin-Tripp & Gordon, 1986). Similarly, we noted that preschoolers use longer utterances with more frequent complex forms when talking to adults than when talking to 2-year-olds (Shatz & Gelman, 1973). In that sense, we should expect that school-age children adjust their use of cohesion markers and the syntactic complexity of their utterances when sharing stories with listeners of different ages or with different experiences.

A study by Liles (1985) confirms this assumption. As in Liles' 1987 study, each participant in the present study was asked to retell a story based on a movie they had seen, and then to retell the story two times—once to an adult who had seen the movie and once to an adult who had not. One finding of this complex study was that the students did indeed adjust their use of language in consideration of the listeners. Specifically, they used a higher proportion of cohesive ties involving personal reference and conjunctives when communicating with adults who did not see the movie than when communicating with those who did. Students also produced more complete ties when telling their story to an adult who did not see the movie and more incomplete ties when telling their story to an adult who did. A **complete tie** is one in which the relationship between the referent and the cohesion marker is unambiguous and clear (e.g., *Katrina is a black cat. When it's dark outside, she is difficult to find*). An **incomplete tie** is one in which the relationship is ambiguous (e.g., *Ken and Jonathan went shopping. He bought a computer game.*).

Children's sensitivity to their conversational partner was also demonstrated in a study by Hislop, Zaretsky, and Vellman (2007). These researchers examined language adjustments by six children between the ages of 3 years, 5 months to 8 years, 6 months during a storytelling task. Each child was asked to tell a story from a picture book to his or her younger sibling (27 to 67 months) and then to his or her mother. Results showed that all children made adjustments based on the age of their communicative partners. When telling the story to their younger siblings, they spoke in a different tone of voice, used fewer and shorter sentences than when telling the story to their mothers. This study should be replicated with a larger number of participants and with attention to an expanded range of variables reflecting narrative language. However, the present results do suggest that preschoolers and young school age children are sensitive to differences in their communication partners and modify their narrative language accordingly.

Sensitivity to a communicative partner is tied to the larger social-cognitive domain known as **Theory of Mind (ToM)** (Johnston, 2008). As indicated previously, ToM refers to the understanding that each individual has a unique set of perspectives and agendas, and that an individual's behavior can be predicted and explained (in part) by reference to these mental states (Baron-Cohen, 2000; Baron-Cohen, Tager-Flusberg, & Cohen, 1993, 2000). Understanding the perspectives of other speakers can aid listeners in the comprehension of narratives. Narratives, especially stories, involve goals and motivations, internal responses to key events, and plans consistent with an agenda. For this reason, we trace some key milestones in the continuing development of ToM at school age.

Recall that ToM development begins at preschool with milestones such as joint attention during the first year of life; the use of desire-based vocabulary (e.g., *want, wish, hope*) in reference to self and others at about 18 months; and the use of cognitive verbs (e.g., *think, know*) at 30 months. By 3 years, children seem to appreciate simple causal relations among desires, outcomes, emotions, and actions, recognizing. For example, they recognize that people will feel good if they get what they want and feel bad if they do not (Bartsch & Wellman, 1995). By 4 years they demonstrate the important understanding that people may believe something that is not true (false belief). Additionally, children develop sensitivity to the visual perspective of others (Flavell, 2004).

At school age, children and youth continue to expand their understanding of other people's internal states. According to Flavell (2004), one new insight acquired at this age is that people do not always actually feel what they appear to feel. Furthermore, children learn that people's emotional reactions to an event may be influenced by an earlier emotional experience with similar events or by their current mood (Flavell & Miller, 1998). Likewise, they come to understand that a person's interpretation of an ambiguous event may be influenced by pre-existing bias or expectations (Pillow & Henrichon, 1996). They learn that the mind is an interpreter rather than just a recorder of experience, and that information must be present in adequate amounts in order to be useful. For example, if a person sees only a part of an object they may come to an incorrect conclusion about what it is.

Three major theories exist regarding the mechanisms underlying ToM development. Some researchers consider ToM to be a domain-specific cognitive module that is distinct from other cognitive functions (e.g., Baron-Cohen, 1995; Leslie, 1994; Scholl & Leslie, 1999). Others conceptualize it as acts of simulation or role-taking (Langdon & Colthart, 2002), and another group views it as acts of theorizing which result in successive revisions through experience (e.g., Gopnik & Meltzoff, 1997; Perner, 1991; Wellman & Gelman, 1998). All recognize that the environment has some influence on children's ToM development. Detailed information about each theory can be found in Flavell (2004) and Astington and Gopnik (1991).

Many environmental factors are likely to encourage the growth of ToM, including certain patterns of child-caregiver interaction (e.g., Adrian, Clemente, Villanueva, & Rieffe, 2005; Peterson & Slaughter, 2003). For example, Peterson and Slaughter reported significant correlations between mothers' preferences for talk about mental states and their children's ToM performance. **Causal talk** was found to be especially relevant. This was characterized by the verbalization of an explanation when referring to a person's mental state or feelings as in the following example: "*The baby is crying because she misses her Mommy*."

A more general environmental factor may be the range of conversational partners experienced by children and youth in elementary, middle, and high school as compared with those experienced by preschoolers. At preschool, conversational partners include a relatively small number of individuals (i.e., parents, siblings, and a teacher) who share a great deal of information and experience with a child and require fewer contextual explanations to understand a young child's utterances. However, by school age, students communicate with a more diverse group of teachers and peers with whom they share far fewer experiences. To accommodate the needs of these less familiar conversational partners, students must learn to use a more explicit vocabulary, more complex syntax, and linguistic cohesion markers. At the very least, they must be prepared to use these strategies in response to requests for clarification.

As children and youth progress through the school years, a wide variety of other environmental factors further encourages reflection on others' mental states. In fact, it is difficult to think of situations that do not invite the consideration of other people's perspectives. At school age children and youth are increasingly exposed to literature (e.g., history books, biographies, dramas) and academic classes (e.g., psychology, sociology, history, anthropology, political science, religion) which highlight the concerns, perspectives, and behavior of others. They are encouraged to read the newspaper, learn about community leaders, and track political elections. Some participate in sports and drama classes that require reflection on the goal-oriented strategies and personal agendas of others. The development of friendships, participation in clubs, and association with peer groups is a routine part of the high school experience, and many students begin dating during their high school years. Learning to drive a car is another major milestone for high school students, and becoming a successful driver requires continuous monitoring of other motorists, their intentions on the road, and their behavior behind the wheel

To the extent that their agendas differ from those of their parents or siblings, children and youth learn the art of verbal negotiation, and many do so by taking the perspectives of others into consideration. All of these social experiences can yield insight into other minds, and language is an all-pervasive thread in the fabric of participation as well as reflection.

Integration of Narratives into Conversational Discourse

Children begin to embed narratives of various types into their conversations with others as soon as they begin talking about past events and especially when they reach school age. Preece (1987) observed the conversations of three children over an 18-month period during daily 30-minute car trips to and from school. The three children (2 girls, 1 boy) were 5 years old at the beginning of the study (entering kindergarten) and 7 at the end (midway through first grade). Almost 90 hours of audio-taped conversation yielded 599 narratives which were analyzed for frequency and type. Results indicated that the children produced an average of four narratives per trip during their kindergarten year and six narratives per trip during first grade. Fourteen different narrative types were identified. The most frequent were personal anecdotes, and anecdotes of vicarious experience, which accounted for 52% and 20%, respectively, of the entire sample.

Twelve percent of the stories generated by the children in Preece's (1987) study were classified as **collaborative narratives**. This form of narrative is constructed as each conversational partner takes his or her turn in contributing information to the construction of the narrative. One of the most complex and sophisticated narratives found in the sample was formed collaboratively by the three children in Preece's study. The formation of collaborative narratives is also known as **story chaining** and was reported in a study by (Schober-Peterson & Johnson, 1993) who observed thirty 8- to 10-year-olds during casual conversation with their peers.

The importance of narrative development and its appearance in conversational speech cannot be overestimated. Narrative language is a means of connecting with others. At adolescence, it is one of the primary tools used to gain entry into a peer group (e.g., Nippold, 1993). Decontextualized narratives are valued in school settings during classroom exercises such as "sharing time" (Bliss & McCabe, 2008), and narrative language is a crucial important bridge to literacy as indicated in the next section.

Relationship of Narrative Language Development to Literate Language Style

Clearly, narrative language has a number of features in common with literate language style. Narrative language is **monologic**, even though it is often embedded within conversation. Like literate language, most narratives are **planned** in that the narrator draws his or her narrative elements from pre-existing narrative and content schemas. Narrative

language requires the use of syntactic **cohesion devices** to establish intersentential relationships and other linguistic devices to mark the macrostructure. As in the case of literate language, narratives include greater **lexical diversity**, **density, and complexity** than conversational speech. Narrative content is based on script knowledge and **content schemas** for its themes and (in part) for its comprehension. Literate language also relies on content schemas albeit at higher levels of abstraction. As with all forms of language, narrative language **must be adjusted** in tune with the perspectives of the conversational partner, and, as in the case of literate language, this requires particular attention to the use of **unambiguous referential language** and endophoric pronoun reference. In that sense, narrative language is **decontextualized**.

Narrative language accounts for a marked portion of the language heard by children in first and second grades. Proficiency in the use of narratives continues to expand throughout school age in conjunction with the continued growth of content schemas, theory of mind, and opportunities to hear and read stories told and written by others.

Of the various narrative forms (recounts, accounts, event casts, stories, verbal scripts), verbal scripts may be the closest in content to the expository forms of literate language style. Recall that verbal scripts require a speaker to describe a general event sequence rather than a specific event as when a child is asked to *Tell Daddy how we check books out of the library* (versus *Tell Daddy how we checked the book out of the library yesterday*). This adds a level of abstraction to the narrative task, and is what brings it closer to the expository forms. In the next section, we address the topic of expository language development.

Development of Oral Expository Discourse

Expository discourse is used to inform. In contrast to narrative language, which is used to communicate personal experiences or fictional events within a temporal context, expository discourse communicates nonfiction content organized along logical rather than temporal lines. The key characteristics (e.g., decontextualization, monologic style, high clausal density, high semantic density, generalized informational stance) were described earlier in connection with literate language style.

Although expository discourse is used extensively in formal settings, less formal variations occur in everyday situations when people respond to requests for information (e.g., *Explain to your mother what a podcast is, What are the steps for making chocolate chip cookies?, How can I get from here to the post office?*). Here, the discourse is embedded within a dialogic framework where each partner in the dialogue contributes an element to the expository text structure. The person asking the question initiates the topic and the person responding provides the elaboration. Some degree of contextual support may be available. For example, if asked to give directions, the speaker may draw a map to support his or her verbal description. Informal expositions of this sort require relatively little reflection or planning since the content is typically familiar to the person giving the information.

In academic settings, expository discourse is highly valued and often embedded within classroom discussions, such as when a teacher asks a student to describe a science experiment. This will place greater processing demands on the student because the information is likely to be more challenging and less well rehearsed. The teacher introduces the topic, the student elaborates. Scaffolding may be provided by the teacher or by peers as needed. In this case, the overall text is generated collaboratively through dialogue. However, when expository discourse is used during a monologic oral presentation, it has all of the characteristics of literate language style.

Milestones in the development of oral expository discourse are even less well established than those representing the development of narrative language. This limitation is due in part to a once held assumption that most aspects of language acquisition were completed by the age of five years (e.g., Lenneberg, 1967). More recently there has been a dramatic increase of interest in all aspects of school-age language development, including the development of extended discourse and literate language style (e.g., Berman, 2004; Berman & Verhoeven, 2002; Bliss, 2002; Nippold, 1998, 2007; Nippold & Scott, 2010). This emerging literature shows that, expository discourse, like narrative discourse, is a complex genre. There are various subgenres

(e.g., enumerative, compare-contrast, cause-effect, argumentation, etc.) which may be used individually or in combination in any given text. Furthermore, there are considerable variations in performance within the same individual depending on the modality (e.g., oral, written) in which expository discourse is assessed, the kinds of tasks that are used to assess it (e.g., conversation vs. monologue; comprehension vs. production), and the specific aspects of expository discourse being targeted (e.g., macrostructure, text cohesion, signaling devices, clause structures, levels of abstraction, etc.). Still, developmental patterns are emerging. In the remainder of this section we summarize three studies representing developmental trends in expository discourse during oral communication tasks.

The first study examined referential specificity within a dialogic, expository speaking task (Lloyd, in Nippold, 2007). The participants were 48 children ages 7 and 10 years. Twelve adults served as the control group. The task involved same-age partners giving and receiving directions from each other over the telephone. Each member of the pair was located in a different room with a table and a telephone. The tabletop in each room contained an identical map depicting a community with a school, churches, shops, garages, and rows of houses. To give directions, the speaker was provided with an overlay to the map which defined a route from the school to a particular house. When receiving directions, the listener was provided with a toy vehicle for use to follow the route. If directions were unclear, the listener was permitted to request clarification.

Results showed that the 10-year-olds and the adults outperformed the 7-year-olds as both direction givers and followers. When giving directions, the 7-year-olds often used ambiguous language. For example, there were several garages on the map, and 7-year-old direction-givers sometimes failed to specify which garage the listener should target (e.g., *Go all the way to the garage*). As listeners, the 7-year-olds often failed to reach the target location, in part because they often failed to request clarification when directions were ambiguous. The 10-year-olds and adults, on the other hand, provided information with more referential specificity (e.g., *Go to the one without the chimney*). They also provided information in more manageable chunks and waited for the listener to confirm understanding before continuing. There were also some differences between the 10-year-olds and the adults. For example, the adults used directional terminology more often (e.g., *left, right, strait on*) and embedded more information into an individual statement (e.g., *Carry on from there, still going right to the building with the yellow flash under the window*). Overall, this study indicates that the ability to give referentially clear spatial directions and to request clarification may not be stable until the age of 10 years. Additionally, it suggests that the ability to speak succinctly continues to develop even after the age of 10 years, and that further research is needed to determine the age at which referentially clear and succinct directions are stable within repertoire (Nippold, 2007).

In another study, Nippold, Hesketh, Duthie, and Mansfield (2005) compared the use of certain syntactic forms in conversational and expository discourse by speakers between 7 to 49 years of age. Each participant was engaged in two speaking tasks: (1) social conversation about familiar topics (family, friends) and (2) exposition about the rules and strategies for playing a favorite game or a sport. Results indicated that speakers of all ages consistently used more complex syntax during the expository speaking task than during social conversation, including a higher proportion of relative, nominal, and adverbial clauses. Expository texts also included a higher clausal density and a higher average number of words per T-unit. (Recall that a T-unit is an independent clause plus all subordinate clauses and nonclausal structures that are related to or embedded within it) (Hunt, 1970). Nippold et al. associated the higher proportion of embedded clauses in expository discourse with an increase in the complexity of the reasoning required by the task. For example, one of the participants used *if-then* clauses when describing strategies for playing poker, but he never verbalized conditional reasoning during social conversation about his dogs or stepsisters. Observations of this type suggest that it is the complexity of thought that drives the use of more complex syntax in expository discourse.

Nippold et al. (2005) also found a significant age-related increase in the use of relative clauses and in the average number of words per T-unit within the expository speaking task. This pattern may be correlated with the increasingly more complex

thought processes and larger knowledge base of the older participants. For example, an 8-year-old boy and a 40-year-old man both chose basketball as the topic of their exposition, and each was asked to describe the strategies that a good basketball player would need to know in order to win a game. The 8-year-old gave a 15-word reply indicating that the winning team would have to score more points, while the 40-year-old used 10 sentences with an average of 12.18 words per T-unit to describe three specific scoring strategies.

Despite the clear pattern of results obtained by Nippold et al. (2005) and despite the finding that even the youngest children used all three of the targeted clause structures (nominal, relative, adverbial), Nippold et al. cautioned that the results of this research cannot be taken as normative. A much larger and more representative sample of the population is needed to establish normative data. Furthermore, the nature of the expository task is crucial. In this study, the participants were asked to inform a listener about a familiar and motivating topic. It is possible that the complexity of the expository text may have been less advanced if the topic had been less familiar and more neutral with respect to each participant's interests. There is a close relationship between an individual's familiarity with a topic and the complexity of the discourse used to describe the topic to others. As with narrative language formulation, a tradeoff may exist between the resources needed to process the logical content and structure of the information and the degree of syntactic complexity or verbal fluency with which it is expressed.

In the third study, Katzenberger (2004) examined the use of hierarchical text structures by five groups of Hebrew-speaking individuals between 9 years and adulthood. Katzenberger conceptualized expository text (regardless of macrostructure) as consisting of a **nucleus** (the essential information conveyed) and its **complements** (additional or supporting information). Additionally, she proposed that text elements can be classified in relation to three kinds of functions: (1) **Move-on** (introducing a new topic), (2) **Expand** (developing a topic currently under discussion), and (3) **Unitize** (summarize information previously mentioned). A move-on assumes a global function when it introduces the overall topic, and a unitize assumes a global function when it summarizes the overarching content of the entire text. All nonglobal elements are considered to have local (more specific or subordinate) functions. Using this model, Katzenberger identified **four stages of expository text development** in the narratives produced by Hebrew-speaking individuals in four age groups: 9 to 10 years, 12 to 13 years, 16 to 17 years, and adults. Although the expositions in this study were produced in writing, the stages of development can be applied to oral exposition as well. Below are the characteristic features of each stage:

1. Minimal—the text consists of a nucleus followed by at least one complement.

2. Partially hierarchical—the text contains global and local level elements. The global elements introduce or summarize the main ideas, but the local level elements lack local organization.

3. Fully hierarchical—there is a graded interplay of information between the global and local elements

4. Fully developed expository rhetoric—the global text organization and the flow of elements are explicitly indicated by linguistic markers.

In a follow-up study, Katzenberger (2004) analyzed the oral and written expository texts of 80 Hebrew-speaking individuals within the same age groups as in the study described previously. Each participant was asked to give a talk and write an essay about the general topic of interpersonal conflict. Half of the participants in each age group wrote the essay before giving the talk and the other half wrote the essay afterward. The data were analyzed to assess modality (oral vs. written) and age-based differences in the use of clause packages and clause markers (to be defined). Our discussion is limited primarily to age-related differences.

A **clause package (CP)** was defined as a text unit that typically consists of several clauses linked by syntactic, thematic, and/or discursive criteria, where each criterion supersedes and incorporates the next. CPs go beyond syntactically defined structures (e.g., clauses), discursively defined elements (e.g., thematic units), or stanzas to form the building blocks of discourse. An **explicit global CP** is one that contains an explicit abstract generalization

(e.g., *There are problems between people which can build the connection and problems that can destroy the connection between them.*) Explicit global CPs can be distinguished from CPs with meanings that are tied more specifically to the speaker (e.g., *I think that lots of people don't respect each other).* Based on earlier findings regarding the development of expository text, Katzenberger predicted that the use of explicit, generalized CPs would increase with age in both oral and written expository discourse. This is exactly what the data showed. These forms occurred in 0%, 10%, 100%, and 100%, of the spoken expository texts of 9- to 10-year-olds, 12- to 13-year-olds, 16- to 17-year-olds, and adults, respectively. Interestingly, the conceptualization of a generalized framework for an oral exposition did not occur during this speaking task as a consistent pattern until midadolescence.

The second target of Katzenberger's (2004) analysis was the use of **discourse markers**. A discourse marker is a word or phrase that specifies a discourse segment or CP. Two types (general and specific) were distinguished by the degree of explicitness. **General markers** indicate either the genre of the text (e.g., *in my opinion*) or the general progression of information (e.g., *so/then*). **Specific markers** were defined as those that signal the discourse function of the CP by indicating the nature of the connection between text segments. For example, a specific marker (e.g., *furthermore)* could be used to signal the relationship between a move-on and its expansion. Results showed that approximately 25% of the CPs produced by participants at all ages were introduced by discourse markers, both in oral and written discourse. However, there is a decrease in the use of general discourse markers and a rise in the use of specific discourse markers with age in both spoken and written text.

Overall, the results of Katzenberger's (2004) study support the prediction that the expository narratives produced by 16- to 17-year-olds and adults are hierarchical while the structure of narratives produced by younger children are not. The younger age groups produced expository texts that included a pair-wise ordering of segments (i.e., a nucleus followed by one or more complements), with the 12- to 13-year-olds providing more complementary information than the 9- to 10-year-olds. However, the two older age groups formulated texts that were hierarchical, including both global and local elements with the use of specific markers to indicate the function of CPs within the hierarchy of the text as a whole. Katzenberger attributes the adolescents' and adults' representations of more complex text structures to the more mature cognitive system associated with these ages. Specifically, she notes that the shift from pair-wise to hierarchical organization may be consistent with Piaget and Inhelder's (1969) framework of cognitive development, which predicts a shift from concrete to formal operations at adolescence. In that sense, the ability to create hierarchical expository language suggests the development of metatextual awareness on a more abstract level.

The studies reviewed here indicate that, although the development of expository discourse overlaps with the development of narrative discourse, the former involves a more protracted period of development. Some of the critical skills that continue to emerge are still developing into adolescence, including: (1) the use of unambiguous referents, (2) the use of syntactic forms to represent increasingly complex relational meanings, and (3) the hierarchicalization of text structures. These developments have been correlated with ongoing cognitive developments such as the emergence of formal operations and advances in social cognition such as theory of mind. However, research on this topic is relatively new. Additionally, performance is dependent in part on the nature of the speaking task and on a speaker's knowledge of a specific domain (Nippold, 2010). For example, if expository output is measured by syntactic complexity, higher levels of performance are observed when speakers are asked to describe strategies for winning a game than when they are asked to describe a relative or a pet. More research is needed to develop a clearer picture of developmental trends in all aspects of narrative development across different speaking tasks.

Factors Associated with Development of Expository Discourse

We have already mentioned that aspects of cognitive development and environmental experience may impact the development of expository discourse. Here we consider these influences in more detail.

Cognitive Development

In an earlier chapter we defined cognition as the processes and products of mind. Within a Piagetian framework, the cognitive developments associated with elementary and high school years include preoperations, concrete and formal operations. A single theme running through each of these stages is the **cognitive distancing principle**, which holds that through development, children learn to explore, perceive, and think about the world in ways that are increasingly more removed from concrete experience. Recall that during the **sensory-motor stage** (0–2 years), infant thought is limited to direct sensory experience and action on the environment. The ongoing development of cognitive tools during the preoperational, operational, and formal operational stages allows thinking to become increasingly removed from the here and now. We briefly summarize the characteristics of these stages. However, we begin with an important note: Current research indicates that Piaget grossly underestimated the ages at which skills are acquired and calls into question the entire concept of discrete developmental stages. We now know that children are able to perform many skills that would not be predicted by Piagetian stage characteristics when given simplified tasks that are relevant to their everyday experiences. Therefore, although we include the age-ranges specified by Piaget in relation to each stage, it is best to consider the stage characteristics as overlapping at the extremes rather than as discrete within the age ranges given. The following information is based primarily on Berk (2000) and Ginsberg and Opper (1969).

During the **preoperational stage** (2–7 years), children are learning to represent ideas through make-believe play, drawing, spatial maps, and especially through language. They can talk about events that they experienced previously or that they may experience in the future. Language becomes one of the tools for thinking about the world without directly manipulating it. However, there are limitations in the logic of children's thinking, especially early in this stage. They **lack conservation**, which is the recognition that certain physical characteristics of objects remain the same despite changes in outward appearance. For example, if water is poured from a short wide glass into a tall narrow glass, the amount of water remains the same even though its level appears higher in the tall narrow glass. However, the reasoning of children at this stage is **perception bound** in that they are distracted by concrete appearances and ignore other relevant dimensions of an event. In our conservation example, children reason that if it looks like there is more water in the glass (due to the higher water level in the taller glass) then there must be more water in the glass. They fail to notice that changes in the height of the water level are compensated by changes in the width of the container. Additionally, they engage in **transductive reasoning**, which proceeds from the particular to the particular. For example, events that occur closely together in time are assumed to have a cause-effect relationship. A child interviewed by Piaget noted that clouds move when people walk, so she reasoned that the movement of people causes the movement of clouds (Piaget, 1926/1929). A final characteristic of preoperational thought is **difficulty with hierarchical classification**. This is illustrated by children's responses to Piaget's class inclusion task. In this task, preoperational children were presented with pictures of 16 flowers: 12 yellow and 4 blue. When asked whether there are more yellow flowers or more flowers, children at the preoperational stage stated that there were more yellow flowers. They failed to recognize that the category "flower" includes both blue and yellow flowers (Berk, 2000).

The period of **concrete operations** (7–11 years) is associated with a shift from reasoning based on perceptual salience to **reasoning based on logic**. Included at this level are reasoning skills associated with the logico-arithmetic operations and spatial operations. Progress in **logico-arithmetic operations** is demonstrated in at least three ways. One is success on **conservation** tasks requiring simultaneous attention to more than one attribute. For example, children at this stage recognize that when water is poured from a small, wide glass to a tall, narrow glass, the amount of water is the same and that the resulting elevation in water is due to a difference in width of the second glass. This understanding also includes **reversibility**, or "the ability to imagine water being returned to the original container as proof of conservation" (Berk, 2000, p. 249). Second, children demonstrate **hierarchical classification** skills. This is demonstrated, for exam-

ple, by their successful performance on Piaget's class inclusion task, by their tendency to develop collections (e.g., stamps, balls, baseball cards, etc.), and by their ability to participate in board games (e.g., Uno) that require a player to exploit the shifting criteria on which the same set of objects (e.g., cards) can be classified. A third manifestation of logico-arithmetic operations is **seriation**. This is the ability to arrange items in order based on a physical quality such as length or weight. By the age of 9 or 10, children can seriate mentally to engage in **transitive inference**. To illustrate this, Piaget showed children pairs of sticks in which A was longer than B and B was longer than C. Children with transitive inference could predict (without direct observation) that A was longer than C.

Children at the operational stage also demonstrate more logic in thinking about **spatial operations** related to distance, direction, and space between objects. To illustrate reasoning about **distance**, consider a situation in which children are presented with two toy cars 12 inches apart. When a miniature stop sign is then placed at an equal distance on the line between the two cars, children at this stage will say that the distance between the two cars remains the same while younger children will say that the distance has become smaller. Improvements involving **directions** emerge at the age of about 7 or 8 years when children begin to perform **mental rotations**. For example, if an adult facing the child asks the child to *name an object on my right*, the child will do so successfully in reference to the other person's perspective of right, which is the opposite of their own (Roberts & Aman, 1993). By approximately 8 to 10 years, children can give relatively clear directions for how to proceed from one familiar place to another (in a small observable space) by using a **"mental walk" strategy** (Berk, 2000, p. 251). Younger children can give directions only after first walking through the route (Plumert et al., 1994). Finally, children at this age are also beginning to develop **cognitive maps**, or mental representations of large-scale places that must be inferred from experience because they cannot be seen all at once. This could include, for example, a mental representation of their neighborhood or of their school. Cognitive maps have been studied by asking children to draw routes. Whereas preschoolers' maps tend to contain familiar landmarks without the organizational relationships, older children form an overall configuration of large-scale space with interrelated landmarks and routes (Newcombe, 1982; Siegel, 1981).

The major limitation of the concrete operational period is that, while children are learning to subordinate perceptual distractions when performing logical mental operations, they can do so only with access to information that is directly perceptible. Their ability to engage in logical thought is challenged when they are asked to consider ideas without tangible props. For example, if they are told (without being shown the visual pairing) that building A is taller than building B, and building B is taller than building C, they are not able (at the stage of concrete operations) to infer that building A is taller than building C. So, although concrete operational thought is more logical, flexible, and organized than preoperational thought, it is not yet distanced from concrete experience. Additionally, concrete operational reasoning is often delayed in non-Western societies and is strongly subject to situational conditions. In other words, it depends in part on experience and may not emerge universally in middle childhood as Piaget proposed (Berk, 2000).

The stage of **formal operations** (11 years to adulthood) is characterized by the capacity for abstract thinking. This includes hypothetico-deductive reasoning and propositional thought. **Hypothetico-deductive reasoning** is characterized by the process of scientific problem solving. It begins with a general **theory** of various factors that may be contributing to a particular outcome and deduces hypotheses or predictions about what might happen. The predictions are then tested in a systematic manner to see which one is confirmed by concrete experience. In a sense, this process is just the opposite of concrete operations, in which children reason from the particular to the general. It is more flexible than concrete operations, because if one prediction is not confirmed, then another can be considered. Piaget demonstrated this shift in thinking by describing differences between teenagers' versus preoperational children's responses to a pendulum problem. All children were given strings of different lengths, objects of different weights, and a bar from which to hang the strings. Their task was to use these materials to determine what influences the speed with which a pendulum swings through its arc. The adolescents identified four hypotheses (length of the string; weight of the object; height of the object before release; force of release) and then they tested each hypothesis systematically by varying one factor at a time. However, the concrete operational children could not separate the effect of each variable by holding other factors constant, and they were not able to identify all relevant variables. As a result, their experimentation was unsystematic.

Propositional thought allows children to evaluate the logic of a proposition without referring to concrete circumstances. For example, Oscherson and Markman (1975) studied propositional reasoning by asking adolescents and younger children to evaluate statements made about a set of red and green poker chips. During one task the examiner hid a chip in her hand and asked the participants to evaluate two propositions as true, false, or uncertain: (1) *Either the chip in my hand is green or it is not green* and (2) *The chip in my hand is green and it is not green.* During another task the experimenter held either a red or a green chip in full view and asked children to evaluate the same statements. The younger children said that they were uncertain about both statements when the poker chip was hidden in the experimenter's hand. When the chip was held in view, they judged each statement to be true if the chip was green and false if the chip was red. However, the adolescents evaluated the statements in terms of their logic, recognizing that the "*either/or*" statement is always true and that the "and" statement is always false, regardless of color. Formal operational thought also includes verbal **reasoning about abstract concepts** that are represented by words in relation to various subject matters such as philosophy (e.g., consciousness, freedom) and science (time, space).

In her review of Piagetian theory, Berk (2000) noted that the ability to think abstractly is not a universal trait for all people across all cultures. In fact, people are most likely to think abstractly about issues with which they have had considerable experience. Approximately 40% to 60% of college students fail Piaget's formal operations problems (Keating 1979), but they can be trained to perform at high levels on such tasks (Kuhn, Ho, & Adams, 1979). Moreover, in tribal and village societies, where people lack opportunities to engage in hypothetical problem solving, formal operational tasks are not mastered at all (Cole, 1990).

From this review of cognitive development, we can see that there is a developmental sequence in the emergence of decontextualized logical thinking of the type that is central to expository discourse, including cause-effect relationships, directions, procedures, and argumentation. Additionally, there is a strong suggestion that schooling may play a major role in promoting the skills needed to organize expository discourse around scientific thinking. For additional information about later cognitive development, see Kamhi and Lee (1988).

Domain Knowledge

Although cognitive processes are clearly important, the depth of accumulated knowledge about a topic also has a clear impact on expository language production. Nippold (2010) described several studies which indicated that the amount, quality, and content of expository discourse is related to the degree of a speaker's or writer's knowledge of a specific domain. She described a study by Jones and Read that examined the oral narratives of college students with comparable verbal abilities but different levels of knowledge about major international events. The latter was assessed by a political knowledge test and awareness scales. The scores received by the students on these measures were used to classify them as experts, intermediates, or novices on the topic. Each student was then interviewed about a political issue, and asked to provide information about its history, including details such as the countries, key individuals, and key groups involved. Results showed that the experts produced more sophisticated expository language than the other two groups. Specifically, "the experts provided significantly longer and more complicated explanations than the intermediates or novices, reflecting greater organization and coherence and a deeper appreciation of underlying causal relationships, critical details, and historical focus on the topic." (Nippold, 2010, p. 53). We turn now to the role of the environment in the developmental process.

Environmental Support

Although Piaget conceptualized cognitive development as an interaction between a child and his or her environment, he excluded systematic consideration of social mediators in this process. In contrast, Vygotsky viewed cognitive development as an outgrowth of interactions between a child and more knowledgeable tutors who scaffold the child's performance by challenging him or her within the zone of proximal development (ZPD) to increasingly higher levels of thinking and talking. This developmental model predicts that the expository discourse, like other forms of language, is scaffolded by adults, teachers, and other individuals who can serve in the role of expert tutors.

Studies examining specific patterns of environmental support for the development of oral expository discourse are limited and difficult to find. A pilot study by Burns-Hoffman (1993) suggests that the roots of oral expository discourse may be found in the scaffolding provided to children by adults in preschool if not earlier. She observed 12 children, including four at ages 3, 4, and 5-years, respectively, during interactions with three teachers in several activities (free play, building a Lego model, making paper flower, making sandwiches). All verbal interactions were recorded and transcribed. Later, interactive segments in which a child's expository proposition was followed by contingent adult responses were extracted for analysis. An expository proposition was defined as an utterance that makes a claim (e.g., *Both slices have big holes in the middle*) or asks a factual question (e.g., *Why is it there are no brakes?*). Contingent teacher responses were then categorized and tallied. Response categories included shaping the child's utterance through content feedback (e.g., affirming, negating), reinforcing the use of a key phrase (e.g., repeating, expanding), maintaining joint attention (e.g., asking for clarification, asking a reflective question), linking propositions to experience (e.g., *You saw one yesterday*), and extending the proposition to a greater number of implications (e.g., *[The Lego] looks like a robot toy*). Results indicated that while the three teachers displayed differed communicative styles, they provided the same range of contingent response types. The study also found that 5-year-olds received fewer contingent responses to their expository propositions than did 3- and 4-year-olds, regardless of the teacher with whom they interacted. This was assumed to reflect the children's development of independence in expository discourse. Unfortunately, no measures of the children's performance were reported.

Once children reach school age, teachers, exposure to literacy, and schooling play a major role in shaping expository thought and talk throughout the school years. This is, after all, an explicit part of the curriculum. Still, it is difficult to find information about the specific patterns of scaffolding that support specific aspects of oral expository discourse. We look forward to further research in this area.

In sum, we have reviewed cognitive and environmental features that are associated with the development of oral expository discourse. Advances in cognitive development support the increasing complexity that is observed in the structure and content of oral expository language by children in elementary school through the high school years. We now turn our attention to the ways in which all aspects of oral language development may be viewed as support for the development of literacy, another important linguistic achievement.

LITERACY DEVELOPMENT

Oral language and literacy are part of the same language tapestry in use and in development. Our description of literacy development begins with a brief summary of the basic reading and writing processes demonstrated by mature language users. We then trace milestones associated with emerging literacy and conventional literacy skills, including environmental conditions that encourage these skills. Information about emerging literacy could very well have been included in the previous chapter within the discussion of early language development. We chose to present this information here under the general heading of literacy development to present key oral and literate process within a single, interrelated framework.

Conventional Literacy Skills

Graphic Symbol Systems

Different languages use different types of visual systems to represent language. For example, Chinese uses a **pictographic system** (also known as a **logo-**

graphic system) in which small picture-like symbols represent entire words. Some forms of Japanese use a **syllabic system** in which individual symbols represent syllables, and words are composed of syllable sequences. However, English and many other languages (e.g., German, French, Italian, Spanish, and Korean) use an **alphabetic system**. Individual letters or letter combinations are used to represent individual phonetic forms, and each word is represented by an alphabetic sequence corresponding to the phonological sequence of the spoken word. The remainder of our discussion is limited to the acquisition of reading of language represented by the **English alphabetic system**.

Reading

The term **conventional literacy** refers to reading and writing. For mature readers, **reading** is "thinking guided by print" (Kamhi & Catts, 1989, p. 4). A skilled reader uses mental processes to convert written symbols into meaningful words, interprets word-meanings in relation to the sentences and discourse structures of which they are a part, and reflects on the message. These multilayered processes are based on a complex set of **simultaneous bottom-up and top-down components**. The **bottom-up** component leads to **decoding**, which is a data-driven process whereby a printed word is used as a signal to be interpreted. The **top-down** component leads to **comprehension**, which is a conceptual process by which the reader draws from several sources of knowledge (e.g., linguistic context, metalinguistic knowledge, text structure knowledge, content schemas, world knowledge) to select and reflect on the probable meaning. Though processes normally work in synchrony, there are times when one is more dominant than another.

Kamhi and Catts (1989) distinguished between two kinds of decoding: the indirect phonetic route and the direct visual route. The **indirect route** is one in which individual letters or sets of letters are converted to speech sounds, blended, recognized as the phonological representation of a word, and associated with meaning. The **direct route** is one in which a word is recognized directly from the visual representation and associated with meaning. The indirect route is the first route available to children who are learning to decode. However, through experience, readers develop an increasing store of visual representations which allow them to by-pass the indirect route, thereby increasing the speed of decoding.

When words are understood in the context of sentences, extended discourse structures, and established themes, meaning is interpreted by using the same hierarchical comprehension frameworks that are involved in the comprehension of decontextualized oral discourse. One of these is the **overriding topic** often based on a reader's **choice of reading material**. For example, if I choose to read a book about strategies for mountain climbing, I will expect an expository text pertaining to a particular content area. **Knowledge of text structure** will lead me to expect a certain type of information (e.g., nonfiction, descriptive, procedural). Similarly, my **knowledge of content schemas** will help me extract meanings more efficiently by narrowing down the range of likely referents. For example, my expectations about the referents for words like *slope, endurance, rate,* and *oxygen saturation* will be different when I am reading about mountain climbing than when I am reading about a stress test to be performed at the cardiologist's office. While I read, I will be thinking critically about the information being presented. Does it make sense? Is it validated by other information in my knowledge base? Does it appear that relevant categories of information have been included or ignored? Does the information that is presented suggest other information that I need to explore? How does this text compare to other texts on the same topic? These are just a few of the questions that may come to mind. Far from being a passive experience, reading is an active search for information through simultaneous bottom-up and top-down patterns of information processing.

Writing

Our description of writing will be limited to the **encoding** process rather than to modality (e.g., printing, handwriting, typing, etc.). Within this framework, **writing** can be viewed as the process of using the **alphabet**, **orthographic rules**, and **conventional formatting** (e.g., punctuation, text segmentation), to generate words, sentences, and organized text structures for communicating intended ideas

in a particular context to a target audience. If reading is thinking guided by print, perhaps writing can be viewed as thinking with a pencil (Applebee, 1977). The power of writing develops from the ability to communicate in a variety of situations to a diverse group of readers (International Reading Association, 1998).

Similar to reading, writing is also a process involving simultaneous bottom-up and top-down components. Top-down components are dominant when the writer conceptualizes a message, selects a text structure to organize the message, and formulates sentences to express the message content using words appropriate to the backgrounds of intended readers. Bottom-up processes may be dominant in aspects of the editorial process to confirm that words are selected and spelled correctly, sentences are formulated properly, the organization of information is presented logically, ideas are expressed clearly and succinctly, and the overall text communicates the topic appropriately from the perspective of intended readers. This is a recursive process and will lead to revision at multiple levels until the text is completed.

Writing is a deliberate, metalinguistic process that draws from an individual's oral language base for vocabulary, sentence structure, text structure, and metalinguistic awareness. The exact components of the process will depend on the nature of a particular writing task. If the task requires research, then it also may draw vocabulary from external sources. Furthermore, it requires knowledge of orthographic and text formatting conventions. Varying degrees of planning may be involved, again, depending on the task. For example, a list of items to buy at the grocery store may be relatively short, require little in the way of sentence structure or orthographic markers, and can be constructed over a period of days by more than one person on a single piece of paper attached to the refrigerator door. Spelling errors may occur but do not matter if the writer(s) are the only reader(s). At the other extreme, the formulation of written expository text requires considerably more planning. Such a task may begin with a review of research about a chosen topic. Once the information is gathered, writers can select one or more text structures to organize the intended content using a decontextualized language style tuned to the intended audience, while at the same time monitoring each part of the process and revising as needed.

Scardamalia and Bereiter (1987) distinguished between two types of writing processes known as knowledge telling and knowledge transforming. **Knowledge telling** is more straightforward as it may require some research but mostly involves the documentation of the writer's knowledge. The **knowledge transforming** process is more effortful, since the writer is using the writing process to discover new thoughts or to view some topic from a different perspective. This type of writing takes longer, involves more revision, and more extensive note-taking than knowledge telling.

Interdependence of Reading, Writing, and Oral Language

As indicated earlier, reading, writing, speaking, and speech comprehension all rely on and contribute to a common language base. Experience in one feeds the other, and growth in each modality is an ongoing interdependent developmental process without an end-point. Acquisition of new vocabulary, exposure to new social experiences, refinement of special interests, and expansion of one's world knowledge all continue to enhance the top-down processes in each modality. Frequent and diverse reading contributes to the continued acquisition of linguistic knowledge (vocabulary, variations in sentence formulation, variations in text structure, metalinguistic knowledge, etc.) and to the store of a reader's world knowledge, both of which provide substance for written and oral language formulation. Moreover, the practice of writing narrative and expository texts leads to increased awareness of text structure, sentence variations, word choices, cohesion devices, stylistic variations, and decontextualized referential patterns. This, in turn enhances comprehension skills in both oral language and reading modalities.

Emergent Literacy

As recently as 20 years ago, experts assumed that literacy development begins with formal instruction at school age (Scarborough, 2003). Educators conceptualized "**reading readiness**" skills as entirely distinct from conventional literacy. More recently, literacy development has been reconceptualized as occurring on a continuum rather than as an all-or-none phenomenon that begins with direct instruction (Whitehurst & Lonigan, 1998, 2003). There is no clear demarcation between pre-reading and reading skills. Instead, reading, writing, and oral language emerge concurrently and interdependently at an early age through children's exposure to literacy activities prior to any formal instruction. This continuum of development is characterized as a period of emergent literacy followed by conventional literacy. The term **emergent literacy** refers to the skills, knowledge, and attitudes that support conventional forms of reading and writing. We now summarize the components of emergent literacy based on a review by Whitehurst and Lonigan (1998).

Learning Literacy Conventions

In American culture, print typically appears in books, magazines, journals, and other reading materials. There is a title on the cover, pages are sequenced from the front of the book to the back, and are turned from right to left. Words are sequenced on a page from left to right and in rows from top to bottom. Orthographic conventions are used to organize the print. There are spaces between words, punctuation marks at the ends of sentences, and other conventions for segmenting paragraphs. Some pages have pictures, but pictures communicate a different kind of information than print.

The process of learning literary conventions is known as **literary socialization** and it typically occurs during joint book-reading as children learn through interactions with their caregivers how to hold a book, how to turn the pages, and how to point to the flow of words from left to right. Eventually children demonstrate this understanding independently by the way in which they hold books on their own, leaf through the pages, and point to items on a page. They also learn that print consistently represents words as the caregiver says the same words each time a particular page is read, and since reading stops if part of the print is hidden from view (Paul, 2007).

Children with fewer opportunities to engage in literary socialization as preschoolers will be at a disadvantage at school age. Clay (1979) reported that children who demonstrated an understanding of literary conventions at the beginning of first grade performed better at the end of second grade on measures of decoding and reading comprehension than children who demonstrated fewer of these conventions when they entered school.

Knowledge of Letters

Knowledge of the alphabet at the beginning of first grade is a strong predictor of later literary success (Stevenson & Newman, 1986). Fortunately, children are often introduced to letters long before first grade. In homes that value literacy, letters are made salient in a variety of ways. For example, magnetic letters may be attached to the refrigerator door. Building blocks may display alphabet letters on the sides. Many aspects of the general environment also highlight the alphabet. T-shirts contain written words. Children's television programs feature "the letter of the day." Songs are sung about the alphabet. Children's computer keyboards often display letters in a colorful array, computer games feature alphabet themes, and hundreds of children's books present the 26 letters in a starring role around a great variety of themes (e.g., the animal alphabet, the sign language alphabet). Child-caregiver interaction routines involving the alphabet also invite children's awareness of alphabet letters.

Metalinguistic Awareness

Earlier in this chapter we noted that **metalinguistic awareness** refers to one's ability to reflect on language as a topic of knowledge in its own right and to use language for talking about language. Metalinguistic awareness emerges gradually during the preschool period and its growth continues through adulthood. During the preschool period, metalinguistic awareness is mostly centered on phonology. For that reason, we refer to it as **metaphonological awareness**. This involves an awareness of the syllable and phoneme structures internal to words. Evidence of metaphonological emergence is observed when children can clap the number of syllables and

sounds in a word. **Phonemic awareness** is a more narrow term referring to the identification of specific sounds within words, such as when a child can say that the word *apple* begins with /æ/. This ability develops later than syllable and sound awareness. Clearly, to learn the correspondence between a letter of the alphabet and a sound in the English language, children must become as aware of the sounds in their language as they are of alphabet letters. In fact, a growing body of literature shows that children who are better at indicating their awareness of syllables, rhymes, and phonemes are quicker to learn to decode words (e.g., Bryant, McLean, Bradley, & Crossland, 1990; Wagner, Torgesen, & Rashotte, 1994). Moreover, learning to decode also increases phonological awareness (e.g., Perfetti, Beck, Bell, & Hughes, 1987; Wagner et al., 1994). There also is evidence that phonological awareness is related to children's spelling abilities (e.g., Bryant et al., 1990).

Note that although metaphonological and phonemic awareness are key features of emerging literacy, the growth of metalinguistic awareness expands throughout elementary school to include other aspects of language. This expansion supports the comprehension process in both oral language and reading. For example, recall the study by Anglin, Miller, and Wakefield (1993) during our discussion of semantic development. These researchers found a marked growth in children's acquisition of derived words in fifth grade, suggesting that **metamorphological awareness** (i.e., the awareness of morphological structures) is emerging at this time, and that children make use of this awareness to guess the meanings of unfamiliar words with familiar morphological components. For example, once they have become aware of the meaning of "un" in a familiar word (e.g., *unhappy)* they are better equipped to infer the meanings of a less familiar word (e.g., *uninhibited, unsparing).*

Metagrammatical awareness allows children to make predictions about word meanings based on the positions of words within the structures of sentences or phrases. For example, if they read a sentence like, "*The slithy toves did gyre and gimble in the wabe*" (Carroll, 1871/1987), awareness of sentence structure supports the understanding that *slithy* is an adjective describing entities called *toves,* that *gyre* and *gimble* refer to the actions of the toves, and that *wabe* is probably the name of a location.

Another level of metalinguistic awareness was discussed in relation to extended discourse development. For example, in our discussion of narrative development, it was proposed that children develop text schemas through repeated exposure to narratives, which have a similar structure regardless of whether they are personal or nonfiction. When children develop **metatextual awareness** (i.e., an awareness of text schemas) they can use this awareness to predict the kind of information that is likely to follow in a narrative (e.g., Garner & Bochna, 2004). Similarly, awareness of expository text schemes (e.g., enumeration, compare-contrast) can help a listener to predict the type of information likely to be presented. In both cases (i.e., narrative and expository discourse), metatextual awareness can increase a child's focus on the listening task and enhance his or her comprehension.

Grapheme-Phoneme Correspondence

The understanding that alphabet letters can be used to represent speech sounds is known as the **alphabetic principle**. This understanding may be viewed as either one of the most advanced emergent literacy skills or as one of the least advanced conventional literary skills (Whitehurst & Lonigan, 1998). The recognition of letter-phoneme correspondences begins during emerging literacy and continues during the first stages of conventional reading and writing.

Oral Language Skills

The importance of solid oral language skills as a foundation for the emergence and development of literacy skills cannot be overstated (e.g., Butler, Marsh, Sheppard, & Sheppard, 1985; Catts, Fey, Zhang, Tomblin, 1999; Pikulski & Tobin, 1989). One important influence early in the process is children's oral **vocabulary** development. When children are first learning to decode, they begin by identifying individual speech sounds (/k/ + /æ/ + /t/) and blending them into a single word (*cat*). Children with larger stored vocabularies (including phonetic representations) have greater top-down resources for recognizing blended phonological forms from the decoded sound sequence and for linking the form with its meaning.

Although the size of a child's vocabulary provides important support for early decoding, other aspects of oral language development support reading comprehension, once decoding has become more fluent. One of these is **oral narrative development** (e.g., Bliss & McCabe, 2008). For example, kindergarten narrative performance is significantly correlated with seventh grade vocabulary and reading comprehension (Dickinson & McCabe, 2001; Tabors, Snow, & Dickson, 2001), and certain features of oral narrative production at kindergarten (e.g., plot structure, plot elaboration) are significantly correlated with reading comprehension at the age of 8 years.

Emergent Reading

When very young children handle books they often pretend to read by flipping through pages, pointing to words, and producing language that resembles a narrative. They also may demonstrate recognition of words that are frequent or salient in their environment (e.g., *Toys-R-Us, McDonalds, Exit, UPS*, and other environmental print). However, research has not supported a direct causal link between early sight-word vocabularies and later word-identification skills (Whitehurst & Lonigan, 1998).

The recognition that print corresponds to words appears to evolve gradually. In fact, Ferreiro and Teberosky (1982) suggest that it develops in stages. These researchers found that Argentinian 4- to 6-year-olds initially think that print is a visual representation of an object, similar to a picture or an icon. Later, the children believe that only some kinds of words (e.g., nouns) are represented in printed symbols, and eventually, they understand that all words in print correspond to words in connected speech. Once children understand that print represents words, they also begin to appreciate its **intentionality**, the fact that print can be used to convey messages (Purcell-Gates, 1996; Purcell-Gates & Dahl, 1991). Eventually children understand that print can have many different communicative functions (e.g., to give directions, to tell a story, etc.).

Children also gradually learn that the style of language used in print (literate style) is different from the style used in oral conversations. Sulzby (1985) asked 24 children to "read" one of their favorite storybooks at the beginning and end of their kindergarten year. Initially, approximately half of the children used an oral language style to produce storylike "readings" that were guided primarily by pictures. By the end of the year, the children's stories were still guided by pictures, but they used a more literate language style.

Emergent Writing

According to Whitehurst and Lonigan (1993), emergent writing commences when children begin to understand that writing carries meaning. This is demonstrated, for example, when they make scribbles or draw pictures on paper and then ask an adult to read the results. Their use of idiosyncratic forms is characterized as a **logographic pattern** since one scribble or one picture represents an entire word. The use of logographic patterns shows that children understand the function of writing if not the conventional form.

As children gain more experience with print, they begin to demonstrate an **alphabetic pattern** of writing by using conventional letters, numbers, and letterlike forms. However, these symbols are produced in unconventional combinations. Additionally, letters may take on properties of the word they represent. For example, if the letter "B" is used to refer to a bee (a relatively small animal) it may be formed with smaller print than a letter sequence referring to a horse (a relatively larger animal), which would be formed using larger print. Later at this stage, children begin to use **invented spelling**, which involves the idiosyncratic use of letters to represent the individual sounds in a word. Often the letters are selected according to the sound of their letter names and vowels are deleted. For example, *Katie* may be spelled *KD*. However, children do not appear to use their own spelling rules to decode what they have written. A conventional **orthographic pattern** of spelling may be used during this period but only for a small number of memorized words such as the child's own name.

Other Cognitive Factors

Two types of cognitive skills have an impact on emerging and later literacy skills. One is **phonological memory**, which is measured by asking children to repeat nonwords or a series of digits. This ability is linked with the rate of vocabulary and conventional reading acquisition (Whitehurst & Lonigan, 1998). The second is **rapid naming**. This is measured, for example, by asking children to name a series of basic geometric shapes, basic colors, or both (e.g., green square, red triangle, etc.) as quickly as possible. Performance on these tasks is considered to reflect the ease of access to phonological information in long-term memory. Rapid naming ability was shown to discriminate poor and good readers, regardless of metalinguistic awareness (McBride-Chang & Manis, 1996). Additional cognitive processes contribute to conventional literacy development and are discussed later.

Print Motivation

Print motivation refers to children's desire to engage in literacy activities (Whitehurst & Lonigan, 1998). Children may demonstrate their motivation by the frequency with which they request shared book-reading and by the amount of time they spend engaged in literacy activities rather than other types of activities. Children with high levels of print motivation are more likely to notice print in the environment, to ask questions about its meaning, and to spend time reading once they have learned to do so (Crane-Thorson, & Dale, 1992; Payne, Whitehurst, & Angell, 1994; Scarborough & Dobrich, 1994; Thomas, 1984). Print motivation predicts reading achievement at school age.

Conventional Literacy Development

Having considered the nature of emerging literacy, we conclude this chapter with a brief summary of conventional literacy development throughout the school years. Our aim is to present a pattern of development that can be recognized as complementary to, reinforcing of, and synergistic with the oral language developments we have discussed so far. Readers who wish to read about conventional literacy development in greater depth may consult the following excellent sources: Kamhi and Catts, (1989; 2005); Kamil, Mosenthal, Pearson, and Barr, (2000); Neuman and Dickinson, (2001); and Stone, Silliman, Ehren, and Apel, (2004).

Development of Conventional Reading

Chall (1983) described reading development in stages reflecting qualitative changes in focus. We summarize this information with a note of caution. While stages lend themselves to an orderly description of developmental changes, they tend to oversimplify the developmental process and blur the fact of individual differences (Kamhi & Catts, 1998). Therefore, consider these stages as a starting point with the recognition that considerable individual variations do occur.

Initial Reading (Decoding). Initial reading or decoding occurs between 5 to 7 years. Children continue to learn the full range of letter-sound correspondences (the **alphabetic principle**) and they begin to apply this knowledge to text. Recall that in our previous discussion the emergence of decoding skills was characterized as either the highest level of emerging literacy or the lowest level of conventional literacy. Children who have greater awareness of such phoneme-grapheme correspondences and a higher ability to blend sound sequences into words demonstrate higher levels of reading achievement (e.g., Whitehurst & Lonigan, 1998).

Two challenges in the learning process were highlighted by Kamhi and Catts (1998). The first is linked with inconsistencies in phoneme production due to **coarticulation** effects. (Recall that coarticulation refers to changes in the production of a target sound due to the effect of neighboring sounds.) For example, when the word *you* is said in isolation, the sound corresponding to "y" is pronounced /j/. However, in the phrase *Did you?* The sound corresponding to "y" is typically produced /dʒ/, owing to the effect of the preceding /d/ in *did*. So, when children learn the correspondence between letters and sounds, they have to resolve inconsistencies in phonological representations that that are not found in print (e.g., there is no /j/ in "Did you?"). The second challenge is linked with irregularities in orthography. The same letter or letter combinations may be represented by different sounds (e.g., "c" can represent /s/, /k/, and /tʃ/), and the same sound may be represented by different letters or letter combinations (e.g., /f/ can be represented by "f," "ff," "ph," or "gh").

Ungluing From Print. The next stage, ungluing from print, is characteristic of developments between 7 to 9 years. By this stage, the accuracy and speed (fluency) of decoding have increased sufficiently to allow for simultaneous attention to meaning. Children progressing normally during this stage will build a store of word recognition skills. Children with developmental problems will remain "glued to print" and lack the fluency needed to focus on meaning. Furthermore, metalinguistic awareness expands across a wider segment of the linguistic system, including narrative text structure. Altogether, these changes support the development of easier text comprehension for normally developing children.

Reading to Learn. Reading to learn becomes the focus between 9 to 14 years. By this time, decoding skills are fully established and automatic. All attentional resources are available to focus on comprehension and learning. Children are motivated to read for content. In academic situations, they are expected to complete reading assignments on curricular content (e.g., history, math, etc.). Vocabulary development accelerates due to increased exposure to text. During the early portion of this stage, children learn to read expository material of adult length, but they cannot yet read adult newspapers or magazines. During the second half of this stage they learn to read newspapers, popular magazines and popular adult fiction. However, literary fiction and newsmagazines like *Time* and *Newsweek* remain beyond reach.

Individual differences in reading ability become increasingly evident during this stage (Hoff, 2009). Children who are initially good readers improve at a faster rate than those who have more difficulty. This is known as the **Matthew effect** because "the rich get richer and the poor get poorer." This effect occurs because good readers like to read, read often, and build up a larger store of visually represented words. This increase in stored representations enhances the ease of reading.

The ability to entertain **multiple viewpoints** characterizes reading between 14 to 18 years. By this time, teenagers have become fluent at comprehending print and are able to reflect and analyze content while reading. They recognize that there are different points of view on any topic, that a writer may be presenting only a single view, and that other views can be constructed. These analytical abilities are consistent with features of cognitive development during formal operations as discussed previously.

Constructing and Judging. Chall (1983) referred to the final stage in reading development as **construction and judgment**, which characterizes the reading patterns of individuals at about 18 years and later. At this point, readers think critically about the material they are reading. They reflect on whether information is logical and supported by external sources of information; how it compares to other strategies for thinking about the topic; whether the ideas are presented to support a particular agenda; how the same information may be constructed from the perspective of different theoretical positions; and so on. In these ways, reading becomes an increasingly active process. This level of reading is expected of college students but may not be developed by those who lack the inclination.

Development of Conventional Writing

Our summary of writing development is based on a review of the literature by Scott (1989). We consider six features of writing (context, cohesion, syntax, literate style, punctuation, process) in the performance of elementary school and secondary school students.

Writing in Elementary School. What children write depends in part on the purpose or context of a writing task. These tasks become increasingly more complex as children progress through school. During the early elementary years, assignments range in length from single words to short narratives. For example, children may be asked to copy words and phrases from the board, generate sentences using

target words, or write stories about themes suggested by a teacher. During the later elementary years, children may be asked to write biographical information, historical narratives, and expository texts (e.g., procedures, descriptions). At home they may write letters, stories, or diaries.

As writing assignments become longer, children have opportunities to use key words and cohesion devices for organizing text structure. Hidi and Hilard (1983) examined the text structures of narratives and expository texts written by third and fifth graders. Results indicated that narrative forms were formulated with better text structure than expository forms. This may be related to experience, since third and fifth graders typically have a longer history of exposure to narrative than to expository discourse. Another study compared the persuasive texts produced by third and fifth graders (Pelligrini, Galda, & Rubin, 1984). Results showed that fifth graders used more advanced strategies for organizing this form of nonnarrative text.

Changes in sentence structure are observed in children's written work. Studies show that sentences in both written and oral language increase in length from 7.5 words per T-unit (WPT) in third grade to 9.5 WPT in fifth grade. However, by fifth grade, written sentences are longer (9.34 WPT) than spoken utterances (8.90 WPT) (O'Donnell, Griffin, & Norris, 1967).

Changes also are observed in the use of syntactic features associated with literate language style (Kroll, 1981). By 9 to 10 years, children begin to use these features differentially in their written work, including more frequent clause subordination, parenthetical constructions, and structures specific to written language (e.g., passive voice, nonfinite verb forms). Additionally, they begin to make word-order changes to emphasize the topic. However, the use of this style is still inconsistent. Elements of oral language style occasionally surface, and there may be residual instances of phonetic spelling (e.g., *privace, thermas, follod*) (Scott, 1989, p. 282). By the age of 12 and later, students move easily between oral and written forms depending on the purpose of the text.

Punctuation errors appear to remain in the written texts of children throughout elementary school. One error pattern includes the overuse of periods, which may reflect children's misconceptions about the structure of sentences. For example, a sixth grader observed by Weaver (1982, p. 442) wrote the following sentence: *I wanted to know one thing. If you would please come with me to the High Wheeler soon* (in Scott, 1989, p. 284).

Developmental changes in the process of planning and organizing text are observed by the age of about 12 years. This was observed by analyzing the notes created by 10- and 12-year-olds in preparation for an expository writing assignment (Bereiter & Scardamalia, 1987). Specifically, the notes of the 10-year-olds tended to include sentences that later appeared verbatim in the final written assignment. However, the notes of the 12- to 14-year-olds tended to consist of bullet points for ideas that were articulated more fully in their final papers. This was interpreted to suggest that while 10-year-olds prepare by <u>rehearsing the content</u>, 12-year-olds prepare by taking a more general stance and <u>thinking about the content</u>.

Writing in Secondary School. Writing in secondary school is done primarily for the teacher in the role of examiner. Most assignments require students to write analyses or summaries. A relatively small percentage of the writing assignments are personal or imaginative. As the topics of written assignments are typically given by the teacher rather than self-selected, students must spend more time becoming fluent with material that may not be familiar to them.

Practice in writing expository texts is extensive at this level. Consistent with an increase in the complexity of expository subgenres is a slow, steady increase in syntactic complexity. As before, this is observed by an increase in the length of T-units and in the degree of subordination (Scott, 1989).

Further changes are observed in the process used by students to plan and work on a written assignment. This has been studied by asking them to think aloud about what they are doing (e.g., Hayes & Flower, 1980). Under these conditions, 18-year-olds comment on a full range of considerations (e.g., spelling, grammar, and text organization) as they plan and review their work, and statements about text structure are explicit (e.g., *I'll start with the idea that . . .*). On the other hand, when com-

pared to adults, secondary students spend relatively less time on revision. Moreover, although revisions made by adults tend to involve the overall theme of the text (e.g., to strengthen an argument), revisions made by secondary school students tend to occur at the sentence level (e.g., to correct spelling, grammar, or punctuation).

As indicated earlier, many writing assignments at the secondary school level require students to summarize the content of reading assignments. Various strategies may be used in this process, including the deletion of redundant or irrelevant information, the use of general category labels to replace specific examples, and the formulation of an original sentence to integrate related features of content from the original text. However, in a study of summaries written by students in fifth, seventh, tenth grades and college, only the first strategy (deletion) was used by all. The third strategy (formulating a new topic sentence) was used minimally by fifth and seventh graders and it was used by college students in only half of the opportunities (Brown & Day, 1983).

Impact of Electronic Media

The world of electronics offers literacy tools (e.g., text-editing software, presentation design) and contexts (e.g., e-mail, text-messaging, Web chats, blogging, Web-based publishing) that are relatively new, and their impact on written communication practices is just beginning to be studied (Abdullah, 2003). Five potentially positive effects are summarized here. First, the nature of web-based communication may increase a student's motivation to write and the amount of writing that is done (Goldberg, Russell, & Cook, 2003; Trupe, 2002). For example, chatroom discourse can bring together individuals with common interests, which increases the value of writing without the fear of losing points/grades (academically) for making spelling or grammatical errors. Second, Web-based publication encourages writers to think about the perspective of audiences that extend beyond the boundaries of their classrooms (Kupelian, 2001). It also encourages the use of decontextualized language and careful editing from a reader's perspective. Third, e-mail encourages written discourse. Fourth, text-editing software increases the ease of revision thereby encouraging the revision process (Leibowitz, 1999). Fifth, e-mail together with text-editing software supports collaboration on individual and group assignments. Students can exchange critiques of each other's work and benefit from feedback. Group work is facilitated by the ease of combining the written products of individuals into an integrated text with supportive multimedia elements (e.g., pictures, video clips). Sixth, Web-based communication encourages linguistic flexibility. For example, college students have been observed to assume multiple identities under different e-mail addresses by systematically varying their word choices and syntactic forms (Trupe, 2002).

Despite these possible advantages, it has also been noted that the electronic communication environment is unique, encouraging a style of writing that is different from conventional forms and may even discourage them. The most obvious example involves the use of acronyms for communicating common phrases such as *BTW* (*by the way*), *IMO* (*in my opinion*), and *LOL* (*laughing out loud*). The conventional use of these symbols has been dubbed as "WebSpeak," "IMglish," "Geekspeak," and "Digispeak" (PC Magazine). Table 5–14 presents a small list of acronyms from *PC Magazine*'s online e-dictionary. For those coming of age within this culture, there is a temptation to use WebSpeak in other forms of writing, as it requires fewer keystrokes. Some parents are concerned because they cannot read their children's texts, and teachers have reported that the use of WebSpeak is trickling into serious writing assignments (Murphy & Allen, 2007). Additionally, observations indicate that, while students may use written language more often in e-mails, the length of their academic writing assignments does not appear any longer (e.g., Kupelian, 2001). Furthermore, the ease of revision may be more attractive in theory than in practice. For example, students will tend to rely exclusively on the spell and grammar check function for proofreading while ignoring other important issues at the text structure level (Leibowitz, 1999). Moreover, words that have scrolled off the screen may be ignored altogether. Finally, although it is easy to assume that e-mail and other forms of e-communication would encourage decontextualization, students actually use a variety of visual strategies (e.g., font variations, icons such as smiley faces and other font combinations) to provide nonlinguistic contextual support for their text, a pattern that does not translate to conventional letter writing (Danet, 2001).

In our roles as university professors, we have received e-mails with short sentences lacking contextual support sent by students, sometimes even by students who failed to sign their names. We also have received term papers in the form of attached e-mails without title pages, author identification, dates, or even course titles. These may be exceptions to the rule. Clearly, further research on the impact of e-media on written language at all ages is of increasing interest to researchers, practitioners, and members of the public who are concerned about literacy trends.

Cognition and Literacy

The same features of cognitive development that support (and are supported by) oral language development at school age also support (and are supported by) the development of conventional literacy skills. One cognitive process that has not yet been mentioned explicitly in this regard is **executive function**, the use of self-regulation skills to structure one's behavior deliberately in the service of a goal. Executive function skills are involved when individuals read text focusing on specific types of information while ignoring others. It is involved when individuals plan and follow through with the construction and formulation of written discourse. Self regulation often involves **private speech** (thinking in words) about one's progress in relation to a task. What needs to be done? How much time is available to do the task? What strategies can be used to complete the task? Self regulation also involves **metacognition**, the ability to think about one's thinking. Metacognition is involved when individuals monitor their comprehension during a reading task, when they identify unfamiliar words, when they distinguish sense-making from nonsense, when they recognize the conditions under which they

TABLE 5–14. Acronyms[1] Used as Shorthand for Phrases in E-Mail, Instant Messages, and Chat

AFAIK	As far as I know.	MYOB	Mind your own business.
AFK	Away from keyboard.	MWA	A kiss (the sound of "mwa.")
A/S/L	Age, sex, location.	N2M	Not too much.
ATM	At the moment.	NALOPKT	Not a lot of people know this.
AYT	Are you there.	NIH	Not invented here.
BBL	Be back later.	OIC	Oh, I see.
BFN	Bye for now.	OMG	Oh my God!
BRB	Be right back.	OTOH	On the other hand.
BTDT	Been there, done that.	OTP	On the phone.
BTW	By the way.	PAL	Parents are listening.
CUL	See you later.	PEBCAK	Problem exists between chair and keyboard
DETI	Don't even think it.		
DQMOT	Don't quote me on this.	PEBKAC	Problem exists between keyboard and chair
EBCAK	Error between chair and keyboard.		
EBKAC	Error between keyboard and chair.	PIR	Parents in room.
F2F	Face to face.	PITA	Pain in the ass.
FOAF	Friend of a friend.	PLBCAK	Problem lies between chair and keyboard.
FWIW	For what it's worth.		
FYI	For your information.	PLBKAC	Problem lies between keyboard and chair.
GAL	Get a life.		
GD&R	Grinning, ducking, and running.	PMJI	Pardon my jumping in.
GMTA	Great minds think alike.	POS	Parent over shoulder.
HB	Hurry back.	PRW	Parents are watching.
HHOK	Ha, ha, only kidding.	PTG&LI	Playing the game and loving it.
IANAL	I am not a lawyer, but . . .	RL	Real life.
IAW	In accordance with.	ROFL	Rolling on the floor laughing.
IMCO	In my considered opinion.	STFU	Shut the f*** up!
IMHO	In my humble opinion.	SUP	What's up?
IMO	In my opinion.	TANSTAAFL	There ain't no such thing as a free lunch.
IOW	In other words.		
JK	Just kidding.	TIA	Thanks in advance.
JOOTT	Just one of those things.	TMTH	Too much to handle.
KK	Okay, all right.	TTFN	Ta, ta for now (goodbye).
KPC	Keeping parents clueless.	TTT	Thought that too.
LMAO	Laughing my ass off.	TTYL	Talk to you later.
LOL	Lots of luck.	TU	Thank you.
LMIRL	Let's meet in real life.	TY	Thank you.
LYLAS	Love ya like a sister.	WFM	Works for me.
		YT	You there?

[1]These acronyms represent a new language called "digispeak," "geekspeak," "Internet Speak," "Webspeak," and "IMglish."

Source: PC Magazine's E-encyclopedia, retrieved August 22, 2008, from http://www.pcmag.com/encyclopedia/

are able to learn as well as those that are too distracting. These skills emerge gradually and should be well established by adolescence. However, there are considerable individual variations, and difficulties with executive function are evident in the case of children with attention and self-regulation problems. For a more detailed description of executive function and metacognition see Brown (1987), Hartman (2001), or Westby (2004).

Final Comments

We leave this topic with three final comments. First, although children seem to learn some aspects of emergent literacy spontaneously through interactions with caregivers in environments where literacy is valued, conventional literacy skills are acquired through deliberate instruction and active participation in the learning process. A discussion about methods of literacy instruction is beyond the scope of this chapter. However, we encourage readers to consult a number of excellent resources on this topic (e.g., Snow, Burns, Griffin, 1998; Strickland, Snow, Griffin, Burns, & McNamara, 2002).

Second, we emphasize the point that reading and writing are developmentally interconnected. This is apparent in ways previously discussed and has been confirmed by various studies. For example, better writers are usually better readers and read more than poor writers (Stotsky, 1983). Also, better readers write with greater syntactic maturity than poor readers. Furthermore, writing tasks can be used to enhance the benefits of reading. For example, when writing activities were used to improve comprehension and retention of new information, participants demonstrated better recall and mastery of the material than when other methods (e.g., repeated reading or oral question/answer tasks) were used (Stotsky, 1983).

Finally, similar to every other language skill, there is no end to literacy learning. Every new writing task comes packaged with its own unique challenges and rewards. Every new reading opportunity offers the possibility of expanding one's horizons. Reading and writing are thinking guided by visual symbols, and the maturation of thought is a lifelong process.

INTEGRATION OF LANGUAGE SKILLS

At school age, children learn to use language in oral and literate channels to exchange a wide range of communicative functions with many communicative partners across a variety of contexts. The integration of language components is evident in almost every communicative act, but especially during the production of extended discourse. Here, a speaker must formulate complete sentences within an organizational macrostructure, using cohesion devices to create intersentential relationships, and selecting vocabulary to achieve referential clarity, while continuously monitoring all levels of output for their intelligibility to the audience. The formulation of written text involves similar levels of integration, but at a metalinguistic level. Writers proceed deliberately by planning texts, organizing ideas, writing sentences, selecting words, and monitoring their print output in consideration of potential readers. Every component of language is involved in this process. To close the circle, we note once again that oral language and literacy reinforce each other. Writers reach into their oral language base to create the text structures, formulate the sentences, and select the words to construct a written text. At the same time, reading increases every aspect of an individual's oral language resources.

CONCLUSION

Later language development is characterized by growth in the ability to communicate in flexible ways for diverse purposes about a wide range of topics independent of context with an increasing range of communicative partners. We have traced this developmental trajectory by considering changes in all components of language and in the acquisition of literacy as another modality through which language can be expressed. Developments in language are paralleled by changes in cognitive processing as well as increases in the accumulation of world knowledge. All of these developments are encouraged by the increasing expectations and support of the academic environment as well as the social community. In the final analysis, language learning is a lifelong process. The acquisition of new vocabulary, pronunciation of unusual words, refinement of grammatical skills, fine-tuning of pragmatic skills, and expansion of literacy skills never stop.

REFLECTION QUESTIONS

1. Define each term and give an example that is different from an example in the chapter.

factive verb	endophoric reference
nonfactive verb	pragmatic inferencing
figurative meanings	logical inferencing
metaphor	expressive elaboration
metalinguistic awareness	text coherence
simile	cognitive distancing
idiom	conservation
proverb	transductive reasoning
phonological awareness	transitive reasoning
phonemic awareness	cognitive map
phrase	hypothetico-deductive reasoning
clause	
complex sentence	decoding
topic shading	encoding
stacked repair sequence	emergent literacy
	literary socialization
decontextualization	alphabetic principle
extraphoric reference	phonological memory
text structure	rapid naming
intrasentential cohesion	Webspeak
	executive function
intersentential cohesion	metacognition

2. In what ways does vocabulary development support literacy development?

3. Distinguish between horizontal and vertical changes in vocabulary development, and give an example of each that is different from the examples in the chapter.

4. What is the difference between convergent and divergent information processing? How do semantic networks support these patterns of thought?

5. Which nonliteral forms emerge earlier? Later? What factors contribute to the development of such forms?

6. Describe different types of word definitions and give an example of each that is different from the examples in the chapter.

7. Summarize the developmental milestones in children's production of word definitions?

8. Describe five factors that support the development of vocabulary.

9. What is the difference between incidental word learning and fast mapping? What percentage of words are children assumed to acquire through incidental word learning?

10. At what ages do children typically acquire phonological and phonemic awareness? What is the relationship between awareness and literacy development?

11. Describe the quantitative changes in children's syntactic development during school age.

12. Characterize the changes in topic maintenance that occur during the school-age years.

13. Describe some ways in which children adjust their language when talking with peers as opposed to adults.

14. What are they key features of contextualized language? Provide examples.

15. What are the key features of literate language style? What is the overall purpose of literate language style? Describe some text structures that support this purpose.

16. What characteristics do story narratives have in common with literate language style? In what ways do these two forms of extended discourse differ?

17. What is the importance of joint book-reading in later language development? Describe five general teaching strategies that caregivers use during joint book-reading. Also, describe six

language-specific strategies that caregivers use during joint book-reading. How do these patterns support the development of literate language style and emergent literacy?

18. What are the informal and more formal contexts in which expository discourse is used?

19. What aspects of expository discourse development demonstrate continued development throughout adolescence?

20. Describe Chall's stages of conventional reading development.

21. Describe the changes in writing skills as children progress through elementary school in relation to the types of written assignments they are asked to write and developmental changes in the writing process.

22. How do students in secondary school compare to adults with respect to the writing process?

APPLICATION EXERCISES

1. Pick a partner and select a topic. Use that topic for the independent construction of two semantic webs. Compare your webs. What are the similarities and differences? What are some possible explanations for differences between your webs?

2. Find 10 proverbs with high transparency and 10 proverbs with low transparency.

3. Look through a high school textbook and identify a low-frequency word whose definition is made apparent by the linguistic context. Write down the word and the linguistic context to show how the word's meaning is implied.

4. Observe a first grade classroom during a joint book-reading activity between the teacher and one or more students. Identify the language-specific interaction strategies that the teacher uses during the activity.

5. This activity requires collaboration with a partner. Each person will observe and record two same-age school children (one pair of first

graders and one pair of fifth graders) during a social conversation for 10 minutes. Transcribe and analyze each conversation in relation to the variables listed below. Then compare the performance of each dyad. Variables: average number of words per conversational turn, different topics, turns per topic, utterances with topic shading, requests for clarification, and successful responses to clarification requests.

6. Observe a sixth and twelfth grade classroom during a period of direct instruction. Describe each observation with respect to the following: teachers' use of narrative discourse, teachers' use of expository discourse, number of "structured school lessons," students' use of narrative discourse, students' use of expository discourse.

7. Find a partner to collaborate in this activity. Each of you will tape-record a conversation between yourselves and a school-aged child (a first grader and a fifth grader). During the conversation, each child should be asked to tell about a recent experience (e.g., birthday celebration) and explain how to play a favorite game or sport. Transcribe the conversation and conduct the following analyses: (a) For each child, compare dialogue discourse, narrative discourse, and expository discourse with respect to the average length of T-units. (Remember, one T-unit is equal to the total number of words in a main clause plus all of the subordinate clauses connected to it). (b) For each child, narrative discourse and expository discourse with respect to the total number of words, the total number of different words, total number of T-units, average number of clauses per T-unit, types and numbers of cohesion devices (refer to Table 5–11), total number of complete ties, and total number of incomplete ties. (c) Compare the results of each analysis across the two children.

8. Find a sixth and twelfth grade textbook. Compare a representative paragraph from each book with respect to the following: number of sentences, average number of T-units, average number of clauses per T-unit, number of different words, number of cohesion devices, and types of cohesion devices.

9. In his dissertation research, Rawlinson (1976) found data to suggest that skilled readers pay little attention to the internal details of words when they are reading. To highlight this point, an anonymous person extracted three sentences from Rawlinson's dissertation, falsely inserted a reference to Cambridge University, and publicized it through e-mail. Maybe you have seen this paragraph before. See if you can read it: "Aoccdrnig to a rscheearch at Cmabrigde Uinervtisy, it deosn't mttaer in waht oredr the ltteers in a wrod are, the olny iprmoetnt tihng is taht the frist and lsat ltteer be at the rghit pclae. The rset can be a toatl mses and you can sitll raed it wouthit porbelm. Tihs is bcuseae the huamn mnid deos not raed ervey lteter by istlef, but the wrod as a wlohe." Although it is easy to read these sentences, current research shows that Rawlinson's theory and the message conveyed by the paragraph is actually incorrect. Researchers from the Cambridge Cognition and Brain Sciences Unit have offered an alternative explanation for the readability of the above text (and other texts containing words with scrambled letters). Can you guess what makes this passage easy to read?

REFERENCES

Abdullah, M. H. (2003) *The impact of electronic communication on writing*. The Clearinghouse on Reading, English, and Communication, Digest 188. Retrieved August 22, 2008, from http://www.indiana.edu/~reading/ieo/digests/d188.html

Adrian, J. E., Clemente, R. A., Villanueva, L., & Rieffe, C. (2005). Parent-child picture-book reading, mothers' mental state language and children's theory of mind. *Journal of Child Language, 32*(3), 673–686.

Anglin, J. M., Miller, G. A., & Wakefield, P. (1993). Vocabulary development: A morphological analysis. *Monographs of the Society for Research in Child Development, 58*(10), 1–166.

Applebee, A. N. (1977). Writing and reading. *Language Arts, 20,* 534–537.

Astington, J. W., & Gopnik, A. (1991). Theoretical explanations of children's understanding of the mind. *British Journal of Developmental Psychology, 9,* 7–31.

Baker, L., Scher, D., & Mackler, K. (1997). Home and family influences on motivations for reading. *Educational Psychologist, 32,* 69–82.

Baron-Cohen, S. (1995). *Mindblindness: An essay on autism and theory of mind.* Cambridge, MA: MIT Press.

Baron-Cohen, S. (2000). Theory of mind and autism: A fifteen year review. In S. Baron-Cohen, H. Tager-Flusberg, & D. J. Cohen (Eds.), *Understanding other minds: Perspectives from developmental cognitive neuroscience* (pp. 3–20). Oxford: Oxford University Press.

Baron-Cohen, S., Tager-Flusberg, H., & Cohen, D. J. (Eds.). (1993). *Understanding other minds: Perspectives from autism.* Oxford, NY: Oxford University Press.

Baron-Cohen, S., Tager-Flusberg, H., & Cohen, D. J. (Eds.). (2000). *Understanding other minds: Perspectives from Developmental Cognitive Neuroscience* (2nd ed.). Oxford, NY: Oxford University Press.

Bartsch, K., & Wellman, H. (1995) *Children talk about the mind.* New York, NY: Oxford University Press.

Bereiter, C., & Scardamalia, M. (1987). *The psychology of written composition.* Hillsdale, NJ: Erlbaum.

Berk, L. E. (2000). *Child development* (5th ed.). Needham Heights, MA: Allyn & Bacon.

Berman, R. A. (2004). *Language development across childhood and adolescence: Psycholinguistic and crosslinguistic perspectives: Trends in language acquisition research (TILAR)* (Vol. 3). Amsterdam, The Netherlands: John Benjamins.

Berman, R. A. (2007). Developing linguistic knowledge and language use across adolescence. In E. Hoff & M. Shatz (Eds.), *Blackwell handbook of language development.* Victoria, Australia: Blackwell.

Berman, R. A. & Nir-Sagiv, B. (2007). Comparing narrative and expository text construction across adolescence: A developmental paradox. *Discourse Processes, 43*(2), 79–120.

Berman, R. A., & Slobin, D. I. (1994). *Relating events in narrative: A crosslinguistic developmental study.* Hillsdale, NJ: Lawrence Erlbaum.

Berman, R. A., & Vaerhoeven, L. (2002). Cross-linguistic perspectives on the development of text-production abilities: Speech and writing. *Written Language and Literacy, 5,* 1–43.

Bernstein, D. K. (1986) The development of humor: Implications for assessment and intervention. *Topics in Language Disorders, 6,* 65–71.

Bieber, J. (Producer). 1994. *Learning disabilities and social skills with Richard Lavoie: Last one picked . . . first one picked on.* Washington, DC: Public Broadcasting Service.

Bierwisch, M., & Kiefer, F. (1970). Remarks on definitions in natural language. In F. Kiefer (Ed.), *Studies in syn-*

tax and semantics (pp. 55-79). Dordrecht, The Netherlands: Reidel.

Bliss, L. B., & McCabe, A. (2008). Personal narratives: Cultural differences and clinical implications. *Topics in Language Disorders*, 28(2), 162-177.

Bloom, L., Lahey, M., Hood, L., Lifter, K., & Feiss, K. (1980). Complex sentences: Acquisition of syntactic connections and the semantic relations they encode. *Journal of Child Language*, 7, 235-261.

Botvin, G., & Sutton-Smith, B. (1977). The development of structural complexity in children's fantasy narratives. *Developmental Psychology*, 13(4), 377-388.

Brinton, B., & Fujiki, M. (1984). Development of topic manipulation skills in discourse. *Journal of Speech and Hearing Research*, 27, 350-358.

Brinton, B., Fujiki, M., Loeb, D., & Winkler, E. (1986). Development of conversational repair strategies in response to requests for clarification. *Journal of Speech and Hearing Research*, 29, 75-81.

Brown, A. (1987). Metacognition, executive control, self control, and other mysterious mechanisms. In F. Weinert & R. Kluwe (Eds.), *Metacognition, motivation, and understanding* (pp. 65-116). Hillsdale, NJ: Erlbaum.

Brown, A., & Day, J. (1983). Macrorules for summarizing texts: The development of expertise. *Journal of Verbal Learning and Verbal Behavior*, 22, 1-14.

Bryant, P. E., McLean, M., Bradley, L. L., & Crossland, J. (1990). Rhyme and alliteration, phoneme detection, and learning to read. *Developmental Psychology*, 26, 429-438.

Burns-Hoffman, R. (1993) *Scaffolding children's informal expository discourse skills*. Paper presented at the biennial meeting of the Society for Research in Child Development, New Orleans, LA, March 25-28.

Butler, S. R., Marsh, H. W., Sheppard, M. J., & Sheppard, J. L. (1985). Seven-year longitudinal study of the early prediction of reading achievement. *Journal of Educational Psychology*, 77, 349-361.

Cain, K. (2003). Text comprehension and its relation to coherence and cohesion in children's fictional narratives. *British Journal of Developmental Psychology*, 21, 335-351.

Cain, K., & Oakhill, J. (2003). The ability to learn new word meanings from the context by school age children with and without language comprehension difficulties. *Journal of Child Language*, 30, 681-694.

Carlisle, J. F., & Katz, L. A. (2005). Word learning and vocabulary instruction. In J. Birsch (Ed.), *Multisensory teaching of basic language skills* (2nd ed.). Baltimore, MD: Paul H Brookes.

Carroll, L. (1871/1987). *Jabberwocky*. New York, NY: Harry N. Abrams.

Catts, H., Fey, M., Zhang, X., & Tomblin, B. (1999). Language basis of reading and reading disabilities. Evidence from longitudinal investigations. *Scientific Study of Reading*, 3(4), 331-361.

Chall, J. (1983) *Stages of reading development.* New York, NY: McGraw Hill.

Chall, J. (1987). Two vocabularies for reading: Recognition and meaning. In M. G. McKeown & M. E. Curtis (Eds.), *The nature of vocabulary acquisition* (pp. 7-18). Hillside, NJ: Lawrence Erlbaum Associates.

Chomsky, C. S. (1969). *The acquisition of syntax in children 5 to 10.* Cambridge, MA: MIT Press.

Clay, M. M. (1979). *The early detection of reading difficulties* (3rd ed.). Portsmouth, NH: Heinemann.

Cole, M. (1990) Cognitive development and formal schooling: The evidence from cross-cultural research. In L. C. Moll (Ed.), *Vygotsky and education* (pp. 89-110). New York, NY: Cambridge University Press.

Corrigan, R. (1975). A scalogram analysis of the development of the use and comprehension of "because" in children. *Child Development*, 46, 195-201.

Crane-Thorson, C., & Dale, P. (1992). Do early talkers become early readers? Linguistic precocity, preschool language, and emergent literacy. *Developmental Psychology*, 28, 421-429.

Crowhurst, M. (1980). Syntactic complexity in narration and argument at three grade levels. *Canadia Journal of Education*, 5, 6-13.

Crowhurst, M., & Piche, G. L. (1979). Audience and mode of discourse effects on syntactic complexity in writing at two grade levels. *Research in the Teaching of English*, 13, 101-109.

Cunningham, A. E., & Stanovich, K. E. (1997). Early reading acquisition and its relation to reading experience and ability 10 years later. *Developmental Psychology*, 33, 934-945.

Danet, B. (2001). *Cyberplay: Communicating online.* Oxford, NY: Berg Publishing.

Dickinson, D., & McCabe, A. (2001). Bringing it all together: The multiple origins, skills, and environmental supports of early literacy. *Learning Disabilities Research and Practice*, 16, 186-202.

Dorval, B., & Eckerman, C. O. (1984). Developmental trends in the quality of conversation achieved by small groups of acquainted peers. *Monographs of the Society for Research in Child Development*, 49(2), 1-72.

Duchan, J. F. (2004). The foundational role of schemas in children's language and literacy learning. In C. A. Stone, E. R. Silliman, B. J. Ehren, & K. Apel (Eds.), *Handbook of language and literacy: Development and disorder* (pp. 380-397). New York, NY: Guilford Press.

Eisenberg, S. L., Ukrainetz, T. A., Hsu, J. R., Kaderavek, J. N., Justice, L. M., & Gillam, R. B. (2008). Noun phrase elaborations in children's spoken stories. *Language, Speech, and Hearing Services in the Schools, 39*, 154–157.

Emerson, H. F. (1979). Children's comprehension of because in reversible and nonreversible sentences. *Journal of Child Language, 6*, 279–300.

Engel, S. (1995). *The stories children tell: Making sense of the narratives of childhood.* New York, NY: W. H. Freeman.

Ervin-Tripp, S., & Gordon, D. (1986). The development of requests. In R. Schiefelbusch (Ed.), *Language competence: Assessment and intervention.* San Diego, CA: College-Hill Press.

Fenson, L., Marchman, V.A., Thal, D., Dale, P., Reznick, J. S., & Bates, E. (2007). *MacArthur-Bates communicative development inventories: User's guide and technical manual* (2nd ed.). Baltimore, MD: Paul H. Brookes.

Ferreiro, E., & Teberosky, A. (1982). *Literacy before schooling.* Exeter, NH: Heinemann.

Flavell, J. H. (2004). Theory-of-mind development: Retrospect and prospect. *Merrill-Palmer Quarterly, 50*(3), 274–290.

Flavell, J. H., & Miller, P. H. (1998). Social cognition. In W. Damon (Series Ed.), D. Kuhn & R. S. Siegler (Eds.), *Handbook of child psychology: Vol. 2, Cognition, perception, and language* (5th ed., pp. 851–898). New York, NY: Wiley.

Flood, J. E. (1977). Parental styles in reading episodes with young children. *Reading Teacher, 30*, 864–867.

Fowles, B., & Glanz, M. E. (1977). Competence and talent in verbal riddle comprehension. *Journal of Child Language, 4*, 433–452.

Gallagher, T. (1977). Revision behaviors in the speech of normal children developing language. *Journal of Speech and Hearing Research, 20*, 303–318.

Garner, J., & Bochna, C. (2004). Transfer of a listening comprehension strategy to independent reading in first grade students. *Early Childhood Education Journal, 32*, 69–74.

Garvey, C. (1977). The contingent query: A dependent act in conversation. In M. Lewis & L. A. Rosenblum (Eds.), *Interaction, conversation, and the development of language* (pp. 63–94). New York, NY: Wiley.

Ginsburg, H., & Opper, S. (1969). *Piaget's theory of intellectual development: An introduction.* Englewood Cliffs, NJ: Prentice-Hall.

Goldberg, A., Russell, M., & Cook, A. (2003). The effect of computers on student writing: A meta-analysis of studies from 1992 to 2002. *Journal of Technology, Learning, and Assessment, 2*(1), 1–51. Retrieved December 15, 2003, from http://www.bc.edu/research/intasc/jtla/journal/pdf/v2n1_jtla.pdf. Link no longer active.

Goodsitt, J., Raitan, J. G., & Perlmutter, M. (1988). Interaction between mothers and preschool children when reading a novel and familiar book. *International Journal of Behavior Development, 11*, 489–505.

Gopnik, A., & Meltzoff, A. N. (1997). *Words, thoughts, and theories.* Cambridge, MA: MIT Press.

Gregg, N. (1986). Cohesion: Inter and intra sentence errors. *Journal of Learning Disabilities, 19*(6), 338–341.

Halliday, M., & Hasan, R. (1976) *Cohesion in English.* London, England: Longman.

Harris, G. (1998). American Indian cultures: A lesson in diversity. In D. Battle (Ed.), *Communication disorders in multicultural populations* (2nd ed., pp. 117–156). Stoneham, MA: Butterworth-Heinemann.

Hartman, H. J. (2001). *Metacognition in learning and instruction: Theory, research and practice.* Dordrecht, The Netherlands: Kluwer Academic.

Hayes, J., & Flower, L. (1980). Identifying the organization of writing processes. In L. Gregg & E. Steinberg (Eds.), *Cognitive processes in writing: An interdisciplinary approach* (pp. 3–30). Hillsdale, NJ: Erlbaum.

Heath, S. B. (1982). What no bedtime story means: Narrative skills at home and school. *Language and Society, 11*, 49–76.

Heath, S. B. (1983). *Ways with words: Language, life, and work in communities and classrooms.* New York, NY: Cambridge University Press.

Heath, S. B. (1986). Taking a cross-cultural look at narratives. *Topics in Language Disorders, 7*(1), 84–95.

Hemmings, A. (2000). The hidden curriculum corridor. *High School Journal, 83*, 1–10.

Hidi, S., & Hildyard, A. (1983). The comparison of oral and written productions in two discourse types. *Discourse Processes, 6*, 91–105.

Hislop, G. G., Zaretsky, E., & Vellman, S. (2007, November). *Who am I talking to? Children's sensitivity to the listener: Evidence from the sibling-to-sibling and sibling-to-parent interaction.* Poster presentation at the Annual Convention of the American Speech-Language and Hearing Association, Boston, MA

Hoff, E. (2009). *Language development* (4th ed). Belmont, CA: Wadsworth.

Hoffner, C., Cantor, J., & Badzinski, D. M. (1990). Children's understanding of adverbs denoting degree of likelihood. *Journal of Child Language, 17*, 217–231.

Hoover, J. J., & Patton, J. R. (1997). *Curriculum adaptation for students with learning and behavior problems: Principles and practices.* Austin, TX: Pro-Ed.

Hughes, D., McGillivray, L., & Schmidek, M. (1997). *Guide to narrative language: Procedures for assessment.* Eau Claire, WI: Thinking Publications.

Hunt, K. W. (1965). *Grammatical structures written at three grade levels* (Research Report, No. 3) Champaign, IL: National Council of Teachers of English.

Hunt, K. W. (1970). Syntactic maturity in school children and adults. *Society for the Research in Child Development Monograph, 134*(1), 1–67.

Huttenocher, J., Levine, S., & Vevea, J. (1998). Environmental input and cognitive growth: A study using time-period comparisons. *Child Development, 69,* 1023–1029.

International Reading Association (IRA). (1998). *Learning to read and write: Developmentally appropriate practices for young children.* Position statement retrieved January 14, 2010, from http://www.reading.org/resources/issues/positions_appropriate.html

Johnson, C. J. (1995). Expanding norms for narration. *Language, Speech, and Hearing Services in Schools, 26*(4), 326–331.

Johnson, C. J., & Anglin, J. M. (1995). Qualitative developments in the content and form of children's definitions. *Journal of Speech and Hearing Research, 38,* 612–629.

Johnston, J. (1982). Narratives: A new look at communication problems in older language-disordered children. *Language, Speech, and Hearing Services in Schools, 13,* 1454–1155.

Johnston, J. (2008). Narratives: Twenty-five years later. *Topics in Language Disorders, 28*(2), 93–98.

Jones, R. (1996) *Emerging patterns of literacy: A multidisciplinary perspective.* London, England: Routledge.

Justice, L., & Ezell, H. (2002). *The syntax handbook.* Eau Claire, WI: Thinking Publications.

Kamhi, A. G., & Catts, H. W. (1989). Language and reading: Convergences, divergences, and development. In A. G. Khami & H. W. Catts (Eds.), *Reading disabilities: A developmental language perspective.* Boston, MA: Little Brown and Company.

Kamhi, A. G., & Catts, H. W. (2005) *The connections between language and reading disabilities.* London, England: Routledge

Kamhi, A. G., & Lee, R. (1988). Cognitive development in older children. In M. Nippold (Ed.), *Later language development: Ages nine through nineteen* (pp. 127–159). San Diego, CA: College-Hill Press.

Kamil, M. L., Mosenthal, P. B., Pearson, P. D., & Barr, R. (Eds.). (2000). *Handbook of reading research* (Vol. 3). Mahwah, NJ: Erlbaum.

Karmiloff-Smith, A. (1986). Some fundamental aspects of language development after age 5. In P. Fletcher & M. Garman (Eds.), *Language acquisition* (2nd ed., pp. 455–474). New York, NY: Cambridge University Press.

Katzenberger, I. (2004). The development of clause packaging in spoken and written texts. *Journal of Pragmatics, 36,* 1921–1948.

Keating, D. (1979). Adolescent thinking. In J. Adelson (Ed.), *Handbook of adolescent psychology* (pp. 211–246). New York, NY: Wiley.

Kernan, K. (1977). Semantic and expressive elaboration in children's narratives. In S. Ervin-Tripp & C. Mitchell-Kernan (Eds.), *Child discourse* (pp. 91–102). New York, NY: Academic Press.

Kessel, F. (1970). The role of syntax in children's comprehension from ages six to twelve. *Monographs of the Society for Research in Child Development, 35*(6), 1–95.

Klecan-Aker, J. S., & Hedrick, L. D. (1985). A study of the syntactic language skills of normal school age children. *Language, Speech, and Hearing Services in Schools, 16,* 187–198.

Kroll, B. (1981). Developmental relationships between speaking and writing. In B. Kroll & R. Vann (Eds.), *Exploring speaking-writing relationships: Connections and contrasts* (pp. 32–54). Champaign, IL: National Council of Teachers of English.

Kuder, J. (2008). *Teaching students with language and communication disabilities* (3rd ed.). Boston, MA: Pearson.

Kuhn, D., Ho, V., & Adams, C. (1979). Formal reasoning among pre- and late- adolescents. *Child Development, 50,* 1128–1135.

Kupelian, M. (2001). The use of e-mail in the L2 classroom: An overview. *Second Language Learning and Teaching, 1.* Retrieved December 15, 2003, from http://www.usq.edu.au/opacs/cllt/sllt/1-1/Kupelian 01.htm. Link no longer active.

Kurland, B. F., & Snow, C. E. (1997). Longitudinal measurement of growth in definitional skill. *Journal of Child Language, 24,* 603–625.

Labov, W. (1972). *Language in the inner city.* Philadelphia, PA: University of Philadelphia Press.

Labove, W., & Waletzky, J. (1967). Narrative analysis. In J. Helm (Eds.), *Essays on the verbal and visual arts* (pp. 12–44). Seattle, WA: University of Washington Press.

Langdon, R., & Coltheart, M. (2001). Visual perspective taking and schizotype: Evidence for a simulation-based account of mentalizing in normal adults. *Cognition, 82,* 1–26.

Langford, D. (1981). The clarification request sequence in conversation between mothers and their children. In P. French & M. Maclure (Eds.), *Adult-child conversation* (pp. 159–184). New York, NY: St. Martin's Press

Larson, V. L., & McKinley, N. (1998). Adolescents conversations: A longitudinal study. *Clinical Linguistics and Phonetics, 12,* 183–203.

Lazar, R. T., Warr-Leeper, G. A., Nicholson, C. B., & Johnson, S. (1989). Elementary school teachers' use of multiple meaning expressions. *Language, Speech, and Hearing Services in Schools, 20,* 420–430.

Leadholm, B. J., & Miller, J. F. (1992). *Language sample analysis: The Wisconsin guide.* Madison, WI: Wisconsin Department of Public Instruction.

Leibowitz, W. R. (1999). Technology transforms writing and the teaching of writing. *Chronicle of Higher Education, 46*(14), A67–A68.

Lenneberg, E. H. (1967). *Biological foundations of language.* New York, NY: John Wiley.

Leslie, A. M. (1994). ToMM, ToBy, and agency: Core architecture and domain specificity. In L. A. Hirschfeld & S. A. Gelman (Eds.), *Mapping the mind: Domain specificity in cognition and culture* (pp. 119–147). Cambridge, UK: Cambridge University Press.

Liberman, I., Schankweiler, D., Fischer, F., & Carter, B. (1974). Explicit syllable and phoneme segmentation in the young child. *Journal of Experimental Child Psychology, 18,* 201–212.

Liles, B. Z. (1985). Cohesion in the narratives of normal and language disordered children. *Journal of Speech and Hearing Research, 28,* 123–133.

Liles, B. Z. (1987). Episode organization and cohesive conjunctives in narratives of children with and without language disorder. *Journal of Speech and Hearing Research, 30,* 185–196.

Loban, W. (1976). *Language development: Kindergarten through grade twelve.* (Research Report No. 18). Urbana, IL: National Council of Teachers of English.

Lund, N., & Duchan, J. (1983). *Assessing children's language in naturalistic contexts.* Englewood Cliffs, NJ: Prentice-Hall.

MacLachlan, B. G., & Chapman, R. S. (1988). Communication breakdowns in normal and language learning disabled children's conversation and narration. *Journal of Speech and Hearing Research, 30,* 185–196.

Makau, J. M. (1990). *Reasoning and communication: Thinking critically about arguments.* Belmont, CA: Wadsworth.

Malvern, D. D., Richards, B. J., Chipere, N., & Duran, P. (2004). *Lexical diversity and language development: Quantification and assessment.* Basingstoke, Hampshire: Palgrave Macmillan.

Markowitz, J., & Franz, S. (1988). The development of defining style. *International Journal of Lexicography, 1,* 253–267.

McBride-Chang, C., & Manis, F. R. (1996). Structural invariance in the associations of naming speed, phonological awareness, and verbal reasoning in good and poor readers. A test of the double deficit hypothesis. *Reading and Writing, 8,* 323–339.

McNeill, D. (1970). *The acquisition of language.* New York, NY: Harper & Row.

Mehan, H. (1979). *Learning lessons: Social organization in the classroom.* Cambridge, MA: Harvard University Press.

Melzi, G. (2000). Cultural variations in the construction of personal narratives: Central American and European American mothers' elicitation styles. *Discourse Processes, 30*(2), 153–177.

Mentis, M., & Prutting, C. A. (1987). Cohesion in the discourse of normal and head-injured adults. *Journal of Speech and Hearing Research, 30*(1), 88–98.

Miller, G., & Gildea, P. (1987). How children learn words. *Scientific American, 257,* 94–99.

Minami, M., & McCabe, A. (1995). Rice balls and bear hunts: Japanese and North American family narrative patterns. *Journal of Child Language, 22,* 423–445.

Moffett, J. (1968) *Teaching the universe of discourse.* Boston, MA: Houghton Mifflin

Moss, B. (2004). Teaching expository text structures through information trade book retellings. *Reading Teacher, 57*(8), 710–718.

Murphy, A. P., & Allen, J. (2007) Webspeak: The secret language of teens. Retrieved August 24, 2008, from http://abcnews.go.com/print?id=2820582

Myles, B. S., Trautman, M. L., & Schelvan, R. L. (2004). *The hidden curriculum.* Shawnee Mission, KS: Autism Asperger Pubishing Co.

Nagy, W., & Herman, P. (1987). Breadth and depth of vocabulary knowledge: Implications for acquisition and instruction. In M. G. McKeown & M. E. Curtis (Eds.), *The nature of vocabulary acquisition* (pp. 19–35). Hillsdale, NJ: Erlbaum.

Nagy, W., Herman, P., & Anderson, R. (1985). Learning words from context. *Reading Research Quarterly, 22,* 233–253.

Nelson, K. (1986). *Event knowledge: Structure and function in development.* Hillsdale, NJ: Erlbaum.

Nelson, K., & Gruendel, J. (1981). Generalized event representation: Basic building blocks of cognitive development. In M. Lamb & A. Brown (Eds.), *Advances in developmental psychology* (pp. 131–158). Hillsdale, NJ: Erlbaum.

Nelson, N. (1993). *Childhood language disorders in context: Infancy through adolescence.* New York, NY: McMillan.

Neuman, S. B., & Dickinson, D. K. (2001). *Handbook of early literacy research. Volume 1.* New York, NY: Guilford Press.

Newcombe, N. (1982). Development of spatial cognition and cognitive development. In R. Cohen (Ed.), *Children's conceptions of spatial relationships* (pp. 65–81). San Francisco, CA: Jossey-Bass.

Ninio, A., & Bruner, J. (1978). The achievement and antecedents of labeling. *Journal of Child Language, 5,* 1–15.

Ninio, A., & Snow, C. (1999). The development of pragmatics: Learning to use language appropriately. In T. K. Bhatia & W. C. Ritchie (Eds.), *Handbook of lan-*

guage acquisition (pp. 347–383). New York, NY: Academic Press.

Nippold, M. A. (1990). *Idioms in textbooks for kindergarten through eighth grade students.* Unpublished manuscript. University of Oregon, Eugene.

Nippold, M. A. (1993). Developmental markers in adolescent language: Syntax, semantics, and pragmatics. *Language, Speech, and Hearing Services in Schools, 24*, 21–28.

Nippold, M. A. (1995). School age children and adolescents: Norms for word definitions. *Language, Speech, and Hearing Services in Schools, 26*, 320–325.

Nippold, M. A. (1998). *Later language development: The school age and adolescent years* (2nd ed.). Austin, TX: Pro-Ed.

Nippold, M. A. (2007). *Later language development: School age children, adolescents, and young adults* (3rd ed.). Austin, TX: Pro-Ed.

Nippold, M. A. (2010). Explaining complex matters: How knowledge of a domain drives language. In M. A. Nippold & C. M. Scott (Eds.), *Expository discourse in children, adolescents, and adults.* New York, NY: Psychology Press.

Nippold, M. A., & Haq, F. S. (1996). Proverb comprehension in youth: The role of concreteness and familiarity. *Journal of Speech and Hearing Research, 39*, 166–176.

Nippold, M. A., Hekseth, L., Duthie, J. K., & Mansfield, T. C. (2005). Conversational versus expository discourse: A study of syntactic development in children, adolescents, and adults. *Journal of Speech, Language and Hearing Research, 48*, 1048–1064.

Nippold, M. A., Martin, S. A., & Erskine, B. J. (1988). Familiarity and transparency in idiom comprehension: A developmental study of children and adolescents. *Journal of Speech and Hearing Research, 36*, 728–737.

Nippold, M. A., Moran, C., & Schwarz, I. (2001). Idiom understanding in preadolescents: Synergy in Action. *American Journal of Speech-Language Pathology, 10*, 169–179.

Nippold, M. A., & Rudzinski, M. (1993). Famliarity and transparency in idiom explanation: A developmental study of children and adolescents. *Journal of Speech and Hearing Research, 36*, 728–737.

Nippold, M. A., Schwarz, L., & Uhden, L. (1992). Use and understanding of adverbial conjuncts: A developmental study of adolescents and young adults. *Journal of Speech and Hearing Research, 35*, 108–118.

Nippold, M. A., & Scott, C. (2010). *Expository discourse in children, adolescents, and adults.* New York, NY: Psychology Press.

O'Donnell, R., Griffin, W., & Norris, R. (1967). *Syntax of kindergarten and elementary school children: A transformational analysis.* Champaign, IL: National Council of Teachers of English, Research Report No. 8.

Oetting, J. B., Rice, M. L., & Swank, L. (1995). Quick incidental learning (QUIL) of words by school age children with and without SLI. *Journal of Speech and Hearing Research, 38*, 434–445.

Oscherson, D. N., & Markman, E. M. (1975). Language and the ability to evaluate contradictions and tautologies. *Cognition, 2*, 213–226.

Owens, R. (2008). *Language development: An introduction.* Boston, MA: Pierson, Allyn, & Bacon.

Pan, B. A. (2005). Semantic development. In J. B. Gleason (Ed.), *The development of meaning.* Boston, MA: Pearson, Allyn, & Bacon.

Paul, R. (2007). *Language disorders from infancy through adolescence* (3rd ed.). Philadelphia, PA: Mosby.

Payne, A. C., Whitehurst, G. J., & Angell, A. L. (1994). The role of literacy environment in the language development of children from low-income families. *Early Childhood Research Quarterly, 9*, 427–440.

PC Magazine's Encyclopedia. Retrieved August 22, 2008, from http://www.pcmag.com/encyclopedia/

Pelligrini, A., Galda, L., & Rubin, D. (1984). Context in text: The development of oral and written language in two genres. *Child Development, 55*, 1549–1555.

Perera, K. (1986). Language acquisition and writing. In P. Fletcher & M. Garman (Eds.), *Language acquisition: Studies in first language acquisition* (2nd ed., pp. 494–519). Cambridge, NY: Cambridge University Press.

Perfetti, C., Beck, I., Bell, L. C., & Hughes, C. (1987). Phonemic knowledge and learning to read are reciprocal: A longitudinal study of first grade children. *Merrill-Palmer Quarterly, 33*, 283–319.

Perner, J. (1991). *Understanding the representational mind.* Cambridge, MA: MIT Press.

Peterson, C., & McCabe, A. (1983). *Developmental psycholinguistics: Three ways of looking at a child's narrative.* New York, NY: Plenum.

Peterson, C., & McCabe, A. (1985). Understanding "because": How important is the task? *Journal of Psycholinguistic Research, 14*, 199–218.

Peterson, C., & McCabe, A. (1991). On the threshold of the story realm: Semantic versus connective us of connectives in narratives. *Merrill-Palmer Quarterly, 37*(3), 445–464.

Peterson, C., & Slaughter V. (2003). Opening windows into the mind: Mothers' preferences for mental state explanations and children's theory of mind. *Cognitive Development, 18*, 399–429.

Piaget, J. (1929). *The child's conception of physical causality.* New York, NY: Harcourt, Brace, and World.

Piaget, J., & Inhelder, B. (1969). *The psychology of the child.* New York, NY: Basic Books.

Pikulski, J. J., & Tobin, A. W. (1989). Factors associated with long-term reading achievement of early readers. In S. McCormick, J. Zutell, P. Scharer, & P. O'Keefe

(Eds.), *Cognitive and social perspectives for literacy research and instruction*. Chicago, IL: National Reading Conference.

Pillow, B. H., & Henrichon, A. J. (1996). There's more to the picture than meets the eye: Young children's difficulty understanding biased interpretation. *Child Development, 67*, 803-819.

Plumert, J. M., Pick, H. L., Marks, R. A., Kintsch, A. S., & Wegesin, R. A. (1994). Locating objects and communicating about locations: Organizational differences in children's searching and direction-giving. *Developmental Psychology, 30*, 443-453.

Preece, A. (1987). The range of narrative forms conversationally produced by young children. *Journal of Child Language, 14*, 353-373.

Purcell-Gates, V. (1996). Stories, coons, and the TV Guide: Relationships between home literacy experiences and emergent literacy knowledge. *Reading Research Quarterly, 31*, 406-428.

Purcell-Gates, V., & Dahl, K. L. (1991). Low SES children's success and failure at early literacy learning in skills-based classrooms. *Journal of Reading Behavior, 23*, 1-34.

Raffaelli, M., & Duckett, E. (1989). "We were just talking . . .": Conversations in early adolescence. *Journal of Youth and Adolescence, 18*, 567-582.

Rawlinson, G. E. (1976) *The significance of letter position in word recognition*. Unpublished PhD thesis, Psychology Department, University of Nottingham, Nottingham UK.

Redmond, S. M. (2003). Children's productions of the affix *-ed* in past tense and past participle contexts. *Journal of Speech, Language, and Hearing Research, 46*, 1095-1109.

Reed, V. (2005). Adolescents with language impairment. In V. Reed (Ed.), *An introduction to children with language disorders* (pp. 168-219). Boston, MA: Pearson, Allyn & Bacon.

Reed, V., McLeod, K., & McAlistair, L. (1999). Importance of selected communication skills for talking with peers and teachers: Adolescents' opinions. *Language, Speech, and Hearing Services in Schools, 30*, 32-49.

Reid, D. K. (2000). Discourse in classrooms. In K. Fahey & D. K. Reid (Eds.), *Language development, differences, and disorders* (pp. 3-38). Austin, TX: Pro-Ed.

Rice, M. (1990). Preschoolers QUIL: Quick incidental learning of words. In G. Conti-Ramsden & C. Snow (Eds.), *Children's language* (Vol. 7, pp. 171-196). Hillsdale, NJ: Lawrence Erlbaum.

Rice, M., & Woodsmall, L. (1988). Lessons from television: Children's word learning when viewing. *Child Development, 59*, 420-429.

Richardson, K., Calnan, M., Essen, J., & Lambert, L. (1976). The linguistic maturity of 11-year-olds: Some analysis of the written composition of children of children in the National Development Study. *Journal of Child Language, 3*, 99-115.

Ripich, D., & Panagos, J. (1985). Accessing children's knowledge of sociolinguistic rules for speech therapy lessons. *Journal of Speech and Hearing Disorders, 50*, 333-344.

Roberts, R. I., & Aman, C. J. (1993). Developmental differences in giving directions: Spatial frames of reference and mental rotations. *Child Development, 64*, 1258-1270.

Roth, F. P., Spekman, N. J., & Fye, E. C. (1995). Reference cohesion in the oral narratives of students with learning disabilities and normally achieving students. *Learning Disability Quarterly, 18*(1), 25-40.

Scarborough, H. S. (1998). Early identification of children at risk for reading disabilities: Phonological awareness and some other promising predictors. In B. K. Shapiro, P. J. Accardo, & A. J. Capute (Eds.), *Specific reading disability: A view of the spectrum* (pp. 75-119). Timonium, MD: York Press.

Scarborough, H. S. (2003). Connecting early language and literacy to later reading (dis)abilities: Evidence, theory, and practice. In S. Newman & D. Dickenson (Eds.), *Handbook of early literacy research* (pp. 97-100). New York, NY: Guilford Press.

Scarborough, H. S., & Dobrich, W. (1994). On the efficacy of reading to preschoolers. *Developmental Review, 14*, 245-230.

Scardamalia, M., & Bereiter, C. (1987). Knowledge telling and knowledge transforming in written composition. In S. Rosenberg (Ed.), *Advances in applied psycholinguistics: Vol. 2. Reading, writing, and language learning* (pp. 142-175). Cambridge, MD: Cambridge University Press.

Schober-Peterson, D., & Johnson, C. J. (1983). The performance of eight- to ten-year-olds on measures of conversational skillfulness. *First Language, 13*, 249-269.

Scholl, B. J., & Leslie, A. M. (1999). Modularitym development and "theory of mind." *Mind and Language, 14*, 131-153.

Schultz, T. R., & Horibe, F. (1974). Development of the appreciation of verbal jokes. *Developmental Psychology, 10*, 13-20.

Scott, C. M. (1984). Adverbial connectivity in conversations of children 6 to 12. *Journal of Child Language, 11*, 423-452.

Scott, C. M. (1988). Spoken and written syntax. In M. A. Nippold (Ed.), *Later language development: Ages nine through thirteen* (pp. 49-95). Austin, TX: Pro-Ed.

Scott, C. M. (1989) Learning to write: Context, form, and process. In A. G. Kamhi & H. W. Catts (Eds.), *Reading disabilities: A developmental language perspective*. Boston, MA: College-Hill Press.

Scott, C. M., & Stokes, S. L. (1995). Measures of syntax in school age children and adolescents. *Language, Speech, and Hearing Services in Schools, 26*, 309–319.

Shapiro, L. R., & Hudson, J. A. (1991). Tell me a make-believe story: Coherence and cohesion in young children's picture-elicited narratives. *Developmental Psychology, 27*, 960–974.

Shapiro, L., & Hudson, J. (1997). Coherence and cohesion in children's stories. In J. Costermans & M. Fayol (Eds), *Processing interclausal relationships: Studies in the production and comprehension of text* (pp. 23–48). Mahwha, NJ: Lawrence Erlbaum and Associates.

Shatz, M., & Gelman, R. (1973). The development of communication skills: Modifications in the speech of young children as a function of listener. *Monographs of the Society for Research in Child Development, 38*, 1–37.

Siegel, A. W. (1981). The externalization of cognitive maps by children and adults: In search of ways to ask better questions. In L. S. Lieben, A. H. Patterson, & N. Newombe (Eds.), *Spatial representation and behavior across the lifespan* (pp. 167–194). New York, NY: Academic Press.

Silva, M. J., & McCabe, A. (1996). Vignettes of the continuous family ties: Some Latino American traditions. In A. McCabe (Ed.), *Chameleon readers: Teaching children to appreciate all kinds of good stories* (pp. 116–136). New York, NY: McGraw Hill.

Sinatra, R., & Dowd, C. A. (1991). Using syntactic and semantic clues to learn vocabulary. *Journal of Reading, 35*, 226–227.

Slater, W. H., & Graves, M. F. (1989). Research on expository text: Implications for teachers. In K. D. Muth (Ed.), *Children's comprehension of text* (pp. 140–166). Newark, DE: International Reading Association.

Snow, C., Cancini, H., & Gonzalez, P., & Shriberg, E. (1989). Giving formal definitions: An oral language correlate of school literacy. In D. Bloome (Ed.), *Classrooms and literacy* (pp. 233–249). Norwood, NJ: Ablex.

Snow, C. E., Burns, M. S., & Griffin, P. (1998) *Preventing reading difficulties in young children*. Committee on the Prevention of Reading Difficulties in Young Children, National Research Council. National Academy Press: Washington, DC.

Snow, C., & Ninio, A. (1986). The contracts of literacy: What children learn from learning to read books. In W. H. Teale & E. Sulzby (Eds.), *Emergent literacy: Writing and reading* (pp. 116–137). Norwood, NJ: Ablex.

Spector, C. (1996). Children's comprehension of idioms in the context of humor. *Language, Speech, and Hearing Services in Schools, 27*, 307–313.

Stein, M. L., & Glenn, C. (1979) An analysis of story comprehension in elementary school children. In R. Freedle (Ed.), *New directions in discourse processing.* Norwood, NJ: ABLEX.

Stevenson, H. W., & Newman, R. S. (1986). Long-term prediction of achievement and attitudes in mathematics and reading. *Child Development, 57*, 76–93.

Stone, C. A., Silliman, E. R., Ehren, B. J., & Apel, K. (2004). *Handbook of language and literacy.* New York, NY: The Guilford Press.

Storck, P. A., & Luft, W. R. (1973). Qualitative analysis of vocabulary responses from persons aged six to sixty-six plus. *Journal of Educational Psychology, 65*, 192–197.

Stotsky, S. (1983). Research on reading/writing relationships: A synthesis and suggested directions. *Language Arts, 60*, 627–642.

Strickland, D., Snow, C., Griffin, P. Burns, M. S., & McNamara, P. (2002) *Preparing our teachers: Opportunities for better reading instruction*. National Research Council, Washington, D.C.

Strömqvist, S., Johansson, V., Kriz, S., Ragnarsdottir, H., Aiseman, R., & Ravid, D. (2002). *Writing the frog story: Developmental and cross-modal perspectives* (pp. 359–594). Mahwah, NJ: Lawrence Erlbaum.

Sulzby, E. (1985). Children's emergent reading of favorite storybooks: A developmental study. *Reading Research Quarterly, 20*, 458–481.

Tabors, P. O. Snow, C. E., & Dickson, D. K. (2001). Homes and schools together: Supporting language and literacy development. In D. K. Dickinson & P. O. Tabors (Eds.), *Beginning literacy with language: Young children learning at home and at school* (pp. 313–334). Baltimore, MD: Brooks.

Thomas, B. (1984). Early toy preferences of four-year-old readers and non-readers. *Child Development, 55*, 424–430.

Trupe, A. (2002). *Academic literacy in a wired world: Redefining genres for college writing courses*. Retrieved October 27, 2003, from http://www.bridgewater.edu/~atrupe/AcadLit/WiredWorld.htm

Ukrainetz, T. A., Justice, L. M., Kaderavek, L. A., Eisenberg, S. L., Gillam, R. B., & Harm, H. M. (2005). The development of expressive elaboration in fictional narratives. *Journal of Speech, Language, and Hearing Research, 48*, 1363–1377.

Valdez, G. (1996). *Con respeto: Bridging the distances between culturally diverse families and schools*. New York, NY: Teacher's College Press.

van Kleeck, A. (2004). Fostering preliteracy development via storybook-sharing interactions. In C. A. Stone, E. R. Silliman, B. J. Ehren, & K. Apel (Eds.), *Handbook of language and literacy: Development and disorder* (pp. 175–208). New York, NY: The Guilford Press.

van Kleeck, A. (Ed.). (2006). *Sharing books and stories to foster language and literacy.* San Diego, CA: Plural.

van Kleeck, A. (2008). Providing preschool foundations for later reading comprehension: The importance of and ideas for targeting inferencing in book-sharing interventions. *Psychology in the Schools, 46*(6), 1–17.

van Kleeck, A., Alexander, E., Vigil, A., & Templeton, K. (1996). Modeling thinking for infants: Middle class mothers' presentation of information structures during book sharing. *Journal of Research in Childhood Education, 10*, 101–113.

van Kleeck, A., & Beckley-McCall, A. (2002). A comparison of mothers' individual and simultaneous book sharing with preschool siblings: An exploratory study of five families. *American Journal of Speech-Language Pathology, 11*, 175–189.

van Kleeck, A., Gillam, R., & Breshears, K. D. (1998, November). *Effects of book genre on mother's emphasis on print meaning and form during book sharing.* Paper presented at the 1998 American Speech-Language-Hearing Association Annual Convention, San Antonio, TX.

van Kleeck, A., Gillam, R., Hamilton, L., & McGrath, C. (1997). The relationship between middle-class parents' book-sharing discussion and their preschoolers' abstract language development. *Journal of Speech-Language-Hearing Research, 40*, 1261–1271.

Van Kleeck, A. Stahl, S.A., & Bauer, E. B. (2003). *On reading books to children.* Mahwah, NJ: Erlbaum.

van Kleeck, A., Vigil, A., & Beer, N. (1998, November). *A longitudinal study of maternal book-sharing emphasis on print form and print meaning with preschoolers.* Paper presented at the 1998 American Speech-Language Hearing Association Annual Convention, San Antonio, TX.

Vihman, M. M. (1988). Later phonological development. In J. Bernthal & N. Bankson (Eds.), *Articulation and phonological disorders* (2nd ed., pp. 110–144). New York, NY: Prentice-Hall.

Wagner, R. K., Torgesen, J. K., & Rashotte, C. A. (1994). Development of reading-related phonological processing abilities: New evidence of bidirectional causality from a latent variable longitudinal study. *Developmental Psychology, 30*, 73–87.

Wallach, G. (1988). Oral language and reading: Connections. *A clinical workshop presented in Denver, Colorado, October 8-9.*

Watson, R. (2001). Literacy and oral language: Implications for early language acquisition. In S. B. Neuman & D. K. Dickinson (Eds.), *Handbook of early literacy research* (pp. 43–53). New York, NY: Guilford Press.

Weaver, C. (1982). Welcoming errors as signs of growth. *Language Arts, 59*, 438–444.

Webster's third new international dictionary of the English language. (1981). Springfield, MA: G. C. Merriam.

Wellman, H. M., & Gelman, S. A. (1998). Knowledge acquisition in functional domains. In W. Damon (Series Ed.), D. Kuhn, & R. S. Siegler (Eds.), *Handbook of child psychology: Vol. 2. Cognition, perception, and language* (5th ed., pp. 523–573). New York, NY: Wiley.

Wells, G. (1985). Preschool literacy-related activities and success in school. In D. R. Olson, N. Torrance, & A. Hildyard (Eds.), *Literacy, language, and learning: The nature and consequences of reading and writing* (pp. 229–253). Cambridge, UK: Cambridge University Press.

Westby, C. (1985) Learning to talk-talking to learn: Oral-literate language differences. In C. S. Simon (Ed.), *Communication skills and classroom success: Therapy methodologies for language-learning disabled students* (pp. 181–213). San Diego, CA: College-Hill Press

Westby, C. (1988, October 8). *Oral language and reading: Connections.* A clinical workshop presented in Denver, CO.

Westby, C. (1994). Communication refinement in school age and adolescence. In W. O. Haynes & B.B. Shulman (Eds.), *Communication development: Foundations, processes, and clinical applications* (pp. 341–383). Englewood Cliffs, NJ: Prentice Hall.

Westby, C. (2004). In C. A. Stone, E. R. Silliman, B. J. Ehren, & K. Apel (Eds.), *Handbook of language and literacy: Development and disorder* (pp. 398–427). New York, NY: Guilford Press.

Wheeler, M. P. (1983). Context-related age changes in mothers' speech: Joint book reading. *Journal of Child Language, 10*, 259–263.

White, T. G., Power, M. A., & White, S. (1989). Morphological analysis: Implications for teaching and understanding vocabulary growth. *Reading Research Quarterly, 24*, 283–304.

Whitehurst, G. J., & Lonigan, C. J. (1998). Child development and emergent literacy. *Child Development, 69*(3), 848–872.

Whitehurst, G. J., & Lonigan, C. J. (2003). Emergent literacy: Development from prereaders to readers. In S. Newman & D. Dickenson (Eds.), *Handbook of early literacy research* (pp. 11–29). New York, NY: Guilford Press.

Wiig, E. (1989). *Steps to language competence.* San Antonio, TX: Psychological Corporation.

CHAPTER 6

Language Delays, Disorders, and Differences

INTRODUCTION

In the previous chapters, we described the intricate process of language development. We have observed both the universal nature of language—evident when children attain comparable milestones with respect to the quantity and quality of language they understand and use—and the unique nature of language evident in each and every individual child. The complementary unity and diversity in language development have stimulated our sustained interest in this phenomenon. The parents of children in our clinical practice have celebrated both how their children achieved the language milestones that are expected across children and how they have simultaneously demonstrated those special characteristics that are theirs alone. Sometimes this celebration of language diversity has evolved into concern by parents about whether the language development of their children could best be characterized as "within normal limits."

As clinical practitioners, we have frequently addressed the question of what constitutes the most accurate description of the language development —or nondevelopment—of a child. Parents request a language evaluation with an SLP for a variety of reasons. In some cases, they anticipate a particular timetable and become concerned when the skills of their children do not appear "on time." In other cases, they observe that their children have found some skill areas problematic. Typical of the concerns that parents have shared with us include that parents consider the language of their children difficult to understand, their children do not appear to understand questions and directions, or that their children communicate in a fashion that draws undue attention. When we explore the language status of children, we aim to determine the presence of typical versus atypical language development and, when the language development is typical, whether the pattern is that of a particular language dialect.

In this chapter, we overview the various classification systems that are available to document multiple patterns of language development and discuss the most appropriate applications of these in the clinical service delivery process. We also overview what patterns constitute "language delays" and "language disorders" in children, as well as the variations of language development that, although distinctive, are not problematic and thus constitute "language differences" in children.

IMPORTANCE OF ACCURATE CLASSIFICATION

We hold that the importance of accurate classification of a child's language status is imperative. The clinical practice standards delineated in the ASHA

Code of Ethics (2003) and the relevant ASHA Position Statements mandate that we consider the welfare of those whom we serve to be of paramount importance. These standards and statements also iterate that, as part of our clinical service delivery, we provide the most accurate information possible to the public—which includes our patients and their families—about communication and communication disorders. Thus, our clinical conclusions must be the most accurate possible based on our available clinical evidence. When we, in the process of evaluation, reach the conclusion that a child presents with typical language development, these valid results allow us to provide reassurance to his or her parents. In contrast, when we reach the conclusion that a child presents with atypical language development, these valid results allow us to initiate the most appropriate course of intervention. The process of accurate classification of children is not without complications. When we aim for accurate classification, we have available to us a number of systems from which to select descriptive labels. No system is comprehensive. In fact, some systems are incomplete or internally and/or externally contradictory. The presence of multiple classification systems that reflect various perspectives on language status increases the potential for confusion for families. Because of these considerations, we wish to describe the presently available classification systems and comment on their usefulness in describing the language status of a child.

CLASSIFICATION OF CHILDREN WHO ARE AT RISK

In some cases, the children whom we serve have risk factors that increase their potential for atypical language development. These children are considered "at risk" for language and/or other communication disorders. The classification of "at risk" is further delineated with respect to the nature of the apparent risk factors.

Established Risk

When a child has "established risk," he or she has atypical development in one or more areas that appears relatively soon after his or her birth (ASHA, 1991). This risk is associated with one or more confirmed medical disorders that present documented influence on developmental patterns. In our clinical practice, we have served children with craniofacial anomalies, such as patterns of cleft lip and palate that were present at birth. The compromise of the speech production mechanism and the subsequent impact of these structural limitations on the communication of the child are obvious. In addition, because of the documented occurrence of medical complications that can lead to failure to thrive, children with these anomalies have the potential for multiple developmental complications.

Biological Risk

A child with "biological risk" presents with a personal history that includes events that may have a subsequent deleterious effect on his or her development (ASHA, 1991; Gerber, 1990). These events may have occurred in the preconception period, as well as in the prenatal, perinatal, neonatal, or postnatal periods. Examples include maternal abuse of controlled or even prescribed and over-the-counter substances and maternal exposure to unsafe or toxic conditions. These risk factors may increase the probability of injury to the central nervous system and thus increase the probability of atypical language development at some point in childhood.

Environmental Risk

When a child has "environmental risk," he or she presents with intact neurologic structure and function which may be compromised because of the nature of the immediate environment (ASHA, 1991; Gerber, 1990). Facets of the environment that may not facilitate typical language development include the quantity and quality of health care, interpersonal stimulation, and opportunities for the child to explore and experiment in the environment.

It is imperative to note that a 1:1 linear relationship between risk factors and atypical language development does not exist. Some children present atypical development in the absence of readily apparent risk factors, and vice versa. And some children experience the combined influence of predispositional and environmental factors on their language development. This less than predictable connection between risk factors and developmental outcomes underscores the need for the earliest possible identification of risk factors, followed by the introduction of preventive intervention to minimize their potential adverse effect on language, as well as the need for broad public education about the earliest possible identification of atypical language, even in the absence of obvious risk factors (Cole & Marge, 1985; Kavanagh, 1982; Kilburg, 1985; Marge, 1984; Weiss & Lillywhite, 1981).

TRADITIONAL DEFINITION OF COMMUNICATION DISORDERS

We continue our overview of classification systems with a traditional definition of communication disorders that we have constructed from the inspiration of available definitions (e.g., Anderson & Shames, 2005; Nicolosi, Harryman, & Kresheck, 2004; Owens, Metz & Haas, 2006; Plante & Beeson, 2007):

A communication disorder is present when a person communicates in a fashion that (a) results from or leads to an impairment in the communication mechanism, (b) is well outside the normal developmental expectations for communication, (c) causes substantial interference with the process of communication, (d) draws undue attention to the communicator to shift the focus of interaction from the ideas to the fashion in which these are transmitted, and/or (e) causes substantial discomfort for the communicator in intrapersonal and interpersonal contexts.

We can address each of these components of the definition in our consideration of whether a child presents with typical or atypical language development.

Consider This Scenario

A child, at birth, presents with a syndrome that includes some structural and functional abnormalities in the communication mechanism, such as velopharyngeal incompetence. Because of these abnormalities, the child is unable to formulate the movements needed for correct articulation and combination of speech sounds. The child is unable to communicate in a clear, conventional fashion to others. This scenario thus represents component (a) in the definition, as the disruption in speech production is a consequence of the abnormalities. Consider also that reconstruction of the communication mechanism will occur over an extended period of time and may even mandate the introduction of prosthetic devices to restore as much function as possible. The child, in an attempt to produce understandable speech, may use some compensatory behaviors that prove abusive to the mechanism. This scenario has now come full circle in that the communication disorder that stemmed from a compromise of the mechanism now has the potential for additional compromise of the mechanism.

Consider This Scenario

An adolescent has a substantial lexicon and uses those words to convey descriptions and explanations about a diverse collection of topics. He or she also demonstrates appropriate use of language for varied interpersonal and intrapersonal functions. However, others notice that some kinds of language are problematic for this adolescent—those that involve the comprehension or production of nonliteral language. Such language as humor, proverbs, parables, utterances open to multiple interpretations, and sarcasm represent examples of the nonliteral language that this adolescent has not mastered. Certainly, the development of nonliteral language continues in adulthood. However, someone in late adolescence typically demonstrates at least some appreciation for and appropriate use of this level of sophistication. Because this adolescent does not, our perception is that he or she possesses skills that are not comparable to his or her peers, and this discrepancy is noticeable even to those unfamiliar with him or her. This scenario represents component (b) in the definition of a communication disorder.

Consider This Scenario

Rather than produce conventional words, a child produces nonwords that others find difficult to interpret. We know that children do not always produce words in the same fashion that adults produce them. Sometimes, because a child may find it difficult to produce the speech sound combinations in the words, he or she may produce simplifications of those words. Simplifications such as [wɛd] ("wed") for [rɛd] ("red"), [bæf] ("baf") for [bæθ] ("bath"), and [dot] ("dote") for [kot] ("coat") are familiar to us. Although these are "incorrect" productions, their resemblance to the words they replace enable us to appreciate the ideas that the child wants to share. So do other simplified forms like "kitty" for "cat." However, because the productions of the child are not mere simplifications of adult forms, a potential for substantial interference in communication exists. This scenario thus represents component (c) in the definition. The time invested by the child to express information and the attempt of the communication partner to interpret the ideas results in a breakdown.

Consider This Scenario

An adolescent appears to have an ample, varied lexicon and considerable sophistication in the structures into which he or she combines these words. What the child lacks, however, is the discretion to appropriately match his or her considerable informational content to the communication situation. Instances such as inappropriate topics for the immediate context, inappropriate quantity and/or quality of information for the topics, inappropriate provision of clarification requested from others, inappropriate methods to commence or conclude interactions, and other examples reflect this lack of discernment as to the interactional dimensions of communication. The instances noted here certainly cause breakdowns in communication, as in the previous scenario. To complicate matters, however, the nature of these instances further causes pronounced reactions from actual or potential conversational partners. In some cases, these reactions lead to conclusions, although sometimes unfounded, about the manners, competence, or even character of the adolescent, whose limitations shift the focus from information communicated to the indiscretions committed with respect to language. This reflects component (d) in the definition.

Consider This Scenario

Like a substantial proportion of his or her peers, a child experiences communication apprehension. This condition occurs as *state* apprehension and as *trait* apprehension. In *state* apprehension, a person has fear about a specific communication situation which manifests itself for a specific period of time, for example, someone who has a role in a community theater play may have apprehension about his or her performance. However, removal of the sources of apprehension (e.g., potential lapses in character lines, reactions of local critics, or sparse attendance by audiences) results in cessation of the apprehension. In *trait* apprehension, however, a person has fear as a personal trait that transcends specific communication contexts. In this case, the apprehension can be apparent in fear-influenced, less than effective language productions. These can lead to diminished language performance, which can lead to increased apprehension, and the cycle continues. The ultimate result of this cycle can be a compromise in communication so severe to cause the child to avoid situations, perhaps to the point of selective mutism, and thus lose valuable opportunities for interactions with others, and is thus an example of trait (e).

This definition for what constitutes a communication disorder has been helpful in our clinical practice. In some instances, we are dependent on criteria-based rather than norm-based measurements to determine the presence of a communication disorder in a patient. This definition has provided us with an application of the Socratic method of analysis to reach an accurate conclusion about communication status. In many clinical contexts, this definition has proven sufficient; however, this definition does not contain the differential diagnosis information that may be necessary for some patients or in some contexts. For those, we may select a more standardized, authoritative classification system.

CLASSIFICATION SYSTEM: ASHA

One definition of communication disorders and variations is available from our national professional association, ASHA (1993). Although not a framework that constitutes an "official" classification from the association, this description of the nature and exemplars of communication disorders is a helpful conceptualization of the various dimensions of communication that can be impaired.

Communication Disorder

The definition starts with a description for *communication disorder*, which is characterized as an impairment in receiving, sending, processing, and/or comprehending various symbol systems: oral, written, and/or manual. A communication disorder can be present in hearing, language, and/or speech, with a variable severity level that need not be consistent across these three areas. This disorder may be developmental or a reflection of an interruption of a normal developmental process. A communication disorder also may be the primary concern for a child, or secondary to another condition. The definition continues with specification and elaboration of the broad domains within communication, hearing, processing, speech, and language.

Hearing Disorder

The description of a *hearing disorder* notes that an impairment in auditory sensitivity can limit the development, comprehension, production, and/or maintenance of communication. This limitation of development can stem from problems with detection, recognition, discrimination, comprehension, and/or perception of auditory information. The presence of a hearing disorder does not always lead to the presence of a language disorder. However, because of the disruption of the auditory reception of information, a hearing disorder certainly has the potential to be the basis for a subsequent language disorder, particularly when the hearing disorder has moved from hardness-of-hearing into more severe deafness.

Processing Disorder

The description of a *processing disorder* (also known as a *central auditory processing disorder*) notes that while auditory sensitivity is intact, the processing of auditory information is not. Limitations occur in the reception, interpretation, transformation, retention, and retrieval of information in auditory input. These limitations compromise how well a person attends to, discriminates, identifies, filters, sorts, transmits, and stores auditory input. The presence of a processing disorder does not always lead to the presence of a language disorder; however, the two conditions can present in a child in a similar fashion. Thus, we must differentiate processing disorders from language disorders based on executive functions versus cognitive-linguistic rules related to auditory information.

Speech Disorder

The description of a *speech disorder* notes that an impairment in the physical production of oral communication can limit the clarity or the quality of communication. Within speech disorders, *articulation disorders* present as incorrect productions of speech sounds that can disrupt the extent to which others can understand the speech. In addition to articulation disorders, *fluency disorders* can occur. These present as substantial interruptions in the flow of speech and thus affect the temporal aspects of speech production. Such interruptions can affect the rate of speech and the duration of speech elements and can include unusual repetitions of sounds, syllables, and even words. Excessive tension of the speech production mechanism and secondary behaviors, such as atypical facial expressions, postures, hand movements, and lip positions, can occur in more severe fluency disorders. In addition to articulation and fluency disorders, *voice disorders* can occur. These present as abnormal productions of the voice that may manifest themselves in unusual vocal characteristics in loudness, pitch, and/or resonance.

Language Disorder

With respect to language, the definition of a communication disorder further continues with a description of how disordered language development can be characterized: *A language disorder is impaired comprehension and/or use of spoken, written, and/or other symbol systems. The disorder may involve (1) the form of language (phonology, morphology, syntax), (2) the content of language (semantics), and/or (3) the function of language in communication (pragmatics) in any combination.* The "form" of language includes *phonology, morphology,* and *syntax,* while the "content" of language includes *semantics,* and the "function" of language includes *pragmatics.* Descriptions of these aspects of language are included in Chapter 1. Disorders in language can co-occur with disorders in the other specified areas of communication.

This classification system is helpful to SLPs because it delineates of the broad areas in which communication disorders can occur—hearing, processing, speech, and language. When we can identify these broad areas, we can focus our evaluation and intervention on the information collection tasks that can help us describe the relevant areas in more detail. Like the previous definition, this ASHA statement does not contain the differential diagnosis information that may be necessary for some patients or in some contexts. For those, we may select a more standardized, authoritative classification system.

CLASSIFICATION SYSTEM: ICD

Description

In 1948, the World Health Organization (WHO) assumed control of a reconceptualized version of an 1893 document, the *International List of Causes of Death,* created by the International Statistical Institute (ISI), which evolved into the *International Statistical Classification of Diseases and Related Health Problems* (ICD). The most recent version of the ICD is the ICD-10, which the WHO endorsed at the World Health Assembly in 1990. Since the late 1990s, this version has been the basis for reports of mortality data from death certificates. However, a version that continues widespread present use in clinical practice environments in the United States is the ICD-09, Volume I, which is available only in electronic form. A related document, the ICD-9-CM, Volume III (in which CM represents "clinical modification"), is used for inpatient and outpatient health care services. Eventually, the ICD-10-CM will replace this document, and even now an ICD-11 is in preparation for release in the next decade.

Purpose

The ICD is an international standard classification for a broad spectrum of health concerns. Via the use of the ICD, entities such as clinics, can monitor the incidence and prevalence of health problems, as well as maintain standardized medical records across national boundaries. These records can then provide data for scholars interested in clinical epidemiologic studies, who can present their results in a format compatible with the ICD model. Clinical practitioners interested in a common frame of reference can use the ICD for characterization of a broad spectrum of clinical conditions. Because of the medical nature of the conditions represented in the codes, SLPs—who can diagnose speech and language conditions but not diseases—do not use this classification system as often as other health care providers do. However, SLPs consider the information contained in the ICD codes used by medical personnel to describe the conditions of their shared patients to be quite valuable for speech and language diagnostic and prognostic purposes.

Relation to Language

The ICD classification system consists of a Diagnosis Code Index (Table 6–1). The broad categories of diagnoses have three-digit labels, which commence with 001 and conclude with 999. Codes 290-319, Mental Disorders, which include Code 315, Specific Delays in Development, are of particular interest to SLPs because delays in development can be manifested in delays in communication and multiple mental disorders can present disruptions in language as salient traits. In addition, codes that represent other potential causes of communication disorders include the Diseases of the Nervous System and the Diseases of the Respiratory System. Reflected in the Congenital Anomalies section are conditions that can certainly disrupt speech, such as Code 749, Cleft Palate and Cleft Lip, and place a child at risk for subsequent language concerns. Several other divisions within the code also represent conditions that can place a child at risk, such as those that prevent a normal course of language development, such as Conditions in the Perinatal Period, and those that interrupt a

TABLE 6–1. ICD Codes (WHO, 1990). These codes allow for the classification of health statistics related to causes of death, as well as to conditions observed in the course of inpatient and outpatient health care services.

001-139	Diseases: Infectious and Parasitic.
140-239	Neoplasms.
240-279	Diseases: Endocrine, Nutritional, Metabolic, and Disorders: Immunity.
280-289	Diseases: Blood and Blood-Forming Organs.
290-319	Disorders: Mental.
320-389	Diseases: Nervous System and Sense Organs.
390-459	Diseases: Circulatory System.
460-519	Diseases: Respiratory System.
520-579	Diseases: Digestive System.
580-629	Diseases: Genitourinary System.
630-677	Complications: Pregnancy, Childbirth, and Puerperium.
680-709	Diseases: Skin and Subcutaneous Tissue.
710-739	Diseases: Musculoskeletal System and Connective Tissue.
740-759	Anomalies: Congenital.
760-779	Certain Conditions: Perinatal Period.
780-799	Conditions: Symptoms, Signs, and Ill-Defined.
800-999	Injury and Poisoning.

normal course of language development, such as Injuries and Poisoning. In addition, the Supplementary Classification of Factors Influencing Health Status and Contact with Health Services component of the ICD has implications for clinical practice and the provision of the most efficacious services for children with language issues.

Critique

The fact that this classification system is standardized, authoritative, and international contributes to ease of communication across clinical practitioners who address the needs of children with language issues. The use of this common frame of reference minimizes the risk of confusion with respect to the terms used to describe conditions. This classification system is helpful to SLPs because of its identification of conditions that can cause, complicate, or contribute to atypical language development. This identification enhances the process of differential diagnosis when questions arise about language in that, with these codes, the SLPs possess valuable patient history information. However, once the SLP reaches some conclusion about the nature and extent of atypical language development, this classification becomes much less useful in clinical practice because of the preponderance of medical (as opposed to developmental or rehabilitative) codes.

CLASSIFICATION SYSTEM: DSM

Description

The *Diagnostic and Statistical Manual of Mental Disorders (DSM)* (2000) provides a standardized classification system for mental health professionals to describe mental disorders. In fact, the ICD-9-CM approach inspired the DSM approach to differential diagnosis of conditions. As with the ICD, the broad categories of diagnoses have three-digit labels (001 through 999) and include decimal points to further delineate the labels. Within these categories are the diagnostic inclusion and exclusion criteria for the specific conditions. To complement the conditions, the DSM provides details relevant to subsets, associated disorders, additional considerations, patterns, and prevalence of said conditions. And, as with the ICD, of potential interest to SLPs and of particular relevance to language are several divisions within the classification system. The DSM-V will eventually replace the DSM-IV in clinical practice. Until that point, a revised version of the DSM-IV, known as the DSM-IV-TR, is in use.

Purpose

The present version of this manual, the DSM-IV, is used in inpatient and outpatient venues on an international scale by practitioners in medical, educational, occupational, rehabilitation, social services, and other disciplines. Like the ICD, the DSM is a research tool to collect and convey public health care statistics about conditions that include those typically initially identified in infants, children, and adolescents. And like the ICD, the DSM classification system also consists of a Diagnosis Code Index. Clinical practitioners interested in a common frame of reference can use the DSM for characterization of a broad spectrum of clinical conditions. With respect to these conditions, this classification system includes several language conditions and delineates the language characteristics that are typical of a myriad of disorders. Because of this, SLPs have broader application of the DSM than of the ICD in day-to-day clinical practice that involves diagnosis of conditions. This use is enhanced by the detailed descriptions of the conditions, which provide an expanded basis for clinical conclusions.

Relation to Language

The DSM includes diagnoses for a multitude of mental disorders that are related in some way to language (Figure 6–1). A number of conditions often present disruptions in language as characteristics that define the disorder. Examples include the Cognitive Disorders (249 Codes), Schizophrenia Disorders (295 Codes), Depressive Disorders (296 Codes), Bipolar Disorders (296 Codes), Psychoses (293 Codes), and Conduct Disorders (312 Codes). Some of the broad diagnoses are particularly familiar to SLPs because of the frequency with which SLPs see these co-occur with disruptions in language. Examples include the Autism Spectrum Disorders (299 Codes), Attention Deficit Disorders (314 Codes), Learning Disorders (315 Codes), levels of Mental Retardation (317, 318, and 319 Codes), and Not Otherwise Specified (NOS) Disorders of Infancy, Childhood, or Adolescence. In addition to this diverse assortment of mental disorders that are related in some way to language, the DSM includes several explicit language (or related) conditions. Code 307.9 represents Communication Disorder NOS, which encompasses other communication disorders without their own explicit codes. Codes 315.31 and 315.32 are Expressive Language Disorder and Mixed Receptive-Expressive Language Disorder, respectively. However, the DSM does not include a code for Receptive Language Disorder to correspond with a code for Expressive Language Disorder. Code 315.39, Phonological Disorder, was formerly known as Developmental Articulation Disorder and, even now, retains much of the descriptive information that once applied to articulation rather than to phonological delays and disorders as specific variations of language delays and disorders. Although the focus of the DSM codes is oral language, two are present for written language, 315, Reading Disorder, and 315.2, Disorder of Written Expression. Two additional communication disorders also appear, 307, Stuttering, and 313.23, Selective Mutism.

Critique

Like the ICD, this classification system is standardized, authoritative, and international. Unlike the ICD, this classification system has a broader assortment of conditions that reflect the populations whom

Axis I

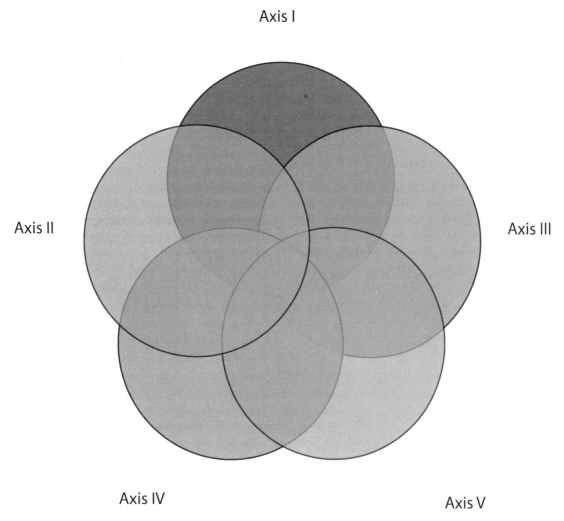

Axis II

Axis III

Axis IV

Axis V

FIGURE 6–1. DSM Codes (APA, 2000). This framework allows for the classification of psychiatric and psychological disorders, which include multiple developmental disorders. Axis I = Clinical Syndromes. Axis II = Developmental and Personality Disorders. Axis III = Physical Symptoms. Axis IV = Psychosocial Stressors. Axis V = Present Level of Function.

SLPs serve in the course of evaluation and intervention for communication disorders. The DSM includes provision for the documentation of specific issues with communication, which is beneficial to mental health professionals who serve patients with communication disorders. The codes related to communication disorders, however, while helpful, have room for improvement. The inclusion of Expressive Language Disorder without the inclusion of a companion code for Receptive Language Disorder renders this system incomplete. And the use of the broad terms *receptive* and *expressive* serve only the purpose of identification rather than also the purpose of description of language disorders. The code for Phonological Disorder, although consistent with current views of the speech sound system, is dated in that, rather than describe phonological skills as aspects of language skills, the code continues to conceptualization of phonological skills only as the physical articulation of speech sounds. The inclusion of broad codes for written language disorders is useful. However, many SLPs will find the need to supplement the DSM codes with considerable descriptive information.

CLASSIFICATION SYSTEM: ICF

Description

Another classification system that can be applied to communication disorders, and language disorders within communication disorders, is the *International Classification of Functioning, Disability, and Health (ICF)*. The WHO endorsed the ICF at the World Health Assembly in 2001 as a complement to the ICD. The ICF is a system that provides a standard for the measurement of health status and the disabilities that occur as a consequence of a decline in health status. The ICF construction reflects the idea that humans have the potential for multiple disabilities across the course of their lives and that these disabilities have social as well as medical and developmental components (Figure 6–2).

Purpose

The focus of the ICF is the status of the systems and/or mechanisms that perform a comprehensive assortment of physical functions. For the SLP, this perspective is quite useful. The ICF sorts codes into four broad areas: Body Functions, Activities and Participation, Environmental Factors, and Body Struc-tures. Information about the physical status has implications for the determination of the cause(s) of a communication disorder, which, in turn, has implication for the potential of a clinic patient to improve over the course of intervention. Information about the physical status is useful in consideration of such clinical questions as to the relative contributions of multiple systems and/or mechanism to an apparent communication disorder, whether and when to initiate treatment, how to coordinate speech and/or language services with services from other providers, which variations of treatment have the potential for additional harm to the mechanism, and which approaches to treatment appear most appropriate.

Relation to Language

Within the Body Functions section of the ICF are specific sections for the physical processes of hearing, speech, and language (Tables 6–2, 6–3, and 6–4). Within Body Functions: Hearing are codes related to how we sense the presence of sounds and discriminate, lateralize, and localize sounds with diverse properties (B230). These codes include a means to record hearing losses and deafness. Within Body Functions: Speech are codes related to how we produce clear, pleasant, fluent speech. Included in this

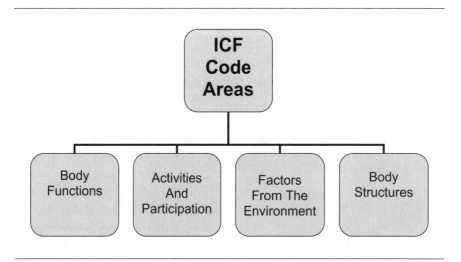

FIGURE 6–2. ICF Codes (WHO, 2001). These codes allow for the classification of the structure and function of physical mechanisms, as well as the impact of structure and function on endeavors such as communication.

TABLE 6–2. ICF Codes (WHO, 2001) related to communication disorders that are contained within the Body Functions: Mental Functions section of this classification system.

BI, Chapter I: Mental Functions.

  B110-B139 Mental Functions: Global.

  B140-B189 Mental Functions: Specific.

   B140 Functions: Attention.

   B144 Functions: Memory.

   B147 Functions: Psychomotor.

   B152 Functions: Emotional.

   B156 Functions: Perceptual.

   B160 Functions: Thought.

   B164 Functions: Higher-Level Cognitive.

   B167 Functions: Mental of Language.

    B1670 Language: Reception.

     B16700 Reception: Spoken.

     B16701 Reception: Written.

     B16702 Reception: Signed.

     B16708 Reception: Other Specified.

     B16709 Reception: Unspecified.

    B1671 Language: Expression.

     B16710 Expression: Spoken.

     B16711 Expression: Written.

     B16712 Expression: Signed.

     B16718 Expression: Other Specified.

     B16719 Expression: Unspecified.

    B1672 Language: Integrative.

    B1678 Language: Mental, Other Specified.

    B1679 Language: Mental, Unspecified.

TABLE 6–3. ICF Codes (WHO, 2001) related to communication disorders that are contained within the Body Functions: Voice and Speech Functions section of this classification system.

B3, Chapter III: Voice and Speech Functions.

  B310 Functions: Voice.

   B3100 Voice: Production.

   B3101 Voice: Quality.

   B3108 Voice: Other Specified.

   B3109 Voice: Unspecified.

  B320 Functions: Articulation.

  B330 Functions: Fluency and Rhythm.

   B3300 Speech: Fluency.

   B3301 Speech: Rhythm.

   B3302 Speech: Speed.

   B3303 Speech: Melody.

   B3308 Speech: Fluency and Rhythm Other Specified.

   B3309 Speech: Fluency and Rhythm Unspecified.

  B340 Functions: Alternative Vocalization.

   B3400 Vocalization: Notes.

   B3401 Vocalization: Range of Sounds.

   B3408 Vocalization: Alternative Other Specified.

   B3409 Vocalization: Alternative Unspecified.

  B398 Functions: Voice and Speech Other Specified.

  B399 Functions: Voice and Speech Unspecified.

---

section is B330, Fluency and Rhythm of Speech, which is further subdivided into Fluency of Speech (B3300), Rhythm of Speech (B3301), Speed of Speech (B3302), and Melody of Speech (B3303). Within Body Functions: Voice is B310, Voice Functions, which is further subdivided into Production of Voice (B3100) and Quality of Voice (B3101), and is complemented with B340, Alternative Vocalizations. In addition to the speech functions, the ICF includes a Body Functions: Language section with B167, Mental Functions of Language. The examples within B167 are diverse and include language reception versus language expression and spoken language versus written language. In addition to the Body Functions section, the Activities and Participation section of the ICF contains multiple references to participation in communication in code D3, with attention to reception versus expression, spoken versus written versus sign language, and other dimensions of interaction. In addition to these two sections, the Body Structures section includes codes for the physical structures that are crucial to the functions of hearing and speaking in codes S2 and S3.

TABLE 6–4. ICF Codes (WHO, 2001) related to communication disorders that are contained within the Activities of Communication section of this classification system.

D3, Chapter III: Communication.
 D310-D329 Communicating: Receiving.
  D310 Receiving Messages: Spoken.
  D315 Receiving Messages: Nonverbal.
   D3150 Receiving: Body Gestures.
   D3151 Receiving: General Signs and Symbols.
   D3152 Receiving: Drawings and Photographs.
   D3158 Receiving: Nonverbal Messages Other Specified.
   D3159 Receiving: Nonverbal Messages Unspecified.
  D320 Receiving Messages: Sign Language.
  D325 Receiving Messages: Written.
  D329 Receiving Messages: Other Specified and Unspecified.
 D330-D349 Communicating: Producing
  D330 Producing Messages: Spoken.
  D335 Producing Messages: Nonverbal.
   D3350 Producing: Body Language.
   D3351 Producing: Signs and Symbols.
   D3352 Producing: Drawings and Photographs.
   D3358 Producing: Nonverbal Messages Other Specified.
   D3359 Producing: Nonverbal Messages Unspecified.
  D340 Producing Messages: Sign Language.
  D345 Producing Messages: Written.
  D349 Producing Messages: Other Specified and Unspecified.
 D350-D369 Communicating: Communication Devices and Techniques.
  D350 Conversation.
   D3500 Conversation: Starting.
   D3501 Conversation: Sustaining.
   D3502 Conversation: Ending.
   D3503 Conversation: With One Person.
   D3504 Conversation: With Many People.
   D3508 Conversation: Other Specified.
   D3509 Conversation: Unspecified.
  D355 Discussion.
   D3550 Discussion: With One Person.
   D3551 Discussion: With Many People.
   D3558 Discussion: Other Specified.
   D3559 Discussion: Unspecified.
  D360 Communication Devices and Techniques.
   D3600 Devices: Telecommunication.
   D3601 Devices: Writing Machines.
   D3602 Devices: Communication Techniques.
   D3608 Devices and Techniques: Other Specified.
   D3609 Devices and Techniques: Unspecified.
  D369 Other Specified and Unspecified.
  D398 Communicating: Other Specified.
  D399 Communicating: Unspecified.

Critique

Like the ICD and the DSM, this classification system is standardized, authoritative, and international. However, with inclusion of both functions and structures related to hearing, speaking, and language, the ICF provides a more detailed portrait of the current and potential status of the mechanism, which then contribute to conclusions about the potential for the improvement of the communication status of a patient. With respect to communication, the ICF provides a diverse assortment of codes to document the aspects and modalities of communication that are problematic. The inclusion of the umbrella of communication, comprising hearing, speaking, and understanding and using language, is an attractive philosophical model for SLPs. However, like the DSM, the labels related to specific conditions are broad. Although the inclusion and exclusion criteria that are the bases for the use of the labels are somewhat helpful, these are not sufficiently comprehensive to include all variations of communication disorders. And, as these criteria focus on disorders with specific functional or structural bases, the idiopathic disorders are not captured as clearly as other disorders. Even so, the ICF provides useful physical status information about the patients whom the SLPs will serve.

OTHER DESCRIPTIONS: GLI, SLI, AND CHILDHOOD APHASIA

In the current descriptions of language in children are three other terms used to conceptualize language concerns: GLI, SLI, and Childhood Aphasia. The initial terms, *GLI* and *SLI*, indicate specific conditions, while the additional term, *childhood aphasia*, is open to some interpretation and thus is a source of potential confusion. Because of this, an overview of the nature of these terms is in order.

GLI: General Language Impairment

As noted in the previous discussions of codes—in particular, the DSM code—children may present with medical or other conditions that co-occur with language disorders. Whether the relationship of these conditions with language disorders is one of causation, co-occurrence, or causation of both from an independent source, a general impairment in language is present. Consider children with a pervasive developmental disorder. Although each of these children certainly presents an individual pattern of developmental concerns, an impairment that permeates each of the skill areas of language to a considerable extent would not be uncommon in this population. The impairment in language, then, that is concomitant with a broader-based condition is considered a *general language impairment* (GLI) (Plomin, 2002). The presence of this condition would have implications for clinical priorities and certainly for conclusions about the potential of the child for substantial improvement in language skills should the condition continue to exist.

SLI: Specific Language Impairment

In contrast to the conditions under which a GLI is apparent, some children present with language disorders in the absence of disorders that compromise mental and/or physical development. These idiopathic language disorders indicate *specific language impairment* (SLI). Like GLI, SLI can affect each of the skill areas of language, sometimes to a severe extent. Unlike GLI, SLI cannot be associated with another broad based condition, such as autism, blindness, or a learning, hearing, or genetic disorder. Although speculation abounds as to the nature of SLI, no authoritative explanation exists to its causal or contributory factors. However, children who have SLI are quite a diverse assortment in their presentation in terms of the skill(s) affected, the level of severity, and the overall impact of their language status on communication (Lahey & Edwards, 1995; Rice & Warren, 2004; Ron & Robbins, 2003). In addition to the distinction between GLI and SLI in terms of *general* versus *specific*, it is important to note the use of the word *impairment*. The WHO (1980) defines *impairment* as the loss or abnormal status related to psychological, physiological, or anatomical structure or function. In contrast, however, the WHO considers *disability* as the reduced ability to meet daily needs, particularly when compensatory measures are restricted, and considers *handicap* to represent the social consequences of an impairment and its concomitant disability. Given those distinctions, each of the three terms, in theory, could describe the impact of a language disorder on the life of a child.

In addition to this consideration, we would be remiss if we did not note that, for the child who presents with SLI, many SLPs further describe the condition with the terms *delay* and *disorder*. In this distinction, *delayed language development* occurs when a child presents a late onset and a slow rate of development. However, the pattern of development is typical, and the communication of the child is commensurate with the level of children at an earlier point in life (Nicolosi, Harryman, & Kresheck, 2004). In contrast, *disordered language development* occurs when a child presents, in most cases, a late onset and slow rate of development. However, the pattern of development is atypical, and the communication of the child is not commensurate with the level of children at an earlier point in life. Instead, the pattern of development contains exceptions to the usual patterns that are common across children (Nicolosi, Harryman, & Kresheck, 2004). Debate continues as to whether a child can present with both delayed and disordered, as well as whether language can be so delayed as to constitute a disorder, instead. Whatever the ultimate resolution of these questions, the terms *delayed* and *disordered* permeate clinical practice and documentation as standard descriptions of language-related conditions.

Childhood Aphasia

The condition of aphasia occurs when the process of normal language development (or, in the case of adults, the presence of normal language) is interrupted, often because of a cerebral vascular accident (i.e., stroke) or disease or trauma (Obler & Gjerlow, 1999). Children are not immune to these conditions and, as a result, may present an acquired language disorder (aphasia) rather than a developmental language disorder (dysphasia), although the distinction has become blurred in some contexts, with the term *childhood aphasia* used to represent both acquired and developmental conditions. For that reason, the term *acquired childhood aphasia*, which contrasts with the common presumption of aphasia as an adulthood condition, has appeared as an alternative form to stress the acquired nature of aphasia.

LANGUAGE DIFFERENCES

In previous sections of this chapter, we emphasized the existence of language delays and language disorders that can be characterized with a diverse assortment of classifications. Certainly, delays and disorders occur in diverse forms. This diversity in language comprehension and language production also is present within normal language development. Variations within a language are considered *language differences*. The previously noted ASHA definition for communication disorders (1993) notes that, *"(A) communication difference/dialect is a variation of a symbol system used by a group of individuals that reflects and is determined by shared regional, social, or cultural/ethnic factors."* The definition then notes that, *"A regional, social, or cultural/ethnic variation of a symbol system should not be considered a disorder of speech or language."* Multiple variations of language differences exist (Wolfram, 1991; Wolfram, Adger, & Christian, 1999; Wolfram & Fasold, 1974; Wolfram & Schilling-Estes, 1998). Some individuals were born into a non-English environment and thus learned another language before English. Such non-English environments occur both outside and inside the United States. Other individuals were born into an English environment and thus learned English before another language, if attempts to become bilingual even occurred (Holmes, 2001; Hudson, 1980; McWhorter, 2000). Every user of a language uses a dialect of that language. This variation of a language reflects the influence of diverse factors: location, status, age, gender, ancestry, ethnicity, personal communication style, models, and experiences. A dialect can influence each skill area within language. When a dialect influences the production and combination of speech sounds, the condition that results is known as an *accent*. One of the position papers from ASHA states the status of language differences (ASHA, 2003) with the assertion a dialect is "adequate" as a functional and effective variation of English, a contributor to social networks and constructs, and a representation of the culture of its speakers. With respect to clinical service provision, SLPs coordinate elective services, such as accent modification, for those individuals who choose to alter their patterns of language.

CONCLUSION

Codes to define and describe communication disorders—and language delayed and disorders within communication disorders—are varied. The standardized codes have both advantages and disadvantages. These codes are not identical, and even if they were, would only be as useful as those who use them allow them to be. This would include strict adherence to the definitions, as the exclusion and inclusion criteria, even when other codes are personal preferences for SLPs and practitioners from other disciplines. As practitioners consider the extent to which the presentation of a child is compatible to a specific code before acknowledging that code, and as this consideration is based on available evidence from the child, a way exists to enhance the usefulness of standardized codes. The supplement of the numbers and labels from the codes with detailed description across the areas of language skill would prove invaluable in comparisons of the skill of a child at multiple points in time, as well as minimize the confusion inherent in the provision of varied codes across varied clinical practice contexts.

REFLECTION QUESTIONS

1. What are the most important reasons that SLPs and their partners should aim for the most accurate classification and description of the language conditions that children present?

2. What factors can explain the creation of such an assortment of classification for language and other health-related conditions?

3. How are the classification systems overviewed in this chapter similar and dissimilar to each other? What are the advantages and disadvantages that result for these systems?

4. What are the distinctions across language delays, language disorders, and language differences that can occur in children?

5. Why are language differences not considered problems in need of clinical intervention, with the exception of elective clinical services?

APPLICATION EXERCISES

1. The parents of a child have secured multiple opinions as to the status of the language of their child. The clinical service providers have determined that the child has a communication disorder but have conceptualized this disorder with multiple classifications. The parents are concerned and confused. The parents have asked your opinion as to whether it is more important to simply know that a disorder is present or, instead, to know the exact disorder, that is present. How would you respond to their question?

2. A child communicates in a fashion that, in some respects, is consistent with delayed language development and disordered language development. What kinds of information would be helpful to the clinical service provider who wants to determine which classification is the better description of the status of the child? What would be the implications of a particular classification for clinical service delivery for the child?

3. A learner of English as a second language is concerned that others cannot easily understand his or her language. This language learner reports that others often ask for repetition or clarification of his or her comments and that, even after these additional productions, others continue to find his or her language unclear. How would you determine whether this language learner presents with a "disorder" versus a "difference" in language? Would it ever be possible for a person to present with both conditions? Under what circumstances?

REFERENCES

American Psychiatric Association. (2000). *Diagnostic and statistical manual of mental disorders (DSM-IV-TR)*. Arlington, VA: Author.

American Speech-Language-Hearing Association. (1991). *Prevention of communication disorders tutorial* [relevant paper]. Retrieved May 12, 2010, from http://www.asha.org/docs/html/PS1988-00228.html

American Speech-Language-Hearing Association. (2003). *American English dialects* [technical report]. Retrieved May 12, 2010, from http://www.asha.org/docs/html/TR2003-00044.html

American Speech-Language-Hearing Association. (2003). *Code of ethics* [ethics]. Retrieved May 12, 2010, from http://www.asha.org/docs/html/ET2010-00309.html

American Speech-Language-Hearing Association. (2007). *Scope of practice in speech-language pathology* [scope of practice]. Retrieved May 12, 2010, from http://www.asha.org/docs/html/SP2007-00283.html

American Speech-Language-Hearing Association Ad Hoc Committee on Service Delivery in the Schools. (1993). Definitions of communication disorders and variations. *ASHA, 35*(suppl. 10), 40–41.

Anderson, N. B., & Shames, G. H. (2005). *Human communication disorders: an introduction* (7th ed.). Boston, MA: Allyn & Bacon.

Cole, L., & Marge, M. (1985). Prevention: A challenge for the profession. In *Prevention of speech, language, and hearing disorders*. Rockville, MD: American Speech-Language-Hearing Association.

Gerber, S. E. (1990). *Prevention: The etiology of communicative disorders in children*. Englewood Cliffs, NJ: Prentice-Hall.

Holmes, J. (2001). *An introduction to sociolinguistics* (2nd ed.). New York, NY: Longman.

Hudson, R. A. (1980). *Sociolinguistics*. Cambridge, UK: Cambridge University Press.

Kavanagh, J. (1982). The prevention of speech-language and hearing problems. *Journal of the National Student Speech-Language-Hearing Association, 10*(1), 16–22.

Kilburg, G. (1985). Communicative wellness model. In *Prevention of speech, language, and hearing disorders*. Rockville, MD: American Speech-Language-Hearing Association.

Lahey, M., & Edwards, J. (1995). Specific language impairment: preliminary investigation of factors associated with family history and with patterns of language performance. *Journal of Speech and Hearing Research, 38*, 643–657.

Marge, M. (1984). Prevention: A challenge for the profession. *ASHA, 26*, 35–37.

McWhorter, J. (2000). *Spreading the word: Language and dialect in America*. Portsmouth, NH: Heinemann.

Nicolosi, L., Harryman, E., & Kresheck, J. (2004). *Terminology of communication disorders: Speech-language-hearing* (5th ed.). Philadelphia, PA: Lippincott Williams & Wilkins.

Objer, L. K., & Gjerlow, K. (1999). *Language and the brain*. Cambridge, UK: Cambridge University Press.

Owens, R. E., Metz, D. W., & Haas, A. (2006). *Introduction to communication disorders: A lifespan perspective* (3rd ed.). Boston, MA: Allyn & Bacon.

Plante, E. M., & Beeson, P. M. (2007). *Communication and communication disorders: An introduction* (3rd ed.). Boston, MA: Allyn & Bacon.

Plomin, R. (October, 2002). *Genetics of language and cognitive impairment: GLI (general language impairment) in addition to SLI (specific language impairment)*. Presented to the workshop on SLI, Genes, Development, and Cognitive Neuroscience, London, UK.

Rice, M. L., & Warren, S. F. (Eds.). (2004). *Developmental language disorders: From phenotypes to etiologies*. Mahwah, NJ: Lawrence Erlbaum Associates.

Ron, M. A., & Robbins, T. A. (2003). *Disorders of the brain and mind* (Vol. 2). Cambridge, UK: Cambridge University Press.

Weiss, L., & Lillywhite, H. (1981). *Communication disorders: Prevention and early intervention*. St. Louis, MO: Mosby.

Wolfram, W. (1991). *Dialects and American English*. Englewood Cliffs, NJ: Prentice-Hall.

Wolfram, W., Adger, C. T., & Christian, D. (1999). *Dialects in schools and communities*. Mahweh, NJ: Lawrence Erlbaum Associates.

Wolfram, W., & Fasold, R. W. (1974). *The study of American dialects*. Englewood Cliffs, NJ: Prentice-Hall.

Wolfram, W., & Schilling-Estes, N. (1998). *American English: Dialects and variation*. Malden, MA: Basic Backwell.

World Health Organization. (1980). The WHO classification of impairments, disabilities, and handicaps. *The WHO Chronicle, 34*, 376–380.

World Health Organization. (1990). *International statistical classification of diseases and related health problems*. Geneva, Switzerland: Author.

World Health Organization. (2001). *International classification of functioning, disability, and health*. Geneva, Switzerland: Author.

CHAPTER 7

Clinical Service Delivery for Children With Language Delays and Disorders

INTRODUCTION

As members of the speech-language pathologist (SLP) discipline, we provide care for individuals with communication disorders, as well as disorders related to the function of the communication mechanism, such as the swallow. Particular areas of specialization within our discipline include language, typical language, atypical language, and clinical service delivery for those who have concerns related to language. The national professional association, the American Speech-Language-Hearing Association (ASHA), states in the Scope of Practice (2007):

As primary care providers for communication, swallowing, or other upper aerodigestive disorders, speech-language pathologists are autonomous professionals; that is, their services need not be prescribed or supervised by individuals in other professions. However, in many cases, individuals are best served when speech-language pathologists work collaboratively with other professionals. (p. 5)

The ASHA Code of Ethics echoes this theme with ethical mandates to consider the welfare of those whom we serve as paramount and to continue to pursue opportunities that will best serve

their needs (ASHA, 2003). Clinical service provision for patients and cooperation with professionals from other disciplines who share our concern for patients are paramount aims for us. Because of that, an overview of standards on which clinical service provision for those with language delays and disorders is based is now in order.

CLINICAL PRACTICE STANDARDS: DEFINITION OF SLP

The United States Department of Labor (2010, classification 29-1127) defines speech-language pathology (SLP) with an overview of the nature of the discipline:

Speech-language pathologists assess and treat persons with speech, language, voice, and fluency disorders . . . Speech-language pathologists work with people who cannot make speech sounds, or cannot make them clearly; those with speech rhythm and fluency problems, such as stuttering; people with speech quality problems, such as inappropriate pitch or harsh voice; and those with problems understanding and producing language. They may also work with people who have oral motor problems that cause eating and swallowing difficulties.

After this overview to the populations whom SLPs serve appears an overview of the nature of interdisciplinary relationships (USDOL, 2010, classification 29-1127):

Most speech-language pathologists and audiologists provide direct clinical services to individuals with communication disorders. In speech, language, and hearing clinics, they may independently develop and carry out a treatment program. In medical facilities, they may work with physicians, social workers, psychologists and other therapists to develop and execute a treatment plan. Speech-language pathology . . . personnel in schools also develop individual or group programs, counsel parents, and assist teachers with classroom activities, to meet the needs of children with speech, language, or hearing disorders.

This overview, extracted from the more extensive definition, establishes SLPs as clinical service providers for people with a diverse variety of conditions related to communication or to the communication mechanism. Various clinical practice standards dictate the nature of the services that SLPs provide to a diverse variety of clinical populations.

CLINICAL PRACTICE STANDARDS: ASHA CODE OF ETHICS

Clinical practice and research are based on a collection of ethical principles that, although not expressed in the same words, are shared across clinical practice disciplines. These principles are the bases for the provisions within the ASHA Code of Ethics (2010). This document contains a preamble, followed by four specific principles of ethics, each of which is exemplified in specific rules of ethics.

Principle I

Individuals shall hold paramount the welfare of persons they serve professionally or participants in research or scholarly activities and shall treat animals involved in research in a humane manner.

From this ideal stems the principles of competence in clinical practice; referral to appropriate professionals, as warranted; nondiscrimination in service provision; accurate representation of professional credentials; appropriate distribution of clinical practice duties to credentialed individuals; disclosure of accurate information about clinical services; incorporation of measurement of treatment effectiveness into service provision; restriction of service provision to appropriate venues; maintenance of confidential, accurate clinical documentation; and withdrawal from clinical practice should situations arise that compromise practice standards. When we consider the partnerships that we establish with parents and professionals, we certainly observe how very applicable this principle of ethics can be, particularly with respect to the referral of our clinical patients to other service providers whose expertise can enhance our own.

Principle II

Individuals shall honor their responsibility to achieve and maintain the highest level of professional competence.

From this ideal stems the principles of clinical service provision commensurate with SLP level of competence; pursuit of professional development over the course of a career; restriction of service provision to appropriate practitioners; and maintenance of current equipment and other clinical materials. Our partnerships with other service providers include aides and SLP assistants, whose involvement in the clinical service delivery process can enhance and expand our services to our clinical patients, provided that we take steps to ensure that the duties of aides and SLP assistants occur within the appropriate professional boundaries and supervision.

Principle III

Individuals shall honor their responsibility to the public by promoting public understanding of the professions, by supporting the development of services designed to fulfill the unmet needs of the public, and by providing accurate information in all communications involving any aspect of the professions, including dissemination of research findings and scholarly activities.

From this ideal stems the principles of accurate representation of credentials, contributions, and competence; avoidance of professional conflict of interest situations; dissemination of accurate information about communication disorders in public venues; and maintenance of acceptable professional standards. This principle of ethics establishes our role as community educators whose role is more expansive than clinical service delivery alone. The mandate to present accurate information about ourselves, our discipline, and our services contributes to prevention of communication disorders, creation of further opportunities for partnerships, protection of the public from inaccurate or incomplete information and inappropriate services, and maintenance of professional standards.

Principle IV

Individuals will honor their responsibilities to the professions and their relationships to colleagues, students, and members of allied professions. Individuals shall uphold the dignity and autonomy of the professions, maintain harmonious interprofessional and intraprofessional relationships, and accept the professions' self-imposed standards.

From this idea stems the principles of maintenance of professional standards; avoidance of personal conflict of interest situations; award of appropriate credit for research contributions, formulate independent clinical decisions; and protection of the intellectual property of others. When we consider the partnerships that we establish with parents and professionals, we certainly observe how very applicable this principle of ethics can be, particularly with respect to the appreciation for both the independence of our discipline and our interdependent relationships with other service providers in endeavors that enhance our collective clinical services for our shared clinical patients. The mandate to formulate independent clinical decisions and, simultaneously, to interact with other service providers can only enhance the protection of all involved.

CLINICAL PRACTICE STANDARDS: ASHA SCOPE OF PRACTICE

The professional Code of Ethics described in the previous section is the philosophical basis for the ASHA Scope of Practice (2007), which delineates the professional boundaries for SLPs with respect to clinical service delivery roles and duties. In addition to this delineation, this document has other important purposes: (a) to educate current and potential clinical patients, as well as their service providers across other professional disciplines, about the nature of SLP clinical services, (b) to inform the sources of clinical rules (such as those in local, state, and federal licensure, certification, or accreditation boards), as well as the sources of clinical reimbursement, about the nature of SLP clinical services, (c) to provide the foundation for evidence-based clinical services for clinical patients across the life span, and (d) to direct the content of professional education curricula in SLP.

With respect to the Scope of Practice, some reminders are in order. Each SLP to whom the Scope of Practice applies has met the minimum standards for independent clinical practice. However, not every SLP demonstrates the same level of experience and competence with every standard inherent in the Scope of Practice. Thus, although an individual SLP may be authorized to practice in accordance with the provisions in this document, not every SLP is able to practice with the same level of competence for each clinical population or each clinical service delineated therein. And, of course, the SLP must practice in accordance with the current state licensure laws in place in the state or commonwealth in which he or she resides, which may or may not be identical to the Scope of Practice. As the depth and breadth of the clinical services approved in this document continues to expand, more SLPs choose to focus their practice in particular areas of expertise. Provided that the clinical practice of any particular SLP resides within the boundaries in the Scope of Practice, then he or she has acted in accordance with the Code of Ethics.

CLINICAL PRACTICE STANDARDS: ASHA PREFERRED PRACTICE PATTERNS

The professional Scope of Practice described in the previous section is the philosophical basis for the ASHA Preferred Practice Patterns Statement (2004a). This document delineates the nature of clinical services to screen, assess, intervene, and consult with respect to potential communication disorders in individuals. This document also delineates the specific considerations to ensure safe clinical practice to maintain the health of our clinical patients, as well as to ensure the confidential nature of our clinical documentation. The Preferred Practice Patterns Statement describes each possible clinical service that an SLP could provide. As a means to describe the depth and breadth of SLP services for a specific population—children with language concerns—we now extract and overview these provisions here. As we have extracted only selected provisions, we have numbered them in a fashion that positions related services in close proximity. Thus, these numbers do not correspond with those in the actual practice statement.

Prevention Services

Process: This clinical task allows the SLP to address the conditions that could cause, contribute to, or complicate communication disorders. In this task, the SLP aims to prevent the onset of a disorder, minimize the impact of risk factors on communication, and provide accommodations to compensate for risk factors. *Initiation:* The SLP initiates prevention when an individual presents with risk factors and when the SLP concludes that prevention will enhance the communication of the patient or at least the extent to which the patient can accommodate to communication limitations. Prevention also involves consultation and education to individual patients and to broader audiences (ASHA, 1988, 1991). *Result:* The expected result will be reduced risk factors and/or the formulation of appropriate referrals to appropriate service providers.

Speech-Language Screening (Children)

Process: This clinical task allows for the identification of infants, toddlers, children, and adolescents who, because of their patterns of communication, require more comprehensive evaluation to determine the present status of their communication and/or referral to other appropriate service providers. *Initiation:* This task is initiated when the families of children have concerns or when children present

with risk factors related to communication disorders (ASHA, 1988). *Result:* The screening result will be Pass/No Pass in nature.

Speech-Language Screening (Adults)

Process: This clinical task allows for the identification of adults who, because of their patterns of communication, require more comprehensive evaluation to determine the present status of their communication and/or referral to other appropriate service providers. *Initiation:* This task is initiated when families of adults—or the adults themselves—have concerns or when adults present with risk factors related to communication disorders (e.g., the presence of a childhood language concern that remains unresolved in adulthood) (ASHA, 1988). *Result:* The screening result will be Pass/No Pass in nature.

Comprehensive Speech-Language Assessment

Process: This clinical task allows for the in-depth description of speech and language status of a clinic patient, as well as the identification of related conditions, functional limitations, and environmental factors that have the potential to enhance communication improvement. *Initiation:* This task is initiated upon request, as well as when the medical and/or the educational status of a patient indicates a potential disorder. *Result:* The assessment result will include a diagnosis of a speech and/or a language condition, as well as an indication of how severe the condition is, descriptions of the speech and/or language characteristics the patient presents, a prognosis for eventual improvement of the condition, recommendations for the eventual intervention process, and referrals to other service providers, as needed.

Communication Assessment— Infants and Toddlers

Process: This clinical task allows for the description of communication skills in children and the status of the precursors that contribute to these skills. *Initiation:* This task is initiated upon request, as well as when identified risk factors exist that mandate sustained attention to the communication development of the child (ASHA, 2004b, 2004c, 2004d, 2004e). *Result:* The assessment result will include a diagnosis of a speech and/or a language condition, or at least identification of risk factors that are related to the presence of such a condition. To supplement this diagnosis, the SLP will discuss recommendations, which include descriptions of the systems that influence the communication of the child and referrals for services from other clinical practitioners.

Communication Assessment—Preschool

Process: This clinical task allows for the description of communication in children to determine the potential impact of communication development level on social interaction and academic performance. *Initiation:* This task is initiated upon request or when the status of other areas (e.g., medical or developmental) appears conducive to the appearance of a communication disorder. *Result:* The assessment result will include a diagnosis of a speech and/or a language condition, as well as prognosis for improvement, recommendations for intervention, and referral for other services when deemed appropriate.

Spoken and Written Language Assessment— Children and Adolescents

Process: This clinical task allows for the evaluation of spoken and written modalities of language and the extent to which function in these areas limits participation in various endeavors and contexts. *Initiation:* This task is initiated upon request or when the status of speech and language appears to compromise educational performance across academic disciplines and/or social interaction with peers in educational and other contexts (ASHA, 2001, 2002a). *Result:* The assessment result will include a diagnosis of a spoken and/or a written language condition, a description of the relative status of spoken versus written modalities as well as skill areas

within the modalities, recommendations for intervention and classroom modifications, and referral for other services when deemed appropriate.

Severe Communication Impairment Assessment

Process: This clinical task involves the evaluation of the clinic patient who presents with severe restrictions on communication. *Initiation:* This task is initiated when unconventional and/or maladaptive communication behaviors severely restrict functional communication competence and thus complete participation in daily interactions. This task also is initiated when the medical status of the clinic patient indicates the potential for further deterioration of communication systems (ASHA, 2002b, 2004f, 2004g). *Result:* The assessment will result in the identification of the effectiveness of behaviors intended to compensate for communication limitations, contextual modifications that could enhance the communication process, and alternate communication systems that could expand the depth and breadth of communication options.

Augmentative and Alternative Communication (AAC) Assessment

Process: This clinical task involves the evaluation of the clinic patient for whom AAC appears to be the most viable communication option, at least at the present time. *Initiation:* This task is initiated upon request, as well as when a clinic patient has presented with structural and functional limitations exist that so severely compromise spoken language production that the prognosis for eventual spoken language is guarded (ASHA, 2002b, 2004f, 2004g). *Result:* The results of this evaluation will inform a recommendation for appropriate AAC procedures and devices to either supplement or replace spoken language across the communication contexts in which the clinic patient is most often a participant. Referral to other service providers whose expertise is crucial for the determination and construction of the most appropriate AAC system also is a result of this assessment process.

Speech-Language Assessment for Individuals Who Are Bilingual and/or Learning English as an Additional Language

Process: This clinical task involves the evaluation of those who possess some level of competence in multiple languages to determine the relative strength of those languages. *Initiation:* This task is initiated upon request, as well as when questions arise as to the level of language competence in one or more languages (ASHA 2004h, 2004i). *Results:* The assessment will provide a comparative description of a first language (L1) with a second or a subsequent language (L2). This description includes establishment of language dominance, as well as the description of the relative functional skill across the areas within each language. This description can inform a conclusion as to whether a language difference or a language disorder exists. This description also addresses the implications of language status for social and educational competence in both languages.

Communication Intervention— Infants and Toddlers

Process: This clinical task allows for the provision of services for children with either documented communication disorders or risk factors that increase the likelihood of such disorders. *Initiation:* This task is initiated upon request, as well as when the results of evaluations indicate a compromise in the status of the language development of the child. This task also is initiated when identified risks are present that have substantial potential to compromise development (ASHA, 1990). *Result:* A successful intervention result includes enhanced status of prelinguistic skills, as well as intact emergence of linguistic skills and enhanced family participation in the language development process.

Communication Intervention—Preschool

Process: This clinical task allows for the provision of services for children with documented communication disorders or risk factors that increase the likelihood of such disorders, particularly in the transition from spoken to written modality. *Initiation:*

This task is initiated upon request, as well as when mandated because of results of previous assessment. Indications such as decreased academic performance and compromised social competence can indicate the need for specific approaches to intervention (ASHA, 2002). *Results:* A successful intervention result includes improvement in the structures and functions that underlie communication development, as well as the enhancement of the participation of the child in the classroom and in social interactions. Modification of contextual factors to enhance communication success may also result, as may referrals to other service providers for assistance to complement the intervention process.

Spoken and Written Language Intervention— Children and Adolescents

Process: This task is initiated on request, as well as when mandated because of results of previous assessment. *Initiation:* Indications such as decreased academic performance and compromised social competence can indicate the need for specific approaches to intervention (ASHA, 2000, 2002). *Results:* A successful intervention result enhances participation of the clinic patient in social, educational, and vocational activities. Intervention also results in enhanced use of language for listening, speaking, reading, writing, and thinking. In addition, intervention equalizes the level of competence between spoken and written modalities and teaches appropriate forms of compensation for deficits that remain in these modalities. Services from practitioners from other disciplines can complement this process of accommodation for deficits.

Severe Communication Impairment Intervention

Process: This task is initiated on request, as well as when mandated because of results of previous assessment. *Initiation:* Indications such as decreased participation in day-to-day interactions, as well as limited expression of basic wants and needs, can indicate the need for this intervention, as can self-injurious and other maladaptive behaviors that can compromise patient health and welfare (ASHA

2002b, 2004f, 2004g). *Results:* A course of intervention can transform present behaviors into more
conventional communication behaviors to results
in more socially effective and appropriate interaction. Intervention also can reveal the need for referrals to other service providers.

Service 15: Augmentative and Alternative Communication (AAC) Intervention

Process: This task is initiated when the results of
a previous AAC assessment indicate that attempts
at production of spoken language should be augmented or replaced with another process. *Initiation:* Indications such as increased effectiveness of
communication with the use of augmented or alternate methods support this course of intervention
(ASHA 2002b, 2004f, 2004g). *Results:* A course of
intervention can expand the contexts for interaction,
as well as expand the scope of content that an AAC
user can comprehend and produce. Intervention
can also educate potential conversational partners
as to the protocol for communication via AAC, as
well as about methods to address communication
breakdowns, either with AAC devices and methods
or factors related to the participants themselves.

Elective Communication Modification

Process: This task is initiated when an individual who
does not present with a communication disorder
wishes to participate in clinical services to enhance
the present status of his or her communication
(ASHA, 1983). *Initiation:* Communication modification is appropriate to address needs related to
communication effectiveness, communication apprehension, and public and interpersonal communication skills. *Results:* Communication modification can
enhance access to communication contexts in which
the clinic patient experiences actual or perceived
difficulty in interactions or presentations. Such
access can, in turn, enhance actual performance
levels across areas of communication skill, which
include self-monitoring and self-correcting, as well
as discerning the needs of specific communication
contexts and adapting the content and structure of
communication to be compatible with these needs.

In addition to these evaluation and intervention services, the Preferred Practice Standards document notes other professional roles for SLPs that
permeate attention to specific disorder conditions.
Two of these roles are *consultation*, which is
described in Chapter 8 as it relates to intervention,
and *counseling.* The opportunities to counsel with
clinic patients and their families are frequent in the
course of clinical service delivery. The SLP may provide *informational counseling* for patients and
families. In this approach, the SLP serves as educa-
tor in the provision and discussion of materials
about normal and non-normal communication, as
well as in the presentation of seminars and other
educational events. The SLP may also provide *supportive counseling* for patients and families.
Because SLPs are not counselors in the traditional
sense, their role in the discussion and resolution of
personal issues is primarily one of referral to appropriate mental health service providers whose expertise encompasses this role. Instead, the SLP serves as
advocate in the process of formulation of creative
solutions to address issues that arise with respect to
clinical service delivery and related areas. In this
role, the SLP may facilitate the involvement of
patients and families in appropriate support circles
and may even serve as a consultant for these circles.
In addition to consulting with and counseling
patients and families, the document also includes a
provision for SLP participation in follow-up procedures. These services, which can be diverse, occur
at predetermined times or on a predictable schedule and may occur by institutional mandate or as
an optional component of evaluation and/or intervention. Participation in these follow-up services
confirms that the care of the SLP for patients and
families does not end once a specific clinical
appointment ends but, instead, extends to the level
needed to ensure appropriate quality of continued
care for the needs of those individuals.

CLINICAL PRACTICE STANDARDS: WHO CONCEPTUAL FRAMEWORK

We would be remiss if we described SLP clinical
service delivery in the United States in a vacuum.
Those who present with communication disorders

do not live only in this country, nor do those who serve their needs. We must position our perspectives on clinical service delivery in relationship with a worldwide perspective, that provided by the WHO (2001). In the WHO ICF (*International Classification of Functioning, Disability, and Health*), which we described in Chapter 6, are the components of a framework that places clinical service delivery into a broader model of *body structures and functions* and *activities and participation*. The concept of *body structures* includes the components of the anatomic structures of the body, whereas the concept of *body functions* includes physiologic and psychological functions of body systems. With respect to structures and functions, SLPs contribute to the identification of structural and functional conditions that influence the communication effectiveness of our clinical patient. The concept of *activities* refers to the performance of tasks and actions, whereas the concept of *participation* refers to the involvement of a clinic patient in the situations that comprise his or her typical way of life. With respect to activities and participation, SLPs contribute to the evaluation of the communication demands present in the environment of our clinical patient; the identification of the extent to which our clinical patient can participate in social, educational, and/or vocational activities; the formulation of means to enhance participation in such activities in the presence of communication limitations; the identification of contextual factors that constitute barriers to or, in contrast, means to enhance successful communication; the formulation of a prognosis for improvement in communication competence and/or the contexts in which communication occurs; the consideration of appropriate referrals to other clinical service providers whose expertise can enhance the participation of our shared clinical patient in selected activities; the measurement of clinical outcomes to ascertain the quantity and quality of care and to enhance the quality of clinical services; and the completion of appropriate follow-up services to measure clinical patient status over a sustained period of time.

The WHO ICF also specifies the difference between *capacity for performance* (i.e., the extent to which a patient can execute tasks and actions within standardized and/or uniform environments) and *performance* (i.e., the level of performance of a patient within his or her current environment). In

addition, the WHO ICF specifies factors that influence whether the performance is indeed equivalent to the capacity for performance. Although the *environmental factors* constitute the environment (physical, social, attitude) in which a clinical patient lives, the *personal factors* include personal characteristics that influence the outcomes of clinical services. A review of the ASHA Scope of Practice and ASHA Preferred Practice Standards documents, as well as the position statements and technical reports that further delineate clinical practice standards, reveal the pervasive influence of the WHO model on our perspective and our approaches for clinical service delivery.

CLINICAL SERVICE DELIVERY: MODELS FOR CLINICAL PRACTICE

The Unidisciplinary Model

Description: In some cases, an SLP may be the sole clinical service provider for a patient. This model is the *unidisciplinary model* for clinical practice. Consider a person for whom English is a second language who presents with an accent. The present clinical practice standards of our discipline do not consider the presence of this accented speech a communication disorder and thus do not mandate the pursuit of intervention services for this person. However, consider that this person may have a specific reason to pursue this option. Perhaps he or she desires multiple options for communication that competence in multiple accents or dialects would provide, such as a person who wishes to become a local theatrical performer. Perhaps he or she desires closer observable identification with peers who communicate with a particular accent or dialect, such as someone who has moved to a new area and wishes to produce a less distinctive language pattern. Perhaps he or she wishes to pursue professional options that consider the presence of a standard dialect to be an asset in communication, such as a person who strives toward a career in broadcast journalism. In cases such as these, the SLP may very well be the sole professional whom the patient consults for assistance.

Discussion: In the event that the SLP is indeed competent to address the communication issues that arise, implementation of a unidisciplinary model may be the most appropriate choice for clinical service delivery. With that said, however, SLPs do not often practice in such an isolated fashion. The demands of our clinical service delivery to our clinical patients underscore our mandate to secure information about the evaluation and intervention services provided to our shared patients by other clinical practitioners, as well as to coordinate our services so that our attempts to enrich the communication of our patients are not at cross-purposes with each other. Toward that end, we now present an overview of three models for clinical practice (Koury, 2007) in which SLPs, by virtue of our clinical practice sites, duties, and/or caseloads, may participate.

The Multidisciplinary Model

Description: In the *multidisciplinary model*, an SLP is one of multiple clinical practitioners who serve the patient in question. In this model, the patient pursues evaluation and/or intervention services from these practitioners. In some cases, the patient has initiated the contact with practitioners based on his or her perception, which he or she formed out of information from varied sources, that this professional can provide appropriate clinical services for his or her needs. In some other cases, however, the patient has initiated the contact with practitioners based on recommendations from one or more practitioners that the patient consult with others. In this model, each practitioner operates in a fashion independent from the others. While each can indeed be aware that the patient has consulted multiple service providers, no process exists for the coordination of care unless the patient himself or herself imposes a framework onto the process that allows him or her to systematically interpret and relate clinical information, recommendations, and services to each other.

Discussion: The *multidisciplinary model* is an appropriate model for the patient who presents with multiple, unrelated conditions that necessitate services from providers whose clinical practices do not tend to intersect. This model, however, is not appropriate for the patient who presents a condition that demands, by its nature, the attention of related disciplines. Sometimes the choice to pursue this model is based on convenience. The administrative structure of many clinical facilities is not conducive to the presence of interdisciplinary or transdisciplinary teams and thus, by default, provide more opportunities for independent appointments with providers than intertwined services. The pursuit of services from such disciplines results in increased potential for redundant services or, in contrast, contradictions in service provision that stem from the various theoretical perspectives and practices of the service providers. The presence of contradictions can then result in confusion for the patient, who may not possess sufficient familiarity with a broad variety of theoretical perspectives that would allow him or her to ascertain the relative value of varied approaches to clinical practice.

The Interdisciplinary Model

Description: In the *interdisciplinary model*, a team of clinical practitioners serves the needs of the clinical patient. Some clinics are home to evaluation and intervention teams, as the existence of teams is representative of the standard clinical service provision of that site. In these clinics, the service providers may be housed in the clinic as staff members or, in contrast, may be available as consultants to the clinic on an as-needed basis. In either case, the presence of specific disciplines in the clinical service delivery process is assured. In contrast to these clinics, some clinics are not home to teams. However, in these instances, either the patient or a professional with expertise relevant to the concerns of the patient takes the initiative to constitute a team with a structural and/or a functional existence.

The team is composed of the professionals whose expertise appears relevant to the most prominent needs of the patient. In one sense, the interdisciplinary team members are independent, in that each one provides the evaluation and/or intervention services in a fashion consistent with the clinical practice standards of his or her discipline. In one sense, however, the interdisciplinary team members are interdependent, as their contributions receive coordination from the professional who serves as the team leader. This leader may be the professional who, in the administrative structure of a clinic, has the authority for team coordination. Or, should the administrative structure have no such provision for authority to be invested in one professional, this leader may be the professional whose expertise is most closely related to the primary concerns of the patient. In either case, this leader coordinates the service delivery process in such respects as the establishment of the appointments, the recommendations with respect to the content of the evaluation appointments, the receipt and review of the evaluation documentation, the presentation and clarification of the evaluation results and recommendations, the resolution of discrepancies in evaluation conclusions, the recommendations with respect to the content of the intervention appointments, the receipt and review of the intervention documentation, the presentation and clarification of the intervention results and recommendations, and the resolution of discrepancies in intervention conclusions. In short, while this model certainly does not preclude direct contact between the patient and individual service providers over the course of evaluation and intervention, the team leader is the primary liaison between the various team members and the patient and his or her family, as appropriate.

Discussion: The *interdisciplinary model* is appropriate for the patient who presents with multiple related conditions or, in addition, a condition for which input from multiple service providers is desirable. If a clinic does not house an interdisciplinary team, the patient and/or a specific service provider are responsible for the creation of a team, which may prove problematic when service providers from particular disciplines are unavailable in local clinics or when appointments with multiple service providers are unavailable within a convenient time frame. As a liaison, the team leader is faced with the task of appreciation for and interpretation of the roles and responsibilities of multiple disciplines, as well as with the resolution of discrepancies in conclusions across service providers. This places a substantial burden on the team leader to interpret and represent ideas and information in as balanced and accurate a fashion as possible.

The Transdisciplinary Model

Description: The *transdisciplinary model*, as was the case for the previous two models, includes a team of clinical practitioners who serve the needs of the clinical patient. As with the previous two

models, the structure of some clinics provides for the creation of such a team on an as-needed basis that consists of service providers internal and/or external to the site. Like the previous two models, the team is composed of the professionals whose expertise appears relevant. However, the approach of these professionals to address the needs of the patient is unique. In this model, the focus shifts from the traditional evaluation and/or intervention services of individual disciplines to a need-centered approach. In this perspective, the team leader and the clinical patient conceptualize the most central needs of the patient, then consider the professionals whose expertise would be most relevant to those specific needs. Thus, the team leader invites the participation of other service providers on the team not because their broad expertise is related to the broad condition of the patient but, instead, because their expertise with respect to a specific area is related to a specific need of the patient, and multiple professionals can provide input as to this specific need. Thus, the task for team participants is not the provision of comprehensive evaluation and intervention services but, instead, the provision of focused information that is combined with the information from other participants to paint the most complete picture of a need that is possible. The team leader collects, compares and contrasts, and conceptualizes the information team participants provide to provide a comprehensive overview of the present status and appropriate recommendations for the patient in a need-by-need approach rather than a discipline-by-discipline approach.

Discussion: The *transdisciplinary model* is appropriate for the patient who presents with multiple related conditions or, in addition, a condition for which input from multiple service providers is desirable. It is most effective when the team leader and the patient can easily identify specific needs which these providers can address in a focused fashion. If a clinic does not house a transdisciplinary team, the creation of a team may prove problematic for the reasons discussed in the overview of the interdisciplinary model. And the coordination of a team may raise the same issues for the team leader discussed in the overview of the interdisciplinary model. In addition to these considerations, the autonomy of the team members can become a serious issue. When a team member receives a request to focus only on a particular concern, he or she may find the request incompatible with his or her own clinical practice standards that mandate that evaluation and intervention services include specific components as standard practice. In this case, the team leader must respect professional autonomy and simultaneously draw from the information of this team member the details relevant to the need at hand. When a team member receives a request to focus on a particular concern about which other service providers will also provide information, he or she may be faced with the issue of shared practice standards and be reluctant to relinquish some of his or her professional autonomy to embrace similar expertise in service providers from other disciplines. In this case, the team leader must respect professional boundaries at the same time that he or she values the perspectives represented in the various disciplines who share the concern for a patient but may approach service delivery differently.

CONCLUSION

For those who are unfamiliar with the depth and breadth of the roles and responsibilities of SLPs, this chapter has provided an overview of the dimensions of clinical practice and the principles which have permeated this endeavor. Although SLPs provide primary care for the speech and language concerns that patients present, this care does not occur in a vacuum. Instead, it occurs as a component of complex relationships across professionals with shared interests and commitments, as well as shared, yet distinctive, areas of experience and expertise. To complement the broad overview of evaluation and intervention in this chapter, Chapter 8 presents some specific elements of these processes to elaborate on the clinical practice endeavors described here.

REFLECTION QUESTIONS

1. What are ethics? Why is it so vital that clinical practice—not only in speech-language pathology, but in any discipline—be based on ethical principles?

2. What is a scope of practice for a discipline? Why is it so vital that the parameters of clinical practice be determined by national or international rather than by local practice standards?

3. What are the broad dimensions of clinical practice represented in a preferred practice standards document? Why is the redundancy inherent in how these standards are presented (both in terms of content and structure) a desirable trait of such a document?

4. What are the central tenets of the models of clinical practice presented in this chapter? What constitute the advantages and the disadvantages of each of these models?

5. If you are a non-SLP, what are your roles in clinical service provision for clinical patients with various communication disorders?

APPLICATION EXERCISES

1. The parents of a child are concerned that their child may have a communication disorder. However, they live in a remote area, and they cannot easily access the services of clinical practitioners whose expertise could be helpful for their child. The parents have approached you for advice. With attention to ethical considerations, how would you advise these parents in their quest to secure appropriate services for their child?

2. The parents of a child have scheduled an evaluation for their child that is multidisciplinary, interdisciplinary, or transdisciplinary in nature. As these approaches to clinical service delivery are unfamiliar to them, they have asked you to describe each of these so that they can know what kinds of interactions to expect. How would you describe each of these approaches in a concrete way to prepare them for the experience?

3. Multidisciplinary, interdisciplinary, and transdisciplinary approaches to treatment typically involve a diversity of services from multiple providers. The coordination of such services is of utmost importance to enhance treatment effectiveness. What factors would you advise a

family to consider with respect to the order of various dimensions of treatment (e.g., simultaneous versus sequential services)?

REFERENCES

American Speech-Language-Hearing Association. (1983). Social dialects and implications of the position on social dialects. *ASHA, 25*, 23–27.

American Speech-Language-Hearing Association. (1988). Prevention of communication disorders. *ASHA, 30*(3), 90.

American Speech-Language-Hearing Association. (1990). The roles of speech-language pathologists in service delivery to infants, toddlers, and their families. *ASHA, 32*(Suppl. 2), 4.

American Speech-Language-Hearing Association. (1991). The prevention of communication disorders tutorial. *ASHA, 33*(Suppl. 6), 15–41.

American Speech-Language-Hearing Association. (2000). *Guidelines for the roles and responsibilities of the school-based speech-language pathologist.* Rockville, MD: Author.

American Speech-Language-Hearing Association. (2001). Roles and responsibilities of speech-language pathologists with respect to reading and writing in children and adolescents (position statement, executive summary of guidelines, technical report). *ASHA Supplement, 21*, 17–28.

American Speech-Language-Hearing Association. (2002a). Knowledge and skills needed by speech-language pathologists with respect to reading and writing in children and adolescents. *ASHA 2002 Desk Reference, 3*, 455–464.

American Speech-Language-Hearing Association. (2002b). Augmentative and alternative communication: Knowledge and skills for service delivery. *ASHA Supplement, 22*, 97–106.

American Speech-Language-Hearing Association. (2004a). *Preferred practice standards for the profession of speech-language pathology.* Available May 14, 2010, from http://www.asha.org/docs/html/PP2004-00191.html

American Speech-Language-Hearing Association. (2004b). Knowledge and skills needed by speech-language pathologists providing services to infants and families in the NICU environment. *ASHA Supplement, 24*, 159–165.

American Speech-Language-Hearing Association. (2004c). *Roles of speech-language pathologists in the neonatal intensive care unit: Guidelines.* Retrieved May 14, 2010, from http://www.asha.org/docs/html/PS2004-00111.html

American Speech-Language-Hearing Association. (2004d). Roles of speech-language pathologists in the neonatal intensive care unit: Position statement. *ASHA Supplement, 24*, 60–61.

American Speech-Language-Hearing Association. (2004e). Roles of speech-language pathologists in the neonatal intensive care unit: Technical report. *ASHA Supplement, 24*, 121–130.

American Speech-Language-Hearing Association. (2004f). *Roles and responsibilities of speech-language pathologists with respect to augmentative and alternative communication: Position statement.* Retrieved May 14, 2010, from http://www.asha.org/docs/html/PS2005-00113.html

American Speech-Language-Hearing Association. (2004g). Roles and responsibilities of speech-language pathologists with respect to augmentative and alternative communication: Technical report. *ASHA Supplement, 24*, 93–95.

American Speech-Language-Hearing Association. (2004h). *Cultural competence.* Retrieved May 14, 2010, from http://www.asha.org/docs/html/ET2005-00174.html

American Speech-Language-Hearing Association. (2004i). Knowledge and skills needed by speech-language pathologists and audiologists to provide culturally and linguistically appropriate services. *ASHA Supplement, 24*, 152–158.

American Speech-Language-Hearing Association. (2007). *Scope of practice in speech-language pathology.* Retrieved May 14, 2010, from http://www.asha.org/docs/html/SP2007-00283.html

American Speech-Language-Hearing Association. (2010). *Code of ethics.* Retrieved May 14, 2010, from http://www.asha.org/docs/html/ET2010-00309.html

Koury, L. N. (2007). Service delivery issues in early intervention. In R. Lubinski, L. A. C. Golper, & C. M. Frattali (Eds.), *Professional issues in speech-language pathology and audiology.* Clifton Park, NY: Thomson Delmar Learning.

United States Department of Labor. (2010). *Standard occupational classification.* Retrieved June 4, 2010, from http://www.bls.gov/soc/2010/soc291127.htm

World Health Organization. (2001). *International classification of functioning, disability, and health.* Geneva, Switzerland: Author.

CHAPTER 8

Evaluation and Intervention for Language Delays and Disorders

INTRODUCTION TO EVALUATION

In the course of our clinical practice, we have served children whose parents have presented us with three distinctive concerns. Sometimes a parent has no particular concerns but welcomes the opportunity to confirm that a child presents with normal language development. Sometimes, in contrast, a parent considers some aspects of language comprehension and/or production problematic and welcomes opinions of whether these are variations of normal or nonnormal language development. Sometimes a parent possesses confirmation of a delay or disorder and desires further descriptive information about particular areas of language skill. Whatever the situation, in each of these an evaluation of language is in order. In this chapter we present an overview of the common processes that constitute such an evaluation.

PROCESS OF LANGUAGE EVALUATION

The principles that dictate the course of an evaluation are constant across clinical practice sites. However, because clinical practice models are influenced, at least in part, by the administrative dictates within these sites, evaluation can unfold uniquely for each

site. Thus, the SLP evaluation within a medical context will contrast with that of an educational context through the professionals involved, procedures incorporated, composition and leadership of the evaluation team, and documentation. The process that we now describe is representative of evaluation in a community-based SLP clinic (Gunter, LeJeune, & Kurfuerst, 2005; LeJeune & Gunter, 2004, 2005; LeJeune, Gunter, & Kurfuerst, 2005, 2006).

Step 1: Review of Patient Concern

When parents schedule an evaluation appointment for their child, their contact includes the provision to the SLP of an encapsulated description of the language concern. Examples of these descriptions include, "Our child does not have a very substantial vocabulary in comparison with other children," "We find the speech of my child very hard to understand, even when we know what my child wants to say," and "Our child does not know how to participate in conversations with others very easily."

Step 2: Formulation of Clinical Hypotheses

As the SLP reviews the patient concern and formulates one or more clinical hypotheses of what the patient's condition could be. Suppose that the parent presented the concern, "I find the speech of my child very hard to understand . . . " The SLP formulates hypotheses as to the nature of the condition. Is this an articulation problem? If so, is this problem secondary to one of the craniofacial anomalies? Is this a phonological problem? If so, is this problem indicative of a broader language problem? Is this an apraxia? A dysarthria? Or even the result of a voice disorder? At this point, the SLP collates every reasonable potential explanation for the perceived status of the child.

Step 3: Review of Patient History

In preparation for the clinical evaluation, the parents provide detailed information related to the medical, developmental, familial, social, and educational history of their child. In some cases, this includes the results of evaluation and intervention services from other clinical service providers. Once the SLP determines the veracity of the history information, he or she reviews these details from the perspective of the clinical hypotheses. That is, the SLP determines which details serve to include or to exclude potential speech-language diagnoses. As the SLP does this, he or she plans evaluation methods that would permit him or her to collect additional information that may include or exclude additional potential diagnoses. In short, the SLP formulates clinical questions, then proceeds to attempt to answer these questions in the course of information collection.

Step 4: Preparation of Evaluation Plan

The SLP has multiple options from which to choose to collect evaluation information to answer the clinical questions: interviewing, sampling, testing, and combinations of these procedures. In addition, for any particular area within the broad scope of communication, the SLP has multiple options from which to choose to explore that dimension of information. Because the constraints of most evaluation appointments (e.g., time available) preclude the use of every possible means to obtain information, the SLP discerns which combination of methods will collect the best quantity and quality of available details, as well as the additional details that other clinical service providers can confirm.

Step 5: Collection of Evaluation Information

In the course of the evaluation appointment, the SLP collects clinical information in the most valid and reliable fashion possible in accordance with the evaluation plan. Although it is vital to structure the appointment in a systematic manner, it should not be so inflexible that it restricts the information collection process. As the appointment proceeds, the SLP may acquire details that necessitate the need to shift the direction of the information collection. At the conclusion of the appointment, the SLP will determine whether additional time, and another appointment, is necessary to collect a sufficient database from which to form clinical conclusions.

Step 6: Review of Clinical Hypotheses

Upon collection of clinical information, the SLP will determine the extent to which evidence supports each of the hypotheses that remain under consideration. At this point, the SLP may be able to systematically exclude every hypothesis except the correct conclusion with little to no difficulty. However, it would not be uncommon if multiple options remain to best describe the patients communication status. To the extent possible, the SLP will ascertain the likelihood of each potential diagnosis and the additional evidence that is necessary to continue to include or exclude each one of these.

Step 7: Formulation of Recommendations

At this point, even if multiple potential diagnoses remain, the SLP should possess sufficient information to formulate clinical recommendations. Certainly these can include the continued accumulation of clinical evidence to identify the correct diagnosis. At the same time, these can include preparing a treatment plan that addresses what appears at this time to be the most salient clinical needs for the patient. Even in the absence of a confirmed diagnosis, the descriptive information the SLP collects in the evaluation can paint a detailed picture of the areas of communication that are and are not intact and thus in need of clinical attention.

COLLECTION OF EVALUATION INFORMATION

It is true that across SLP evaluations, some information collection procedures are common and popular because of their potential to reveal crucial information. However, it is important to note that no standard protocol exists that dictates each specific procedure across every evaluation. Thus, rather than present an established outline for an evaluation, we describe the common evaluation procedures.

Evaluation Procedures: Screening

A screening (also described in Chapter 7) is a procedure that enables an SLP to place a child into one of three broad classifications: normal communication status, nonnormal communication status, or uncertain status at this time. A screening consists of a brief observation and conversation, and/or the administration of a brief screening test to a child. In a conclusion of *normal communication status*, an SLP concludes that evidence exists that a child *does* present communication skills within his or her developmental expectations. This conclusion does not assure those who care about the child that he or she will never present with a communication disorder, but rather indicates a normal status at this point in time. In contrast, in a conclusion of *nonnormal communication status*, an SLP concludes that evidence exists to confirm that a child *does not* present communication skills within his or her developmental expectations. A subsequent comprehensive evaluation is necessary to determine the severity of the communication disorder, as well as the area(s) of communication the disorder impacts. In a conclusion of *uncertain status*, an SLP has insufficient evidence to formulate conclusions about the present status of a child's communication. A number of factors can account for this situation, from such child variables as level of interest and attention to the process, to such situational factors as appointment time allocation. In this case, as with the previous result, a recommendation for a comprehensive evaluation is in order to determine whether a child presents intact communica-

tion. Should this evaluation provide evidence of normal levels, such information could reassure the parents and the teachers about the status of the child. However, should this evaluation reveal causes for concern, the SLP and others who care for the child can initiate appropriate intervention as soon as possible. The earliest possible identification and intervention are crucial components of prevention of the more deleterious effects of a communication disorder on the life of a child.

Evaluation Procedures: Interviewing

Interviews are conversations with the clinical patient (or a child's parents) in which the SLP systematically collects relevant information about the patient, then the specific concerns. SLPs incorporate interviews into evaluations for diverse reasons. They permit the SLP to confirm or to request clarification of information the patient submitted in his or her intake information form, as well as resolve any discrepancies that may have been submitted. Interviews also permit the SLP to request more in-depth information or representative examples about areas that address the heart of the patient's concern. Such details are crucial in the process of differential diagnosis at the conclusion of an evaluation. In addition to these purposes, in an interview the SLP may ask the patient to complete written documents (e.g., open-ended and closed-ended questionnaires) that reveal additional history information about the patient and his or her communication needs. Finally, the SLP also may need to answer questions from the patient.

The format for an interview varies. The SLP can structure the interview as a series of closed questions, or with a broad question that stimulates a response that includes multiple details to which the SLP can respond with requests for elaborated responses, as needed. Sometimes the SLP will incorporate a questionnaire or a related document into the interview to collect further information about a specific aspect of language that is a cause for concern. The content of the interview varies based on the unique characteristics of the patient. The SLP, however, can incorporate discussion of areas that have the potential to be important across a broad population of patients. An overview of these areas follows.

Medical

The SLP poses questions about the medical status of the patient to determine whether the patient presents any medical conditions that have compromised his or her communication development. If this is the case, then the SLP poses questions to determine whether referral(s) to medical service providers is warranted to ascertain whether medical treatment should precede the initiation of SLP services to increase the opportunities for success in subsequent treatment. The SLP also is concerned as to whether conditions exist that would necessitate a guarded prognosis for substantial improvement in SLP services.

Developmental

The SLP poses questions about the developmental status of the patient to determine whether the patient presents any broad developmental conditions of which language issues could be a part. If the developmental status is compromised, the SLP then queries whether the language of the patient reflects the traits that this developmental condition tends to impose or, whether the language comprehension and production are inconsistent with those expectations.

Educational

The SLP addresses this area to determine whether the patient simultaneously presents with language issues and learning issues. In addition, the SLP requests information about how the patient learns best, which has implications for a subsequent treatment plan in terms of the accommodations needed to provide the patient the best chance for success in the intervention process. Information about educational interests can provide the SLP with topics which would motivate the patient in treatment and inform the choices of the SLP for specific methods and materials.

Familial

In questions related to familial status, the SLP is concerned about the extent of the social support the patient would have in the course of intervention.

Descriptions of the family members and their roles in the patient's life inform the SLP about the realistic extent to which these individuals could and would participate throughout the intervention process. Details about the family structure inform the SLP about social service needs a patient can present, such as issues with finances and transportation to and from clinical appointments.

Cultural

Questions about the cultural identification of the patient will allow the SLP to determine whether the presence of a nonstandard dialect influences how well the patient comprehends and produces dialect and whether English or another language is the dominant language for the patient. Questions about culture also can reveal the attitudes of the patient with respect to communication disorders and the individuals who present with these.

Communication

The SLP requests information about the communication history of the patient in an attempt to reconstruct the fashion in which the speech and language skills unfolded. In addition, details about previous evaluation and intervention services will inform the SLP about patient level of familiarity with and prior impressions of clinical services, as well as the extent to which any prior intervention was successful. Overall, at the conclusion of the evaluation, the SLP hopes to have ideas as to factors that caused and/or contributed to a communication disorder, as well as the factors that have a substantial impact on the present life of the patient.

Evaluation Procedures: Sampling

Language samples are collections of language representative of the patient's day to day language. It is crucial that the sample not contain language that could result in *underestimation* of the language level of the patient. For that reason, the SLP will avoid requests that the patient produce language that is, by its nature, restricted, such as responses to Yes/No questions or comments when the patient is preoccupied with a complicated task. Conversely, it also is crucial that the sample not contain language that could result in *overestimation* of the language level of the patient. For that reason, the SLP will avoid requests that the patient produce rote, scripted, or memorized language that could be advanced in comparison with his or her own day to day productions (Miller, 1981). Although the SLP can collect a language sample in any number of contexts, the most common scenario for a child patient is a free play situation, whereas the most common scenario for an adult patient is a free conversation situation. Both situations allow the SLP to follow the lead of the patient and respond to his or her comments in standardized, planned way to elicit the most representative language possible. A sample gives a rich assortment of details about the semantic and structural sophistication of the patient's language. Because of that, numerous language sample analysis procedures are available that permit the SLP to extract a wealth of information about the language of the patient.

Language Sample Procedures Related to Lexicon

The three examples that follow are representative of those procedures SLPs use to measure the extent to which children comprehend and produce the lexicon of their language. Certainly, many other analysis procedures exist besides these, and SLPs may continuously create new, criterion-based procedures as appropriate to describe the quantity and the quality of the vocabulary of a child.

Example 1. A simple analysis of vocabulary involves the identification of the child's words in earlier language development over a series of measurements. The SLP calculates the number of words at each point. Then, he or she compares the lists with each other to determine which words the child maintains from one point to the next, as well as whether the child introduces new or subtracts old words from the lexicon. This, in turn, allows the SLP to determine the introduction, for instance, of superordinate, subordinate, or synonymous words, as well as the removal of redundant or diminuitive lexical items.

Example 2. Another simple analysis of vocabulary involves the description of the child's words in ear-

lier language development with respect to the parts of speech these represent. Details about the number and relative proportion of words that are nouns, verbs, prepositions, and other parts of speech can provide information related to language potential. For instance, if the preponderance of a child's words represent a specific part of speech, the SLP can use that pattern to formulate some predictions as to the semantic, syntactic, and pragmatic tasks that could prove difficult for the child because of vocabulary limitations.

Example 3. In an early analysis of vocabulary that is still popular, Templin (1957) devised a way to measure the diversity of the vocabulary a child produces. This procedure, known as the *Type-Token Ratio*, examines the relationship between the total number of words a child uses versus the total number of *different* words he or she uses. Once the SLP calculates this ratio, he or she can interpret the number with reference to normative data Templin collected, which indicate that a ratio of approximately .50 indicates sufficient but not excessive diversity in the vocabulary of early language development.

Language Sample Procedures Related to Syntax

The three examples that follow are representative of those procedures SLPs use to measure the extent to which children incorporate semantic information into their utterances and coordinate the semantic content with the structural necessities that allow them to convey ideas and information. As noted earlier, many other analysis procedures, both norm-referenced and criterion-referenced, exist to describe this dimension of language skill.

Example 1. Bloom (1973) presented a scheme for the classification of one-word utterances, or those utterances in which a child incorporates implied content into the production of an isolated word. This scheme included three variations of words: names, substantive words, and function words. In this scheme, *names* are words that a child uses to refer to specific items in his or her environment, such as the name of a parent or a pet. In contrast, *substantive words* are words that a child uses to refer to items and events that are not specific to the environment. These include common nouns (such as "ball" or "doll") and common verbs to describe action (such as "eat" or "drive"). In addition to these, *function words* are applied to items and events and elaborate the nature of the relationship the child has or desires with these. Examples are "down" (i.e., the child wants to move or has moved in relation to items) and "nice" (i.e., the child applies a description word to the condition of an item or an event). This scheme will result in the percent of utterances accounted for with one-word utterances, as well as the relative proportion of each kind of word used.

Example 2. Brown (1973) presented a list of what he considered the prevalent semantic relations in the earlier stages of a child's language, those relationships which he contented established the foundation for subsequent language sophistication: *agent*, *action*, *object*, *demonstrative*, *entity*, *locative*, *possessor*, and *possession*. In this scheme, the SLP applies these relations to components of each two- and three-word utterance of the language sample, then determines which combinations are the most prevalent in the language production, at least for the present sample.

Example 3. Bloom and Lahey (1978) created a system to analyze semantic content and its incorporation into structures with increased sophistication. In this system, known as the *Content-Form Interaction* system, the SLP evaluates the content inherent in each utterance via the use of labels for semantic content provided by the system. Once he or she has done so, the SLP then evaluates the structure of each utterance. The presumption within this system is that increased sophistication of content leads to increased sophistication of structure to encode the content. The interpretation of the results are based on the MLU (mean length of utterance) of the child. Once the SLP calculates the MLU (described in Chapter 4), he or she matches that MLU to a "phase" of development. The expectation for a child is that his or her language will reflect the established content-form interactions commensurate with that phase, as well as present or prior mastery of the interactions appropriate for earlier phases. The determination of whether this is the case will be

one basis for recommendations for additional evaluation or a course of intervention.

Language Sample Procedures Related to Phonology

The three examples that follow are representative of those procedures SLPs use to measure the phonological skills in the language. Certainly, as noted earlier, many other analysis procedures, both norm-referenced and criterion-referenced, exist to describe this dimension of language. These procedures focus both on individual phonemes and the patterns of the combinations of these phonemes in individual and combined words.

Example 1. One concern with respect to how well a child produces and combines phonemes is the extent to which others can understand the speech of that child. Toward this end, an SLP may calculate *speech intelligibility*. Bleile (2004) provides multiple variations of this measurement. In the more objective measurements, the SLP determines the percent of individual words or, in contrast, the connected speech that he or she (or another observer) can understand. In the more subjective measurements, the SLP places the speech on a continuum from *increased intelligibility* to *decreased intelligibility*, with such disclaimers as whether the SLP is familiar or unfamiliar with the topic at hand or whether a child can compensate for various interferences.

Example 2. A related concern with respect to the potential of a child to produce and combine phonemes is the extent to which he or she can imitate the models and production cues from others. An SLP can evaluate this skill, known as *speech stimulability*, in a variety of ways. A common procedure involves the use of a hierarchy of phonetic complexity, in which the SLP introduces imitative and nonimitative productions at the phoneme, syllable, word, phrase, sentence, and narrative levels. At each level, the SLP establishes a criterion the child should reach to advance to the next level. This criterion permits the SLP to determine the level of breakdown in phoneme production and thus a potential level for the introduction of speech production skills in intervention.

Example 3. Another procedure that can provide important information is a *phonetic feature analysis*. In this analysis, the SLP ascertains whether the features of *manner of production* and *place of production*, as well as the distinction between *voiced* and *unvoiced* consonants, are intact. If this is not the case, then the SLP ascertains whether patterns of incorrect productions of features are present (i.e., the systematic replacement of one manner or place of production with another option) and whether the features that are present are consistent with developmental expectations. The SLP can also ascertain whether incorrect productions occur because of the use of a feature not only when it is appropriate but also in instances when it is inappropriate.

Language Sample Procedures Related to Morphology

The three examples that follow are representative of those procedures SLPs use to measure the morphological skills in the language. They focus both on individual morphemes and the patterns of the combinations of these morphemes into syntactic structures. As noted earlier, SLPs may employ additional measures to describe the comprehension and production of morphemes besides those featured here.

Example 1. As noted in Chapter 4, Brown described a set of morphemes as *grammatical* morphemes, or morphemes that enhance the structure of an utterance with the addition of sophistication. One analysis method based on the normative information from deVilliers and deVilliers (1973) involves determining the extent to which a child achieves correct production of these morphemes in obligatory contexts in 90% of production opportunities, as well as determining whether the expected morphemes for each stage within Brown's stages are indeed present in the language of the child.

Example 2. As noted in Chapter 1, children learn to comprehend and produce various kinds of morphemes, two of which are *inflectional* and *derivational*. One analysis method involves the comparison of the relative proportion of attempted morphemes and with that of correct productions that reflect each kind. This information will allow the SLP to observe the child's preference for a particular mor-

pheme to enhance the structural sophistication of a word, as well as the relative ease with which a child applies each kind of transformation to the base morpheme of a word. The SLP can further compare these patterns with developmental expectations.

Example 3. Although the mastery of morphemes certainly includes the mastery of bound morphemes, it also includes the child's appreciation for the distinction between *regular* and *irregular* forms. Unlike *regular* forms, which mandate the addition of a bound morpheme to a base morpheme, *irregular* forms mandate that words either remain the same (such as the plural form of "moose") or convert to a new word (such as the plural form of "mouse" as "mice"). The SLP can observe the relative proportion of regular versus irregular forms attempted, as well as the relative proportion of times the child applied the correct morphological rule to the word in question.

Language Sample Procedures Related to Syntax

The three examples that follow are representative of procedures SLPs use to measure a child's syntactic skills These attempt to capture the relative proportion of simple, compound, and complex elements in the language, as well as the narrative structures that a child imposes on combined utterances. As noted earlier, many other analysis procedures are available for the description of various aspects of syntax.

Example 1. One source of information about the complexity of language structure is the *noun phrase*, or a noun with its various modifiers. The SLP can extract the noun phrases from within the sentences a child produces, then divide them into noun phrase examples with descriptions comprised of parts of speech (e.g., article + adjective + noun), location in sentence (e.g., noun phrase within a prepositional phrase), or role in the creation of compound or complex sentences (e.g., noun phrase within the compound subject or the compound predicate). The SLP can then determine the relative proportion of the correct noun phrases the child produces. This particular analysis can be adapted to evaluate other phrases, such as verb phrases and prepositional phrases.

Example 2. Another means to determine the complexity of language structure is through *transformations*. As noted in Chapter 2, transformations are rules that children use to convert a basic syntactic structure (e.g., a declarative statement) into another form. The SLP can extract the declarative and nondeclarative productions from the sample, then systematically compare every production to discern the specific rule a child has applied to his or her productions. From this information, the SLP can determine whether these structures are within normal expectations for the language development of the child and thus evidence of a disorder.

Example 3. In addition to the two previous analyses, the SLP can describe the relative proportion of *simple*, *compound*, and *complex* sentences in the language sample. Within the classification of *compound*, the SLP can differentiate sentences with compound subjects from sentences with compound predicates, as well as those that contain both compound elements. In addition, the SLP can differentiate these variations from the sentences that reflect the traditional compound structure. Within the classification of *complex*, the SLP can differentiate complex sentence variations, such as the infinitive structure, the gerund structure, the relative clauses, and the complements. Identification of the relative proportion of these can inform the SLP about sentence complexity.

Language Sample Procedures Related to Pragmatics

The three examples that follow are representative of those procedures SLPs use to describe the pragmatic skills the child demonstrates. These attempt to capture the social, interactional, and conversational dimensions of language. As noted earlier, many other analysis procedures are available for the description of various aspects of pragmatics.

Example 1. A critical aspect of pragmatic language is the use of language for multiple purposes. A number of lists of communication intentions are available for clinical use. With these lists, the SLP reviews on an individual basis each of the utterances in the language sample. As he or she does so, the SLP determines the purpose(s) each utterance served in the interaction. After this review is completed, the SLP then determines such information as the number and relative proportion of different functions represented in the sample, the number and relative proportion of utterances with multiple functions in the sample, and even the responses to the conversational partner(s) to these utterances.

Example 2. Another dimension of pragmatic language is conversational competence. Within the language sample, the SLP can extract a number of details to describe a child's conversation: the number of child-initiated conversations, child responses to the initiations of others, and utterances per turn in the conversation. In addition to these quantitative data, the SLP can also note qualitative aspects of conversation, such as the methods the child used to initiate, maintain, conclude, and shift topics within a conversation. The SLP can easily create ways to capture the different approaches the child uses for these conversational tasks.

Example 3. Competence in participation in social routines is another vital component of pragmatic language. If the SLP desires, he or she can supplement a traditional play-based language sample with a series of role-play samples. In these scenarios, a child plays various roles in situations that are familiar to him or her in daily life. The SLP can then describe the extent to which the child effectively performs the script, sequences the actions, and produces the related movements associated with a particular interaction. The SLP also can then describe the extent to which the child can adapt his or her communication to alternate variations of a specific social routine.

Evaluation Procedures: Testing

Language testing involves the administration of one or more published and/or clinical practitioner-created standardized tests that, in many cases, also provide such normative scores as *mean score, standard deviation, quotient, stanine score, percentile rank*, and *age-equivalent score*. By their very nature, even the most comprehensive of these tests provides but a snapshot or a sample of the language comprehension and/or production skills of the child. Therefore, their value is more to confirm the presence or absence of a language delay or disorder than for the in-depth description of the status of the language of a child for purposes of formulation and implementation of treatment aims and directions. Their provision of normative scores is useful for the purpose of qualification of a child for public school-based clinical services, as well as for periodic re-evaluation of skills in a noncontext-dependent format. We overviewed a sample of 30 published, standardized test protocols, which are included in the Resources sec-

tion at the conclusion of this chapter. From these, we have formed clinical impressions of the most common test items to use to collect information about the six areas of language skill discussed earlier. Thus, we present these examples as a means to illustrate the diversity of items that can sample the skill of a child in a standardized format.

Lexicon

(Figures 8–1 and 8–2) *Example 1:* The SLP presents a set of multiple pictures of items, then asks the

INSTRUCTION:

"Point to the [indicated term]."

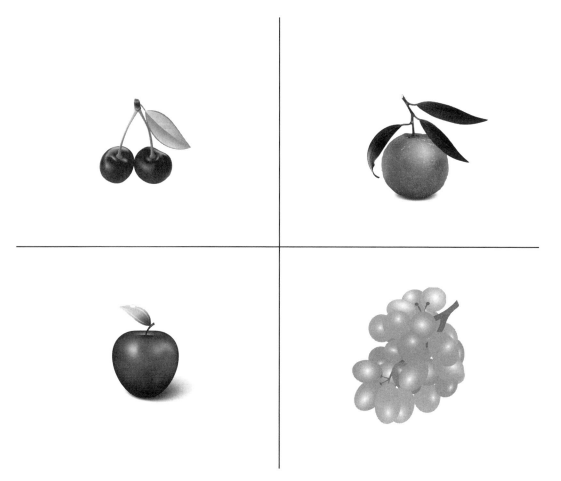

FIGURE 8–1. Test Item: Lexicon. This simulated test item is representative of those used in published tests to evaluate the comprehension of language in the *lexicon* skill area. Images from Shutterstock®. All rights reserved.

INSTRUCTION:

"What is this?"

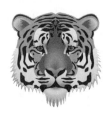 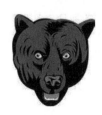 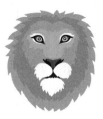

FIGURE 8–2. Test Item: Lexicon. This simulated test item is representative of those used in published tests to evaluate the production of language in the *lexicon* skill area. Images from Shutterstock®. All rights reserved.

child to indicate the picture that the SLP named by pointing or providing the number of the picture. *Example 2:* The SLP provides a word that represents a class of items, such as "animal," and asks the child to name as many examples of related items as quickly as he or she can in a specified time frame. *Example 3:* The SLP produces a word, then asks the child to indicate a word that (a) means the same, (b) means the opposite, or (c) relates to the word. *Example 4:* The SLP presents a word, then asks the child to define what the word means. *Example 5:* The SLP shows a picture and asks the child to name the item (or class of items) represented in the picture. *Example 6:* The SLP presents a set of words, then asks the child to indicate which word does not relate to the other words in the set.

Semantics

(Figures 8–3 and 8–4). *Example 1:* The SLP presents a picture, then asks the child to explain the content of the picture. *Example 2:* The SLP presents pairs of words, then asks the child to provide examples of how these two words are the same and are not the same. *Example 3:* The SLP presents a word with multiple common meanings to a child, then asks the child to provide as many meanings for the word as possible. *Example 4:* The SLP provides analogies with fill-in-the-blank items for the completion of the

analogies, then asks the child to complete these with the appropriate words. *Example 5:* The SLP presents semantic absurdities and asks the child to explain why a statement is nonsensical or incorrect. *Example 6:* The SLP presents a picture of an item or an actual item, then asks the child to provide a description of the item that contains as many traits of the item as possible.

Phonology

(Figures 8–5 and 8–6). *Example 1:* The child produces words that name pictures as the SLP analyzes the quality of those word productions. *Example 2:* The SLP provides a word and asks the child to break this word into its constituent sounds, then provides the child with a set of sounds and asks the child to combine these into a word. *Example 3:* The SLP provides a word to produce, then asks the child to produce the word with a portion of it removed. *Example 4:* The SLP tells a story, then asks the child to re-tell the story so that the SLP can determine the presence of speech sound errors and a measure of speech intelligibility. *Example 5:* The SLP provides words for which the child should produce rhymes. *Example 6:* The SLP produces individual speech sounds, then asks the child to imitate them so that the SLP can determine the speech stimulability of the child.

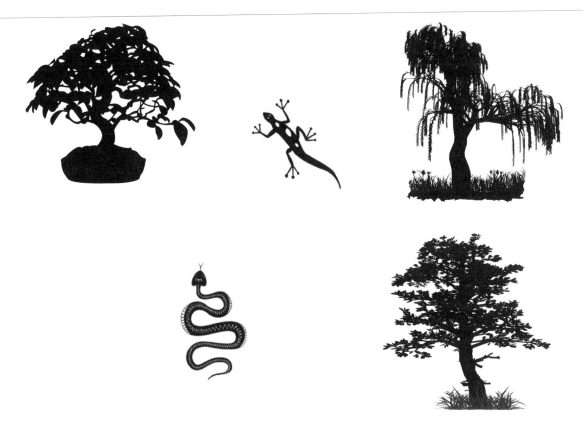

FIGURE 8–3. Test Item: Semantics. This simulated test item is representative of those used in published tests to evaluate the comprehension of language in the *semantics* skill area. Images from Shutterstock®. All rights reserved.

INSTRUCTION:

"How are these the same? Not the same?"

FIGURE 8–4. Test Item: Semantics. This simulated test item is representative of those used in published tests to evaluate the production of language in the *semantics* skill area. Images from Shutterstock®. All rights reserved.

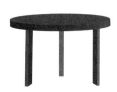
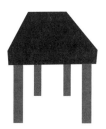

INSTRUCTION:
"Are these words the same or not the same?"

pat-bat
pat-pat
light-right
light-light
far-far
far-par
sink-sink
sink-think
dance-chance
dance-dance
fine-vine
fine-fine

FIGURE 8–5. Test Item: Phonology. This simulated test item is representative of those used in published tests to evaluate the comprehension of language in the *phonology skill* area.

Morphology

(Figures 8-7 and 8-8). *Example 1:* The SLP provides a fill-in-the-blank item that allows the child to add a bound morpheme to the word in the carrier phrase. *Example 2:* The SLP presents a set of pictures, then asks the child to indicate the picture that matches a word with a bound morpheme that the SLP produced.

Syntax

(Figures 8-9 and 8-10). *Example 1:* The SLP provides one or more words, then instructs the child to create a sentence that includes the words. *Example 2:* The SLP instructs the child to imitate the sentences (that rank from easier to systematically harder) that the SLP said. *Example 3:* The SLP presents declarative sentences, then asks the child to transform these into imperatives, exclamations, or interrogatives. *Example 4:* The SLP provides a set of two, three, or four sentences and asks the child to combine those sentences into one sentence.

INSTRUCTION:

"What is this?"

NOTE:
Photos feature the phoneme [l] (Row 01) and [d] (Row 02) in word initial, word medial, and word final positions.

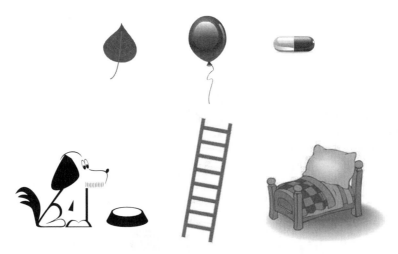

FIGURE 8–6. Test Item: Phonology. This simulated test item is representative of those used in published tests to evaluate the production of language in the *phonology skill* area. Images from Shutterstock®. All rights reserved.

INSTRUCTION:
"How many morphemes does each of these words have, and what are these specific morphemes?"

love
loving
lovingly
hope
hopeful
hopefully
independent
subordinate
walk
walks
walking
walked

FIGURE 8–7. Test Item: Morphology. This simulated test item is representative of those used in published tests to evaluate the comprehension of language in the *morphology skill* area.

INSTRUCTION:
"Here is one (word). Here are two (intended word)."

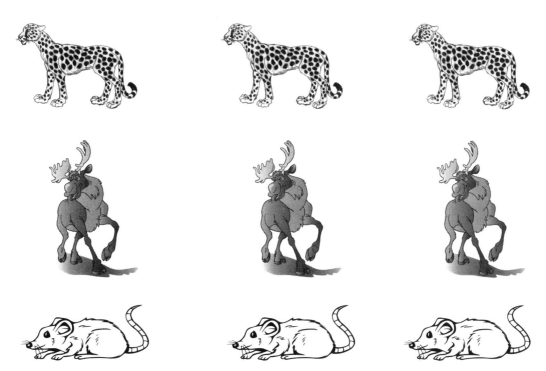

FIGURE 8–8. Test Item: Morphology. This simulated test item is representative of those used in published tests to evaluate the production of language in the *morphology skill* area. Images from Shutterstock®. All rights reserved.

INSTRUCTION:
"Select the two sentences in each set that mean the same."

John ate the pizza.
The pizza was eaten by John.
The pizza was John's.

The car was the father's.
Mary drove her father's car.
The father's car was driven by Mary.

FIGURE 8–9. Test Item: Syntax. This simulated test item is representative of those used in published tests to evaluate the comprehension of language in the *syntax skill* area.

INSTRUCTION:

"Use these words to create a sentence."

BOY THE PIZZA AND DRANK THE **ATE** POP
THE

FIGURE 8–10. Test Item: Syntax. This simulated test item is representative of those used in published tests to evaluate the production of language in the *syntax skill* area.

Example 5: The SLP produces sentences that are semantically and/or syntactically incorrect, then asks the child to determine whether these are correct, and explain the reasons for his or her conclusion. *Example 6:* The SLP asks the child to construct a narrative about a specific event, which the SLP uses to evaluate the child's narrative structure.

Pragmatics

(Figures 8-11 and 8-12). *Example 1:* The SLP provides a series of scenarios, then asks the child to state the appropriate behavior under those conditions or in those situations. *Example 2:* The SLP provides a number of social situations and asks the child to demonstrate the appropriate behavior (such as when a child attempts to compliment someone or provide directions to someone). *Example 3:* The SLP provides a topic to describe. In the course of the description, the SLP asks for clarification and elaboration to determine the extent to which the child can accommodate the comprehension level of a listener. *Example 4:* The SLP provides a puppet, then asks the child and the puppet to role-play common social situations.

REFLECTIONS ON EVALUATION

At this point, we should remember the process of evaluation described at the start of this chapter. This systematic collection and interpretation of informa-

---

INSTRUCTION:

Listen to this short story. One afternoon after school, three friends went to the house of a classmate. The father of this classmate had just finished a batch of home baked chocolate cookies. The cookies looked and smelled wonderful, so of course the friends all wanted to taste them. The 1st friend said, "Those cookies are my favorite kind. My mother's are better than yours." The 2nd friend snatched a cookie off the plate before the father knew what had happened. The 3rd friend said, "May I please have a cookie?" Now, tell me, which of the friends was the most polite? Why?

FIGURE 8–11. Test Item: Pragmatics. This simulated test item is representative of those used in published tests to evaluate the comprehension of language in the *pragmatics skill* area.

INSTRUCTION:

Tell me what you say when:

You need to borrow a pencil from a classmate.
You want to invite a friend to your home for supper.
You need to ask directions to a store.
You want to compliment a friend on a nice outfit.
You do not understand the instructions your teacher provided.
You need to ask the price of an item in a store.
You want to introduce a new classmate to some other students.
You want to order a meal at your favorite fast food restaurant.

FIGURE 8–12. Test Item: Pragmatics. This simulated test item is representative of those used in published tests to evaluate the production of language in the *pragmatics skill* area.

---

tion has as an ultimate aim to determine an accurate and appropriate description of a clinical patient's language status which, in some cases, is supplemented with a specification of the area(s) of language affected, the extent to which each of these areas is affected, and the prognosis for eventual improvement of language skills. The process of diagnosis of language delays and disorders is not always easy. In some cases, for some patients, our conclusions must remain tentative or conditional until such time as we have sufficient information to allow us to conclude with few, if any, reservations that a patient presents with a particular condition. Even so, any information can be only beneficial in the process of intervention, a focus to which we next turn.

INTRODUCTION TO INTERVENTION

When a child presents with delayed or disordered language development, one or more variations of intervention may be valuable for him or her. *Intervention* represents any direct or indirect influence that results in improvement in the language status of the child, including language therapy. However, intervention need not be restricted to this direct service provision for the child. As noted in this chapter, although an SLP provides direct services, he or she also may participate in consultative and collaborative services to broaden the population of professionals who contribute to the intervention process. And, although professionals indeed possess experience crucial to the process, the incorporation of families and friends as partners in the process also is crucial to broaden the extent of the influence on the life of the child day by day. Presently, a diverse assortment of approaches to intervention exists that is complemented by the collection of readily available clinical materials. A discussion of the nature, advantages, and disadvantages of specific intervention approaches is outside the scope of this book, but for such information, consult resource books that overview specific approaches (e.g., McCauley & Fey, 2006). Our discussion focuses on the principles to which we as SLPs attend as we consider our contributions to the intervention process for children with delayed or disordered language development.

PREVENTION OF LANGUAGE DELAYS AND DISORDERS

As SLPs, a substantial proportion of our clinical practice centers on prevention of communication disorders, and particularly, language delays and disorders. The process of *prevention* is multifaceted and consists of *primary*, *secondary*, and *tertiary* elements (ASHA, 1988, 2004b). In *primary prevention*, we take steps to eliminate the onset of a communication disorder. Examples that reflect this level of prevention include creation of informational literature, provision of educational seminars, participation in health promotion events, and consultation with civic associations. In *secondary prevention*, we take steps toward identification of the earliest possible evaluation and intervention of communication disorders in order to eliminate, or at least reduce the complications of, these disorders. Examples that reflect this level of prevention include initiation of events to screen communication for members of civic associations, coordination of parent support circles to enhance parent-child interaction, collaborative events with professionals from other disciplines (e.g., classroom teachers) to enhance communication in children, and provision of direct clinical services to children in assorted clinical practice contexts. In *tertiary prevention*, we take steps to reduce the impact of a communication disorder on the life of a child who has experienced at least some residual effects of that condition. Examples of this level of prevention include provision of augmentative or alternative communication opportunities for children, introduction of compensatory behaviors to maximize present skill levels, inclusion of parents and other care providers in the intervention process to enhance the communication environment for a child, and educational seminars on interaction with those with communication disorders. In whichever variation it occurs, prevention is pervasive in the intervention process for language delays and disorders.

INTERVENTION: ADMISSION TO CLINICAL CASELOAD

Our national professional association, ASHA, has established *admission criteria* (ASHA, 2004a), which reflect the most common reasons that we as SLPs conclude that a child could receive a substantial benefit from intervention, and used when we consider whether we should recommend if a child be admitted to our caseload for language intervention. Such criteria allow the decision in favor of admission to be as systematic and data-based as possible. Note that these criteria are broad standards applicable across clinical practice contexts, as well as across communication disorders areas that include but are not restricted to language. Based on these admission criteria, initiation of SLP intervention services is warranted when an individual cannot communicate in an effective fashion or when reason exists to believe that intervention will prevent or reduce the development of a communication disorder, result in improved functional communication, or prevent the decline of communication (ASHA, 1989, 1998). The criteria that reflect these broad aims for admission are portrayed in Figure 8-13.

INTERVENTION: DISCHARGE FROM CLINICAL CASELOAD

As a companion to the *admission criteria*, ASHA also has established what we know as *discharge criteria* (ASHA, 2004a). After a child has participated

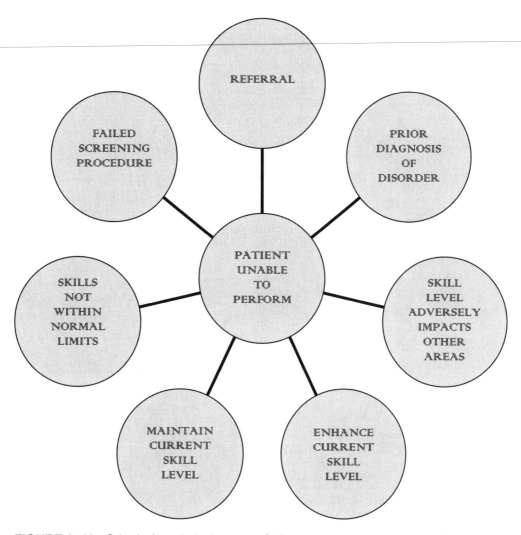

FIGURE 8–13. Criteria for admission to an SLP caseload. Adapted from ASHA (2004).

in a course of intervention, we consider whether we should recommend continuation of these services with the same approach; a shift in methods, materials, model, and/or focus; or discharge. These criteria reflect the most common reasons that SLPs conclude a child would not continue to receive a substantial benefit from intervention and thus should receive a recommendation for discharge. Based on these discharge criteria, discontinuation of SLP intervention services is warranted when the SLP and other relevant individuals conclude that a communication disorder is remediated or that the patient has established sufficient compensation for the condition. The criteria that reflect these broad aims for discharge are portrayed in Figure 8-14.

INTERVENTION: MODELS OF LANGUAGE TREATMENT

Now that we have presented the current criteria relevant to the initiation and conclusion of intervention, we move into a description of the clinical decisions that SLPs confront during intervention. One of the earliest choices that we must deliberate is which model of clinical practice to use as a base for the patient's services. A model is a unified framework that influences our selections of the contexts in which we provide our services, the participants and their respective roles in the intervention process, the methods and materials that we incorporate into our treatment

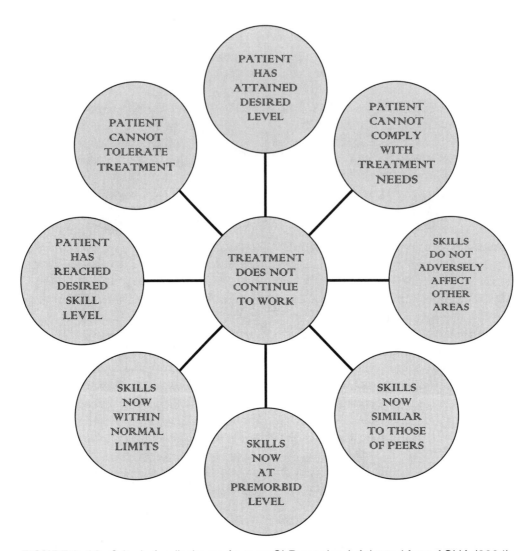

FIGURE 8–14. Criteria for discharge from an SLP caseload. Adapted from ASHA (2004).

sessions, and our conceptualization and measurement of improvement. Three models exist that have provided the bases for clinical practices in language intervention. These include the *consultative model*, *collaborative model*, and *direct services model*. For purposes of description, we place these models within the public school clinical practice context (although they can occur across clinical practice contexts) to illustrate their use with classroom teachers.

The Consultative Model

In the *consultative model*, the SLP provides information and, in some cases, instruction, to other profes-

sionals who serve a child with a language disorder but does not provide direct clinical services to that child (DeKemel, 2003; Hegde & Davis, 1999).

Clinical Example

A director of a preschool observes that a child does not initiate conversations and interactions with the other children. While the child does respond to contact from other children, he or she does so in a reserved fashion, with minimal expansion of the comments of other children. In addition to this reluctance towards other children, the child also hesitates to express wants and needs to the preschool staff members. When questioned, the child will affirm desires and preferences, but he or she does not question the staff members about any aspects of the preschool experience. The director has noted several salient traits of the child: the child is the third of five children in the home, lives in a multicultural home with multiple forms of communication in place, and the family has recently moved to this area from another section of the country. In this case, the SLP may conclude that consultation services would be the most appropriate option. The SLP can provide the preschool staff members with information about normal communication development, as well as factors that can enhance this development. The SLP also can demonstrate interactional methods that can increase the opportunities for this child to initiate communication with others, as well as respond in a more elaborate fashion to their overtures. In addition to information and demonstrations, the SLP can provide reminders as to traits of the child that indicate the need for subsequent, comprehensive communication evaluation.

Clinical Example

A teacher in a secondary school composition class has an adolescent student who has previously participated in a course of intervention, which focused on the enhancement of multiple precursors for written language development and the improvement of multiple written language skills related to narrative structures. Because of the demands of the composition class and the implications of composition skills for success across academic disciplines, the teacher is concerned about the status of written language for this adolescent. Although the student has exhibited no particular difficulties with the submission of inside and outside class written papers, the teacher desires to prevent problems even before these arise. In this case, the SLP can review with the teacher information on narrative language development and can supplement this with reminders of the salient spoken language precursors that strengthen written language. The SLP also can describe characteristics of written language that represent appropriate developmental patterns of composition rather than written language disorders, per se. As the teacher reviews the compositions of the student, as well as the student's reactions to specific methods of instruction, he or she can be alert to any relapse

that the student may present, as well as sensitive to the point at which the student has reached his or her maximum performance level. When either of these situations arises, the teacher can then initiate the process of SLP re-evaluation for the student.

The Collaborative Model

In the *collaborative model*, the SLP enters into a cotreatment relationship with the classroom teacher to address the needs of the child in the classroom and in conjunction with enhancement of communication across the entire classroom population (ASHA, 1991). This relationship is exemplified in various forms (Borsch & Oaks, 1993; DeMil, Merritt & Culatta, 1996), which we describe here.

Supportive Instruction

In supportive instruction (Lue, 2001), the SLP provides in-class demonstrations intended to enhance specific language skills in children. Consider the scenario in which a language curriculum for an academic year includes an introduction to spelling. Important to success in spelling are skills related to word segmentation (i.e., division of a word into its constituent phonemes) and word reconstruction (i.e., formulation of a word from its constituent phonemes). Because of that consideration, the SLP can participate in the classroom-based instruction that addresses the precursors that increase the likelihood of success when the children start to spell words. This involvement can include various tasks that enhance phonological awareness, as well as self-monitoring and self-correcting while matching phonemes to possible graphemes.

Resource Adaptation

In resource adaptation (Lue, 2001), the SLP discusses with the teacher the language aims that are incorporated into the classroom. Based on relevant theoretical and empirical considerations, the SLP will note whether the current language aims are structurally and functionally sound, as well as easily measurable. Should the SLP observe aims that are unclear or incompatible with reasonable expectations for this point in the curriculum, he or she will collaborate with the teacher to reformulate those. To determine whether the classroom instruction is conducive to the attainment of the aims, the SLP observes the lesson and the interaction of the students in response to the lesson. If specific methods and materials appear to be appropriate, the SLP will note that. However, if specific methods and materials appear to be problematic, the SLP will advise the teacher about potential modifications. In this fashion, the teacher instructs in a fashion most conducive to attainment of the skills that will permeate all aspects of the academic curriculum.

Complementary Instruction

In complementary instruction (Lue, 2001), the SLP and the teacher both participate in the act of dissemination of academic information to the students. Although their task is the same, their roles are distinct. For instance, the teacher would assume leadership in the instructional interaction with the selection of the academic goals, the preparation of methods and materials, the formulation of the schedule, and the measurement of student competence with respect to the information presented. As the teacher leads this process, the SLP contributes in a manner that complements and enhances the language elements of the process. For example, when the teacher introduces unfamiliar lexicon, the SLP can offer methods to ascertain the content from the language context and thus comprehend those words with increased ease. Or, when the teacher requests that the children summarize central concepts within the information, the SLP can suggest variations in the construction of narratives.

Team Instruction

In team instruction (Lue, 2001), the SLP and the teacher are both in a shared classroom for a school day or, as an alternative, for the duration of a specific focal area, such as a unit in a language arts curriculum. In this model, the classroom teacher plans and implements the lessons based on the traditional academic curriculum. Although the teacher performs this role, preparing the lesson or series of lessons based on the content, the SLP initiates steps to enrich the lessons. If the lesson were astronomy, the teacher would introduce planets, stars, nebulae, comets, and other astronomical concepts. During

this, the SLP can enhance lexical development through the provision of new vocabulary items, syntactic development using instruction on how the child can formulate the best descriptive narratives to explain the solar system, or even semantic development through discussion of the kinds of lexical items that can appropriately be combined to encode the information contained in the lesson.

The Direct Services Model

In the *direct services model*, although the SLP and the teacher may often communicate about the status of and services for a child, the two professionals address the needs of that child in an independent fashion. In clinical practice in public schools, this model is sometimes described as a "pull-out," as it necessitates the removal of a child from a classroom so that he or she, with the assistance of the SLP, can address communication needs. In direct services, the child may participate in an individual treatment session, as well as in small and large group contexts. In this model, in contrast to the instruction-based models described earlier, a child may receive more individual attention from the SLP. However, in comparison to these instruction-based models, a child may receive a restricted number of opportunities to interact with the SLP because the schedule for clinical sessions may reflect their decreased frequency of occurrence, as well as their decreased duration. Even so, this model permits the SLP to plan and implement individualized services based on the needs of the child, as well as to provide explicit feedback about language comprehension and/or language production that may not be appropriate in the classroom context. One aim, then, is the transfer of skills acquired in this contrived context into the day-to-day actions of the child.

TREATMENT OF LANGUAGE DELAYS AND DISORDERS: PROTOCOL

Another decision with which SLPs are presented relates to the choice of the treatment protocol. A protocol, in a broad clinical sense, is an approach to treatment that is standardized, with specific clinical aims and anticipated clinical outcomes. We do not lack treatment protocols to consider for adoption in our clinical practice, as they are available in a variety of shapes and sizes. While some protocols are intended to address one aspect of language, others are meant to address language in a broader sense. Some are meant for short-term use, others for application over a sustained period of time. They may also center around the participation of the patient or mandate the incorporation of others (such as the parents of a pediatric patient) into the treatment process. In addition to these considerations, some may insist on strict adherence to the protocol rules, while others may allow the SLP to adjust and adapt a protocol to increase its appropriateness for a particular clinical patient. Whatever the circumstances, the choice of the protocol is crucial to the treatment process: it should address the specific needs of the patient, be compatible with the theoretical orientation of the SLP, have minimal (if any) risks for the patient, possess empirical support (if available) for its effectiveness, be easily applicable in the clinical context, and easily shared with the patient and his or her family members. To enhance the decision about the protocol, various sources supplying relevant information can be consulted which, in some cases, provide a framework for clinical decisions.

Gilliam and Gilliam (2006) noted that clinical decisions should stem from the interaction of three factors—current scientific evidence, experience of the SLP who cares for the patient, and desires and preferences of the patient (and the family, if warranted). Other authors have confirmed their support for this approach to clinical decisions (Dollaghan, 2004; Johnson, 2006; Perzsolt et al., 2003). Gilliam and Gilliam further noted that SLPs can approach their clinical decisions with a multistep process that allows them to use the current scientific evidence for the enhancement of their clinical service delivery. A description of each step in their protocols follows.

Step 1: Formulate A Clinical Question. At this point, the SLP forms a question for which he or she needs an answer, for example, in a clinical setting, "Which method would be more effective than the other for the task of enhancement of the language of a child?"

Step 2: Locate External Evidence That Addresses This Question. At this point, the SLP compiles available research literature that will have evidence that he or she can use to answer this question.

Step 3: Determine Level of External Evidence. He or she reviews the results of studies that attempted to address this question, then rank-orders the evidence on a continuum such as "sufficient evidence to support clinical application of this method" to "insufficient evidence to support clinical application of this method."

Step 4: Locate Internal Evidence Related to the Patient That Addresses This Question. The SLP evaluates the personal characteristics of the patient (and of the family, if warranted) that have the potential for a substantial influence on the course of intervention.

Step 5: Locate Internal Evidence Related to the SLP or to the Clinical Practice Site That Addresses This Question. The SLP evaluates the professional characteristics that have the potential to influence the intervention, as well as factors related to the clinic that have the same potential (e.g., schedule considerations, facility limitations, or theoretical approaches).

Step 6: Reach a Decision After Relating and Integrating the Evidence. Based on the available evidence and after a process of induction and deduction, the SLP decides on a course of intervention to pursue.

Step 7: Evaluate Outcome of Clinical Decision. The SLP who wants to maintain a particular level of clinical expertise will welcome the opportunity to evaluate and even to revisit any clinical decision when new evidence becomes available that relates to that decision. This series of steps mandates that the SLP incorporate evaluation of outcomes of decisions into the step-by-step process that led to formation of those decisions.

In the course of their discussion, Gilliam and Gilliam described what constituted valid evidence on which to base clinical decisions with a system of "levels" of evidence. *Level 1* is a randomized clinical trial, in which treatment and no-treatment groups are established to measure the maximum amount of change in a group. *Level 2* is a nonrandomized clinical trial or a systematic review of such clinical trials which, although not as controlled as a Level 1 study, can provide some empirical evidence for reflection. *Level 3* includes base control studies, whereas *Level 4* includes both case studies and systematically reviewed archival data. Then, at the lowest level and thus least strict level of evidence is *Level 5*, which consists of committee reports, conference papers, and the opinions of those who are respected for their expertise.

At the same time that we can access systems that describe levels of evidence, from most to least robust, the state of the art with respect to treatment for language delays and disorders is characterized by relatively few clinical trials completed. SLPs, then, are faced with a dilemma. On the one hand, we are admonished to base treatment decisions on empirical evidence. On the other hand, we are sorely in need of such evidence. Thus, until such time as our discipline accumulates a collection of Level 1 and 2 evidence, we are pressed to employ alternate ways to evaluate potential treatment protocols, particularly with respect to the validity and consistency of their theoretical bases. For this, the overview of theoretical explanations of language development in Chapter 2 would be quite useful for the SLP who wishes to ascertain the extent of the influence of specific theoretical models to specific components of treatment protocols.

Straus and Sackett (1998) echoed the admonitions of Gilliam and Gilliam (2006) in their reminders of the steps to implement in order to practice in a fashion consistent with evidence-based practice: Convert the need for information into clinically relevant, answerable questions. Find, in the most efficient way, the best evidence with which to answer these questions. Critically appraise the evidence for its validity, reliability, and usefulness. Integrate the appraisal with clinical expertise. Apply the results to clinical practice. Evaluate your performance. Implementation of this process will ensure that, even when we are unclear as to the most appropriate protocols to introduce into the process of intervention, we have taken the steps necessary to monitor and adapt the intervention as needed for the welfare of those whom we serve.

TREATMENT OF LANGUAGE DELAYS AND DISORDERS: GOALS

Goals are the aims that we hope to accomplish for and with our clinical patients via the process of intervention. The selection and implementation of appropriate overall goals and short-term goals is essential to protect the enormous investment of time and talent from both the patient and the SLP into the intervention process. Several frameworks are available to influence the perspective that we have with respect to selection of these aims.

In a *theoretical approach* for the selection of overall and short-term goals, the SLP considers the theoretical views of language development. Each of these perspectives defines what it is that children learn (or develop) in the course of language development, as well as how children learn (or develop) language in a particular fashion. Thus, an adherent to the behavioral perspective would select as aims specific language behaviors that he or she could deconstruct into a hierarchy of easier to harder, earlier to later skills. In contrast, an adherent to the psycholinguistic (semantic) perspective would focus on the cognitive-linguistic relationship and it is manifested in the increased quantity and quality of semantic content children learn. The psycholinguistic (structural) perspective would dictate a focus on the appreciation of the superficial, then the deeper, rules of the language and would thus embrace any methods and materials that would stimulate the activation or maturation of these rules. From the perspective that remains, the sociolinguistic view, we note a focus on language competence, with particular attention to the pragmatic language skills that enhance the mastery of language use for a variety of functions across a variety of situations and conditions. Some clinical practitioners embrace the idea that the treatment aims should be consistent with the theoretical perspective to which one subscribes. However, many clinical practitioners who have not entirely embraced a specific perspective or created their own must use an alternate approach when selecting treatment aims. The traditional approaches of developmental (i.e., the focus on skills in the order in which a child would master these skills), categorical (e.g., the focus on a set of interrelated skills, such as all phonemes in a feature class or all sentences with complex structure), and/or functional (e.g., the focus on a set of skills deemed most useful in the contexts in which a child communicates on a day-to-day basis).

REFLECTIONS ON INTERVENTION

As SLPs, our concern is for people who present with language delays, language disorders, and language differences, as well as one or more of the other communication disorders that can have such a profound impact on both intrapersonal and interpersonal communication. This concern is manifested, in part, in our choices and recommendations as to the course of intervention a clinical patient should follow. At the present time, our expertise, both our own and that of our discipline as a professional community, does not provide us with the ultimate answer about the most efficacious treatment for all patients across all contexts. However, this chapter does remind us of some of the principles on which we can base our choices and recommendations, as well as continue our day-to-day quest to provide as best as we can for those who have entrusted themselves to our care.

REFLECTION QUESTIONS

1. What is the process for the completion of a diagnostic evaluation for a child with a suspected speech and language disorder? What is the value of each of the components of such an evaluation?

2. What constitutes a speech and language screening? How would that process change for patients across age levels? Why is this screening a helpful procedure for the SLP?

3. Why is each section of the patient history interview so important in the completion of a speech-language diagnostic evaluation?

4. Describe two methods an SLP can use to analyze each area of language skill within a language sample.

5. Describe two variations of test items an SLP can administer to address each area of language skill.

6. How do primary, secondary, and tertiary forms of prevention of communication disorders manifest themselves within a clinical practice in SLP?

7. What criteria are used as the basis for the decision to initiate or terminate SLP services for a clinical patient?

8. What traits do the models of language intervention share? How is each model distinctive from the others?

9. What are the bases on which an SLP should select a specific treatment protocol to introduce to his or her clinical patient? What factors should the SLP not consider as part of this decision?

10. What are the components that constitute a treatment plan? Within this plan, what information should the SLP include in the long-term and short-term clinical goals?

APPLICATION EXERCISES

1. Sometimes an SLP has a restricted amount of time to complete the evaluation process for a child. When that is the case, what do you consider the most valuable information collection and interpretation elements to include in the evaluation process? Why do you consider these elements the priorities?

2. Sometimes the results of a speech and language screening are inconclusive. That is, the SLP has sufficient evidence to suspect both the potential presence and the potential absence of a communication disorder. In such cases, what do you consider the most appropriate course of action on the part of the SLP? Why?

3. Because the history information is very important in the evaluation process, it is vital that the information be complete and accurate. What steps should the SLP take to ensure that the choice of an informant is the most appropriate one and that the informant provides relevant, reliable history information?

4. A child has multiple communication concerns, each of which needs to be addressed in the course of treatment. However, it is not possible to address all of these concerns simultaneously. How would an SLP determine the treatment priorities for this child? What considerations would be important?

5. The parents of a child have heard news reports about a popular new treatment method and are convinced that this would be the most appropriate method to address the communication concerns of their child. How would an SLP advise these parents to be cautious about treatment methods?

6. The parents of a child with multiple communication concerns want to support the treatment process in an appropriate fashion. How could an SLP incorporate the parents into the process? And how would an SLP and the parents determine what would be appropriate versus inappropriate roles for the parents?

RESOURCES

Bankson, N. W. (1989). *Bankson screen BLT-2S.* Austin, TX: Pro-Ed.

Bankson, N. W., & Bernthal, J. E. (1990). *Bankson-Bernthal test of phonology.* Chicago, IL: Applied Symbolix.

Bankson, M. W., & Bernthal, J. E. (1990). *Quick screen of phonology.* San Antonio, TX: Special Press.

Boehm, A. E. (2000). *Boehm test of basic concepts* (3rd ed.). San Antonio, TX: Psychological Corporation (Harcourt Assessment).

Bowers, L., Barrett, M., Hulsingh, R., Orman, J., & LoGiudice, C. (1994). *Test of problem solving, revised.* East Moline, IL: LinguiSystems.

Bracken, B. A. (1984). *Bracken basic concepts scale.* San Antonio, TX: Psychological Corporation (Harcourt Assessment).

Brownell, R. (2000a). *Expressive one-word picture vocabulary test.* Novato, CA: Academic Therapy Publications.

Brownell, R. (2000b). *Receptive one-word picture vocabulary test.* Novato, CA: Academic Therapy Publications.

Bzoch, K. R., & League, R. (2003). *Receptive-expressive emergent language test* (3rd ed.). Austin, TX: Pro-Ed.

Carrow-Wolfolk, E. (1999). *Comprehensive assessment of spoken language.* Circle Pines, MN: American Guidance Service.

German, D. J. (2000). *Test of word finding* (2nd ed.). Austin, TX: Pro-Ed.

Goldman, R., & Fristoe, M. (2000). *Goldman-Fristoe test of articulation* (2nd ed.). Circle Pines, MN: American Guidance Service.

Hammill, D. D., Brown, V. L., Larsen, S. C., & Wiederholt, J. L. (1994) *Test of adolescent and adult language* (4th ed.). Austin, TX: Pro-Ed.

Hresko, W. P., Reid, D. K., & Hammill, D. D. (1999). *Test of early language development* (3rd ed.). Austin, TX: Pro-Ed.

Huisingh, R., Barrett, M., Zachman, L., Blagden, C., & Orman, J. (1990). *The word test-revised.* East Moline, IL: LinguaSystems.

Kahn, L., & Lewis, N. (2002). *Khan-Lewis phonological analysis* (2nd ed.) Circle Pines, MN: American Guidance Service.

Kaufman, A. S., & Kaufman, N. L. (1993). *Kaufman survey of early academic and language skills (K-SEALS).* Circle Pines, MN: American Guidance Service.

Kirk, S. A., McCarthy, J. S., & Kirk, W. D. (2001). *Illinois test of psycholinguistic abilities* (3rd ed.). Austin, TX: ProEd.

Lippke, B. A., Dickey, S. T., Selmar, J. W., & Soder, A. L. (1997). *Photo-articulation test* (3rd ed.) East Moline, IL: LinguiSystems.

Retherford, K. S. (1993). *Guide to analysis of language transcripts.* Eau Claire, WI: Thinking Publications.

Richard, G. J., & Hanner, M. A. (1995). *Language processing test, revised.* East Moline, IL: LinguiSystems.

Robinson, C., & Salter, W. (1997). *The phonological awareness test* (2nd ed.). East Moline, IL: LinguisSystems.

Rossetti, L. (1990). *The Rossetti infant-toddler language scale.* East Moline, IL: LinguiSystems.

Secord, W. A., & Donohue, J. S. (2002). *Clinical assessment of articulation and phonology.* Greenville, SC: Super Duper Publications.

Semel, E., Wiig, E. H., & Secord, W. A. (2003). *Clinical evaluation of language functions* (4th ed.). San Antonio, TX: The Psychological Corporation (Harcourt Assessment).

Shewan, C. M. (n.d.). *Auditory comprehension test for sentences.* Chicago, IL: Biolinguistics Clinical Institutes.

Shulman, B. B. (1985). *Test of pragmatic skills, revised.* Tucson, AZ: Communication Skill Builders.

Wallace, G., & Hammill, D. D. (2002). *Comprehensive receptive and expressive vocabulary test.* (2nd ed.). Austin, TX: Pro-Ed.

Williams, K. T. (1997). *Expressive vocabulary test.* Circle Pines, MN: American Guidance Service.

Williams Hodson, B. (1986). *The assessment of phonological processes-revised.* Austin, TX: Pro-Ed.

Zimmerman, I. L., Steiner, V. G., & Pond, R. E. (2002). *Preschool language scale* (4th ed.). San Antonio, TX: Pearson Education.

REFERENCES

American Speech-Language-Hearing Association. (1988). Prevention of communication disorders. *ASHA, 30*(3), 90.

American Speech-Language-Hearing Association. Committee on Language Learning Disorders. (1989, March). Issues in determining eligibility for language intervention. *ASHA, 31,* 113–118.

American Speech-Language-Hearing Association. (1991). A model for collaborative service delivery for students with language-learning disorders in the public schools. *ASHA, 33*(Suppl. 5), 44–50.

American Speech-Language-Hearing Association. (1998). *Guidelines for referral to speech-language pathologists.* Rockville, MD: Author.

American Speech-Language-Hearing Association. (2001). *Scope of practice in speech-language pathology.* Rockville, MD: Author.

American Speech-Language-Hearing Association. (2004a). *Admission/Discharge criteria in speech-language pathology* [Guidelines]. Retrieved May 19, 2010, from http://www.asha.org/docs/html/GL2004-00046.html

American Speech-Language-Hearing Association. (2004b). *Preferred practice patterns for the profession of speech-language pathology.* Rockville, MD: Author.

Bleile, K. M. (2004). *Manual of articulation and phonological disorders: Infancy through adulthood* (2nd ed.). Clifton Park, NY: Thomson/Delmar Learning.

Bloom, L. (1973). *One word at a time: The use of single-word utterances before syntax.* The Hague, The Netherlands: Mouton.

Bloom, L., & Lahey, M. (1978). *Language development and language disorders.* New York, NY: John Wiley and Sons.

Borsch, J., & Oaks, R. (1993). *The collaboration companion: Strategies and activities in and out of the classroom.* East Moline, IL: LinguiSystems.

Brown, R. (1973). *A first language: The early stages.* Cambridge, MA: Harvard University Press.

DeKemel, K. (2003). Alternative service delivery models: The move toward collaboration and consultation and classroom-based intervention. In K. DeKemel (Ed.), *Intervention in language arts: A practical guide for SLPs* (pp. 109–126). Philadelphia, PA: Butterworth-Heinemann.

DeMil, H., Merritt, D. D., & Culatta, B. (1998). Collaborative partnerships and decision-making. In D. D. Merritt & B. Culatta (Eds.), *Language intervention in the classroom.* San Diego, CA: Singular.

deVilliers, J., & deVilliers, P. (1973). A cross-sectional study of the acquisition of grammatical morphemes. *Journal of Psycholinguistic Research, 2,* 267–278.

Dollaghan, C. A. (2004). Evidence-based practice in communication disorder: What do we know, and when do we know it? *Journal of Communication Disorders, 37,* 391–400.

Gilliam, S. L., & Gilliam, R. K. (2006). Making evidence-based decisions about child language intervention in schools. *Language, Speech, and Hearing Services in Schools, 37,* 304–315.

Gunter, C. D., LeJeune, J. B., & Kurfuerst, S. (March, 2005). *The process of evidence-based practice.* Presented to the Annual Convention, Pennsylvania Speech-Language-Hearing Association, Pittsburgh, PA.

Gunter, C. D., LeJeune, J. B., & Kurfuerst, S. A. (November, 2005). *The scholar-practitioner: Professional development for clinical service providers.* Presented to the Annual Convention, American Speech-Language-Hearing Association, San Diego, CA.

Hegde, M. N., & Davis, D. (1999). *Clinical methods and practicum in speech-language pathology.* San Diego, CA: Singular.

Johnson, C. J. (2006). Getting started in evidence-based practice for childhood speech-language disorders. *American Journal of Speech-Language Pathology, 15,* 20–35.

LeJeune, J. B., & Gunter, C. D. (April, 2004). *Enhancing clinical skills through improving critical thinking skills.* Presented to the Annual Convention, Pennsylvania Speech-Language-Hearing Association, State College, PA.

LeJeune, J. B., & Gunter, C. D. (November 2005). *Critical thinking across the clinical service provision continuum.* Presented to the Annual Convention, American Speech-Language-Hearing Association, San Diego, CA.

LeJeune, J. B., Gunter, C. D., & Kurfuerst, S. (April, 2006). *Scholar-practitioner skills for clinical practitioners.* Presented to the Annual Convention, Pennsylvania Speech-Language-Hearing Association, King of Prussia, PA.

Lue, M. S. (2001). *A survey of communication disorders for the classroom teacher.* Needham Heights, MA: Allyn & Bacon.

McCauley, R. J., & Fey, M. E. (2006). *Treatment of language disorders in children.* New York, NY: Brookes.

Miller, J. F. (1981). *Assessing language production in children: Experimental procedures.* Needham Heights, MA: Allyn & Bacon.

Oxford Center for Evidence-Based Medicine. (2001). *Levels of evidence and grades of recommendation.* Retrieved May 19, 2010, from http://www.cebm.net/index.aspx?o=1025

Perzsolt, F., Ohletz, A., Gardner, D., Ruatti, H., Meier, H., Schlotz-Gorton, N., & Schrott, L. (2003). Evidence-based decision-making: the six-step approach. *American College of Physicians Journal Club, 139*(3), 1–6.

Straus, S. E., & Sackett, D. L. (1998). Getting research findings into practice: Using research findings in clinical practice. *British Medical Journal, 317,* 339–342.

Templin, M. (1957). *Certain language skills in children: Their development and relationships.* Minneapolis, MN: University of Minnesota Press.

Index